Essentials of Dental Hygiene
Clinical Skills

Mary Danusis Cooper, RDH, MSEd
Professor, Dental Hygiene Program
Indiana University Purdue University
Fort Wayne, Indiana

Lauri Wiechmann, RDH, MPA
Coordinator, Dental Hygiene Program
Carl Sandburg College
Galesburg, Illinois

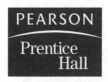

PEARSON
Prentice
Hall

Upper Saddle River, New Jersey 07458

Library of Congress Cataloging-in-Publication Data

Cooper, Mary Danusis.
  Essentials of dental hygiene : clinical skills / Mary D. Cooper, Lauri Wiechmann.
    p. ; cm.
  Includes bibliographical references and index.
  ISBN 0-13-046258-6
1. Dental hygiene—Outlines, syllabi, etc.
  [DNLM: 1. Dental Prophylaxis—methods—Outlines.   2. Dental Care—methods—Outlines.
3. Dental Hygienists—Outlines.]   I. Wiechmann, Lauri.   II. Title.
  RK60.7.C66 2006
  617.6'01—dc22

                                                    2005004462

Publisher: Julie Levin Alexander
Publisher's Assistant: Regina Bruno
Executive Editor: Mark Cohen
Associate Editor: Melissa Kerian
Editorial Assistant: Jaquay Felix
Director of Manufacturing and Production: Bruce Johnson
Managing Editor for Production: Patrick Walsh
Production Liaison: Christina Zingone
Production Editor: Karen Berry/Pine Tree Composition, Inc.
Manufacturing Manager: Ilene Sanford
Manufacturing Buyer: Pat Brown
Creative Director: Cheryl Asherman

Senior Design Coordinator: Christopher Weigand
Cover Designer: Christopher Weigand
Director of Marketing/Marketing Manager: Karen Allman
Channel Marketing Manager: Rachele Strober
Marketing Coordinator: Michael Sirinides
Media Product Manager: John Jordan
Media Production Manager: Amy Peltier
Media Production Project Manager: Stephen Hartner
Composition: Pine Tree Composition, Inc.
Printer/Binder: Courier Companies
Cover Printer: Lehigh Press

Credits and acknowledgments borrowed from other sources and reproduced, with permission, in this textbook appear on the appropriate page within text.

Pearson Education LTD.
Pearson Education Singapore, Pte. Ltd
Pearson Education, Canada, Ltd
Pearson Education–Japan
Pearson Education Australia PTY, Limited
Pearson Education North Asia Ltd
Pearson Educación de Mexico, S.A. de C.V.
Pearson Education Malaysia, Pte. Ltd
Pearson Education, Upper Saddle River, New Jersey

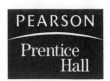

10 9 8 7 6 5 4 3 2 1
ISBN 0-13-046258-6

To George and George IV,
thank you for your ongoing support and love. I couldn't have completed this
project without you.

To Lauri Wiechmann,
words cannot express how much I appreciate and respect you—professionally
and personally. You give one hundred percent of yourself, not only to our
profession, but to your family. Working with you couldn't have been any easier.
Thank you for your confidence in me, and more importantly, for your
faithful friendship.

To all the dental hygiene students I have had the pleasure of teaching,
past and present, I thank you for so many fond memories.
I wish you all continued success.

Mary Danusis Cooper

To Jay, Kendra, and Colleen—
thank you for your patience and love. I thank you for understanding how
important this project was and giving me the time I needed. Your continued
support has truly been cherished. I hope I can someday give to you what you
have given me.

To my parents and family—
Thank you for instilling discipline and dedication in me. The words of
encouragement and wisdom were appreciated.

To Mary Cooper—
words cannot express how I feel about you. Not only are you my mentor but a
professional I truly admire! I am truly honored to have worked on this second
book with you and am blessed to have you as a friend.
Thank you for all you have done for me.
This adventure was wonderful.

To my present and former students—
Each of you has left an etching in my memory. Your desire to attain your goal of
becoming a hygienist is to be commended. May you take your knowledge and
skills as a hygienist and make the world a better place.
I wish only the best for each of you!

Lauri Wiechmann

Contents

Section III: Supporting Services   271

Preface

Essentials of Dental Hygiene: Clinical Skills is written for the dental hygiene student providing direct care for patients. The purpose of the book is to build on skills introduced in the preclinical semester and incorporate higher order thinking skills. This is the second book of two in the *Essentials of Dental Hygiene* series; the first book, titled *Essentials of Dental Hygiene: Preclinical Skills,* is designed for the first year, first semester of the dental hygiene curriculum.

Each chapter is written in an outline format, which offers the student a comfortable style for reading and studying the material, while providing fundamental information. Each chapter provides the dental hygiene student the opportunity to learn information in a step-by-step sequence. Not only are the skills provided—the hows—but also the reasons—the whys.

Objectives are listed at the beginning of each chapter, providing the student with fundamental concepts presented in the chapter. Key terms are bolded in each chapter with definitions provided in the glossary. In addition, text boxes are found throughout providing information that is interesting and useful.

References to current literature are made throughout the book. They reflect current research results and support the philosophy of life-long learning. At the end of the chapter are review questions, which serve as a self-evaluation for the student. Students can review the text, answer the questions, and refer back to the material, if needed, to reinforce the information. Correct answers to the questions may be obtained from the course instructor possessing the supplementary instructor's manual. In addition, a companion CD-ROM supplements the materials presented in the written text through video clips and additional photographs.

Each chapter presents the following information:

Chapter 1: "Clinical Applications of Pain and Anxiety Control: Local Anesthesia and Nitrous Oxide" focuses on local anesthesia techniques while reviewing local anesthetic agents, anatomy, and neuroanatomy of the involved areas along with introducing nitrous oxide–oxygen sedation.

Chapter 2: "Advanced Instrumentation" guides the student to advanced instrumentation and alternative fulcrums while addressing area-specific curettes.

Chapter 3: "Power-Driven Scaling" introduces the student to periodontal debridement with adjunct technology in discussing ultrasonic scalers.

Chapter 4: "Air Polishing" addresses the method used to remove extrinsic stain, plaque, and soft deposits with greater ease with an air polishing unit.

Chapter 5: "Tobacco Cessation" directs the dental hygiene student in assessing, planning, and implementing education sessions for patients who use tobacco products.

Chapter 6: "Dental Sealants" guides the student in placement of pit and fissure sealants using different materials available on the market.

Chapter 7: "Rubber Dams Isolation" launches the second section of the book, where auxiliary procedures are discussed. This chapter discusses the skill of rubber dam placement in a step-by-step sequence.

Chapter 8: "Sutures" introduces students to the different types of sutures placed in the oral cavity and removal methods.

Chapter 9: "Periodontal Dressings" logically follows "Sutures," providing students with continuing information in caring for sutured areas.

Chapter 10: "Pulp Vitality" leads the student through the possible causes of non-vital teeth and methods of determining vitality.

Chapter 11: "Taking Alginate Impressions and Trimming Study Models" discusses the need for replicating the patient's dentition, along with the step-by-step procedure for obtaining impressions, as well as methods of pouring and trimming casts.

Chapter 12: "Marginating, Finishing, and Polishing Dental Amalgam Restorations" guides the student in finishing and polishing a dental amalgam restoration to produce smooth surfaces.

Chapter 13, "Temporary Restorations" introduces the student to the need for and technique of applying temporary restorative materials.

Chapter 14: "Medical and Dental Emergencies" embarks on the final section of the book, Supporting Services. The student will learn about the most common medical emergencies evident in the dental setting and the appropriate management techniques.

Chapter 15: "Dental Implants" discusses various types of implants and the dental hygienist's role in proper maintenance.

Chapter 16: "Perioral Piercings" focuses on the implications of piercings in the oral cavity and surrounding structures as well as the importance of maintaining a clean environment surrounding the piercing(s).

Chapter 17: "Dentin Hypersensitivity" concludes the textbook, showing the student one of the most common conditions evidenced by the dental patient and methods the dental hygienist can incorporate to help eliminate the discomfort.

Mary Danusis Cooper
Lauri Wiechmann

Acknowledgments

We would like to express our sincere appreciation to all the contributors who have dedicated many hours to help develop this textbook. Each of you has made a personal contribution and commitment to helping dental hygiene students attain the knowledge and skills needed to provide direct care for patients.

We would also like to thank Melissa Kerian and Karen Berry for their ongoing support throughout this entire process. You both made the development of this book almost an easy task.

We also acknowledge the support people who helped us with photographs and video for the CD. A special thank you to Kim Norris and Dia McKillip from Carl Sandburg College for the many hours they devoted in taking quality photos and videos. Elmer Denman, from Indiana University Purdue University, we also thank you for your skills and steadfast commitment in helping us with additional photographs.

Acknowledgments for Chapter 16

The author is grateful to those individuals who assisted with the development of this manuscript. Alicia Cardenas of Twisted Sol (Denver, CO) provided invaluable practical and historical information on piercing. The Association of Professional Piercers continues to exemplify their dedication to health, safety, and education within the piercing industry and provided images and material which is included in this chapter. Marc Gagnier of Painful Pleasures (Owings Mills, MD) provided invaluable photo images for use in this manuscript. Without their help, this chapter could not have been produced.

Contributors

Brian R. Crawford, DDS
Assistant Director, Idaho Advanced General
   Dentistry Residency
Idaho State University, Department of Dental
   Sciences
Pocatello, Idaho

Mary Danusis Cooper, RDH, MSEd
Professor in Dental Hygiene
Indiana University Purdue University Fort Wayne
Fort Wayne, Indiana

Debi Gerger, RDH, BS, MPH
Adjunct Faculty
Riverside Community College
Riverside, California

Anne Nugent Guignon, RDH, MPH
Private Clinical Practice
RDH Columnist—Feature Writer, PennWell
   Publications
Houston, Texas

Shirley Gutkowski, RDH, BSDH
Sun Prairie, Wisconsin

Harold A. Henson, RDH, MEd
Assistant Professor in Dental Hygiene
University of Texas Dental Branch at Houston
Houston, Texas

Michelle Hurlbutt, RDH, BS
Adjunct Faculty
Riverside Community College Dental Hygiene
   Program
Moreno Valley, California

Nancy K. Mann, RDH, MSEd
Clinical Assistant Professor in Dental Hygiene
Indiana University Purdue University Fort Wayne
Fort Wayne, Indiana

Elizabeth C. Reynolds, RDH, MS
Adjunct Faculty
Community College of Denver
Denver, Colorado

Sheri Granier Sison, RDH, BS
Clinical Instructor
LSUSHC School of Dentistry
New Orleans, Louisiana

Deb Stuart, CDA, EFDA, MS
Clinical Assistant Professor
Indiana University Purdue University Fort Wayne
Fort Wayne, Indiana

Lauri Wiechmann, RDH, MPA
Coordinator, Dental Hygiene Program
Carl Sandburg College
Galesburg, Illinois

Reviewers

David G. Arreguin, DDS
Director
Dental Programs
Del Mar College
Corpus Christi, Texas

Charmaine P. Godwin, CDA, RDH, MEd.
Assistant Professor
Dental Programs
Santa Fe Community College
Gainesville, Florida

Jamie A. Moss, RDII, MEd.
Professor
Horry-Georgetown Technical College
Myrtle Beach, South Carolina

Rebecca J. Sullivan, MEd., RDH, CDA
Professor
Dental Hygiene Program
Tunxis Community College
Farmington, Connecticut

Anne S. Uncapher, RDH, MA
Instructor
Broome Community College
Department of Dental Hygiene
Binghamton, New York

Chapter 1

Clinical Applications of Pain and Anxiety Control: Local Anesthesia and Nitrous Oxide

Brian Crawford, DDS, and Lauri Wiechmann, RDH, MPA

MediaLink

A companion CD-ROM, included free with each new copy of this book, supplements the procedures presented in each chapter. Insert the CD-ROM to watch video clips and view a large collection of color images that is also included. This multimedia library Is designed to help you add a new dimension to your learning.

KEY TERMS

administration
aspirate
biotransformation
distribution

excretion
leukopenia
local anesthesia
metabolism

sharps container
syringe
uptake
vasodilation (vasodilatation)

LEARNING OBJECTIVES

After reading this chapter, the student will be able to:

- differentiate between local anesthesia and general anesthesia;
- list the qualities of an ideal anesthetic;
- define and discuss the key terms;
- compare and contrast local anesthetic agents in uptake, biotransformation, metabolism, and excretion;
- differentiate methods of administration for anesthetic agents;
- discuss why highly perfused tissues will have higher concentrations of the local anesthetic agent and possible repercussions to these tissues with local anesthesia toxicity;
- describe effects of local anesthetic agents on the central nervous system (CNS) and the cardiovascular system;
- identify mild signs of CNS stimulation and progressive symptoms of CNS stimulation explaining the physiological effects taking place;
- determine when a vasoconstrictor would be indicated in a local anesthetic agent based on benefits the agent provides;

- explain the criteria for selecting a vasoconstrictor in a local anesthetic agent;
- list and explain possible drug–drug interactions that must be examined when reviewing the health history;
- discuss factors that affect duration of a local anesthetic agent;
- differentiate topical anesthetics and local anesthetics, discussing the role of each in pain management and their relationship with each other;
- recognize toxic levels of local anesthetics, categorizing findings into pre-convulsive signs, convulsive stage, and overdose/complications from a given case study;
- implement emergent care for local anesthetic toxicity from a given case study;
- differentiate local anesthetic agent overdose from vasoconstrictor overdose;
- discuss local complications of local anesthetics, including management methods of each complication;
- demonstrate proper record keeping for administration of local anesthesia;

- identify, describe, and discuss problems with the armamentarium for local anesthetic injections;
- label and identify the parts of the syringe, needle, and cartridge used in local anesthetic injections;
- trace the pathway and identify the areas of innervation of each respective nerve associated with the maxillary and mandibular divisions of the trigeminal nerve;
- describe the need for following regimented protocol and the process involved when administering local anesthesia beginning with patient preparation through syringe disassembly;
- identify and verbalize landmarks, injection site, insertion angle, penetration depth, and amount of solution deposited for all local anesthetic injections discussed;
- compare and contrast local anesthesia and nitrous oxide–oxygen sedation, focusing on their roles in pain and anxiety control;

- discuss the physiologic effects of nitrous oxide and the response of the cardiovascular system, respiratory system, and other organs in the body;
- describe the need for following regimented protocol and the process involved when administering nitrous oxide–oxygen sedation, beginning with patient preparation through the recovery phase;
- discuss contraindications for nitrous oxide–oxygen sedation and recognize those contraindications in a given case study;
- discuss issues related to nitrous oxide–oxygen sedation, including indications for use and complications of use;
- identify and describe the parts of the nitrous oxide–oxygen sedation unit;
- demonstrate proper use of the equipment involved with nitrous oxide–oxygen sedation.

I. Introduction

Patients undergoing periodontal debridement commonly receive some type of pain and/or anxiety control through **local anesthesia** and/or nitrous oxide sedation. Local anesthesia, one of the most common procedures in dentistry today, used to reversibly block peripheral nerve conduction, has been available to the dental profession for over 100 years.[1] It is legal in the majority of the states for dental hygienists to administer local anesthesia.[2] The likelihood of a dental hygienist providing care for a patient who would benefit from local anesthesia is high. Prior to administering an injection, it is imperative the dental hygienist have a complete understanding of the complexity of the procedure. This chapter provides information about local anesthetic agents, the anatomy of the oral cavity where injections are administered, injection techniques, and common complications with injections. Delivery of nitrous oxide–oxygen is also discussed along with pharmacology, the equipment used, and complications related to the drug.

II. Local Anesthesia

Local anesthesia produces a loss of sensation in a localized area of the body due to an anesthetic agent which causes depression of the excitation in nerve endings or an inhibition of the conduction process in peripheral nerves. An important feature of local anesthesia is that it produces this loss of sensation without inducing a loss of consciousness; it is in this area where local anesthesia differs dramatically from general anesthesia.[3]

A. Historical fundamentals of impulse generation and transmission.
   1. In the late 1800s, scientists discovered chemicals that could prevent pain in medical and dental procedures without loss of consciousness.
   2. Concept behind the action of local anesthetics.
      a. Prevent the conduction and generations of nerve impulses.
      b. Set up a "chemical roadblock" between the source of the impulse and the brain.[4]
B. Methods for inducing local anesthesia. There are various ways local anesthesia can be accomplished, including:
   1. Mechanical trauma, such as cutting with a scalpel or sharp object.
   2. Lowered temperature, such as applying ice.

3. Anoxia, nerves not getting any oxygen, as when a tourniquet is used to stop the blood flow.
4. Chemical irritants, such as capsaicin, which is found in hot green and red peppers.
5. Neurolytic agents, such as phenol or alcohol.
6. Chemical agents, such as local anesthetics.

C. Qualities of a local anesthetic. Only methods or substances that induce transient and completely reversible anesthesia are acceptable for clinical use.
   1. Local anesthetic agents exhibit the general properties and satisfy the previously mentioned absolute criteria.
   2. These "ideal" agents or methods include all of the following; however, most agents do not completely satisfy all of these variables.
      a. Do not irritate the tissue to which it is applied.
      b. Do not permanently alter the nerve ending.
      c. Show low systemic toxicity.
      d. Are effective injected or applied topically.
      e. Possess as short an onset as possible.
      f. Allow adequate duration for the procedure planned.
      g. Are potent without being a harmful, concentrated solution.
      h. Do not produce an allergic reaction.
      i. Are stable in solution and biotransform (break down) in the body.
      j. Can be sterilized by heat without deterioration.

D. Basic Pharmacology. The major difference between local anesthetics and other common drugs is how they are introduced to the body. Most drugs must reach sufficient concentrations and be absorbed before they begin to work; local anesthetics cease to work when they are absorbed.
   1. **Uptake.** The absorption of the agent or drug through the tissue into which it was introduced in preparation for **distribution** to other parts of the body; local anesthetics generally produce a **vasodilation (vasodilatation).**
      a. Due to vasodilatation, absorption into the bloodstream is increased, thus decreasing the duration of anesthesia and increasing the blood level of the drug, leading to a potential for overdose.
      b. Esters are generally taken up more quickly than amides (amides and esters will be discussed later in this section).
      Note: Cocaine causes a *vasoconstriction.*
   2. **Administration.** Means by which the drug or agent is introduced into the body; methods of administration include:
      a. Oral. Achieved by placing the drug in the mouth and swallowing it; local anesthetics are absorbed poorly from the gastrointestinal tract, except for cocaine.
      b. Topical. Achieved by placing the drug on the skin or mucosa; local anesthetics are absorbed at differing rates by different mucosa.
      c. Injection. Achieved by delivering the drug through penetrating the skin or mucosa; may result in rapid elevation of blood levels.
      d. Intramuscular. Achieved by delivering the drug into muscle tissue; agent is absorbed more quickly than subcutaneous injection because of the greater blood supply to the muscles.
      e. Subcutaneous. Achieved by delivering the drug just beneath the skin; better results for dentistry but results vary depending upon the area's vascularity.
   3. Distribution. Transportation of the drug or agent to all parts of the body by the blood stream; once the local anesthetic is absorbed into the

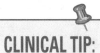

CLINICAL TIP:

Innervating Your Knowledge: Sunburn remedies are effective because they are absorbed through damaged skin.

CLINICAL TIP:

Innervating Your Knowledge: The concentration gradient, the blood flow, and the drug's ability to be absorbed by the target organ all affect the possibility of toxicity of the anesthetic agent.[5]

CLINICAL TIP:

Innervating Your Knowledge: The brain and the heart are the major target organs for local anesthetic toxicity.[5]

CLINICAL TIP:

Innervating Your Knowledge:
Esters are not available in local anesthetic cartridges used in the dental office.

CLINICAL TIP:

Innervating Your Knowledge:
Anesthetic solutions with low lipid solubility include prilocaine, lidocaine, and mepivacaine. Anesthetic solutions with high lipid solubility include bupivacaine and etidocaine.

CLINICAL TIP:

Innervating Your Knowledge:
Patients with pseudocholinesterase deficiency, a genetic condition affecting the biotransformation of esters, metabolize the anesthetic agent at a slower rate.[6]

CLINICAL TIP:

Innervating Your Knowledge:
Between 1 and 10 percent of an anesthetic agent is excreted unchanged in the urine.[5]

CLINICAL TIP:

Innervating Your Knowledge:
Prior to administering any local anesthetic agent, attention must be given to those who have a severe liver dysfunction because they may experience difficulty in the biotransformation of the agent.

blood stream, it is transported to all intended and unintended tissues and organs.[5]

   a. Highly perfused tissues, such as tissues with a high oxygen requirement like the brain, head, liver, lungs, kidneys and spleen, will have higher concentrations of the drug.

   b. Skeletal muscle, while not as well perfused as some other tissues, makes up more body mass; therefore, more drug will be present.

4. **Metabolism** and **biotransformation.** All local anesthetics are lipophilic and hydrophilic and most are tertiary or secondary amines; those with low lipid solubility are less toxic than anesthetics with high lipid solubility; esters and amides are described as:

   a. Esters. A group of anesthetic agents predominantly hydrolyzed by plasma cholinesterase also known as pseudocholinesterase[6]; include cocaine, benzocaine, and procaine; procaine is metabolized the fastest, breaking down to paraminobenzoic acid (PABA), which is excreted in the urine as an alcohol. PABA is a significant allergen.

   b. Amides. A group of anesthetic agents hydrolyzed primarily in the liver by a complex process.

      (1) Include articaine, bupivacaine, lidocaine, mepivacaine, and etidocaine.

      (2) Rate is similar for all amides, hence this breakdown can be significantly affected by abnormal liver function.

5. Difference between esters and amides includes how they are broken down metabolically in the body. Toxicity of a drug is dependent upon the rate of absorption into the bloodstream and its rate of removal.

6. **Excretion.** Removal of the drug and its breakdown products from the body.

   a. Excretion occurs primarily in the kidneys.

   b. Some of the parent drug is excreted into the bile, as well as the metabolites.[7]

   c. Compared to amides, fewer esters are excreted because they are hydrolyzed in the blood; therefore, renal impairment will affect excretion of local anesthetics.[6]

   d. Other problems that may affect excretion include:[5]

      (1) Too much anesthesia for the size of the individual.

      (2) Too rapid an injection: Injecting too much solution in a short time, such as one cartridge of anesthetic solution in 15 seconds.

      (3) Injecting anesthetic solution into the vascular supply (intravascular injection).

      (4) Liver impairment will compromise biotransformation of the agent.

7. Systemic actions of local anesthetics. All drugs, no matter where they are introduced into the body, will have various effects on other parts of the body as a result of the uptake, distribution, and excretion processes. The fundamental process in nerve conduction is a large transient increase in the permeability of the membrane to sodium. Local anesthetics block conduction by interfering with the increase in sodium permeability. The local anesthetic effect is a cascade of electrophysical changes. The first change is an increase in the threshold for electrical stimulation, followed by a reduction in the size of the action potential, a slowing of conduction velocity, and finally the cessation of impulse propagation. The duration of the anesthesia is determined by the redistribution and depends on the ability of the local anesthetic agent to stay within the nerve and block the sodium channels.[6]

   a. Local anesthetics are chemicals that reversibly block action potentials in ALL excitable membranes.

     (1) Central nervous system (CNS) and cardiovascular system (CVS) are extremely susceptible.

     (2) Effect depends upon the plasma level; the plasma level depends upon the drug's uptake rate and distribution rate to the liver.

   b. CNS effect. Denotes the affect the local anesthetic agent has on the CNS; the brain, spinal cord, and nerves.

     (1) Local anesthetics do cross the blood-brain barrier.[5]

     (2) Most signs of CNS stimulation are stimulatory; the pharmacological effect is depression.

     (3) Mild signs of CNS stimulation include slurred speech, localized muscle twitching, apprehension, disorientation, numbness of the tongue and circumoral regions, lightheadedness, dizziness, inability to focus, and tinnitus.[8]

     (4) Progressive symptoms of CNS stimulation include lethargy; slight drop in blood pressure, respirations and pulse; drowsiness and unresponsiveness.[8]

     (5) Further increased plasma levels lead to convulsions.

   c. CVS effect. Denotes how local anesthetics affect the heart and blood vessels of the cardiovascular system; local anesthetics depress the myocardium, slow conduction of impulses, and prolong the refractory period. This is why lidocaine is used in the emergent treatment for arrhythmias such as premature ventricular contractions (PVCs).

E. Local tissue effect. Denotes how the tissues react at the site where the local anesthetic agent is injected; skeletal muscle may be damaged by the injection of local anesthetics; this damaged tissue will regenerate in approximately two weeks.

F. Respiratory system effect. Denotes how local anesthetics affect the lungs and our ability to breathe; minimal respiratory depression is observed with low levels of local anesthesia, significant depression is observed at near-toxic levels.[9]

G. Pharmacology of vasoconstrictive agents. Vasoconstrictors constrict blood vessels and thereby control tissue perfusion; they are added to local anesthetic solutions to oppose the vasodilating effects caused by local anesthetics[5]; benefits include:[5,8,9]

   1. Decreased blood flow to the site of injection. This allows for the local anesthetic agent to retain its concentration and thus its effectiveness, without being diluted or removed from the site of injection by the normal blood flow through the area.

   2. Absorption is slowed causing lower plasma levels. This leads to decreased toxicity, keeping the distribution to other tissues at a minimum and thus decreasing the risk of an overdose, or causing an effect not desired in another tissue, such as the brain or the heart.

   3. More anesthetic agent stays in the tissue, increasing the duration of anesthesia. This translates to a need for less anesthetic agent to achieve the anesthesia adequate to perform the desired procedure.

   4. Decreased bleeding at the site of administration created by a chemical tourniquet that reduces blood loss during the procedure, increasing operator visibility, allowing better restorations and affording the patient greater safety.

CLINICAL TIP:

Innervating Your Knowledge: To achieve the desired duration of the anesthetic agent, all patients require the standard amount of local anesthetic agent regardless of liver function. Duration is determined by redistribution of the agent, not biotransformation.[6]

CLINICAL TIP:

Innervating Your Knowledge: Peak plasma levels of the anesthetic agent are reached within 10 minutes if no vasoconstrictor is used, 30 minutes if the agent contains a vasoconstrictor.[5]

CLINICAL TIP:

Innervating Your Knowledge: A true allergy, i.e., immunoglobulin E mediated allergic reaction, to local anesthesia is rare. It is estimated that less than 1 percent of the adverse reactions are true allergies.[8]

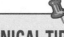

CLINICAL TIP:

Innervating Your Knowledge: Andrew Chen's article describes the actions on the CNS best when he says, "The stimulatory effect is the indirect result of a depression of cerebral inhibitory centers. This results in unopposed facilitatory neurons causing random stimulatory firing of the neurons in the brain. This generalized stimulation of the brain causes generalized tonic-clonic seizures."[8]

CLINICAL TIP:

Innervating Your Knowledge:
The cardiovascular system is more resistant to elevated blood levels of the local anesthetic agent than the central nervous system.[8]

CLINICAL TIP:

Innervating Your Knowledge:
Sympathomimetic drugs have an effect similar to that produced when the sympathetic nervous system is stimulated—fight or flight. Adrenergic drugs release epinephrine or a similar substance.

CLINICAL TIP:

Innervating Your Knowledge:
Catecholamines are compounds, such as norepinephrine and dopamine, that are secreted or are by-products of secretions of the medulla of the adrenal gland and affect the sympathetic nervous system.

CLINICAL TIP:

Innervating Your Knowledge:
Most of the drugs used for vasoconstriction in conjunction with a local anesthetic for use in dentistry are direct-acting drugs.

CLINICAL TIP:

Innervating Your Knowledge:
Local anesthetic agents with a 1:50,000 epinephrine ratio are not recommended in dentistry for controlling pain but may be used sparingly when hemostasis is needed.[5]

5. Vasoconstrictors used with local anesthetics are similar to the sympathetic nervous system mediators and cause such a similar reaction in the adrenergic nerves response to stimulation that they are classified as sympathomimetic or adrenergic drugs.

H. Chemical structure. Vasoconstrictors are categorized as catechols and catecholamines. The distinction is based upon the presence of a hydroxyl group attached to the aromatic ring (catechol) or an amine group attached as well as the hydroxyl group (catecholamine).

I. Modes of Action. How these drugs cause the receptors to respond.
   1. Direct-acting drugs. Exert their action directly on adrenergic receptors.
   2. Indirect-acting drugs. Act by releasing norepinephrine from adrenergic sites.
   3. Mixed drugs. Can have both actions.

J. Dilution. How much of a specified drug is dissolved in a solution, such as sterile water. For epinephrine and other vasoconstrictors used in conjunction with local anesthetics for dentistry, the dilution is denoted as a ratio; 1:100,000 is calculated as one gram of drug in 1000 ml of solution. This means that there is increasingly less drug per ml in the most common dilutions or concentrations used in dentistry today, which are 1:50,000, 1:100,000, and 1:200,000.

K. Characteristics of specific vasoconstrictors.
   1. Epinephrine. Best example of a drug that mimics the reaction of sympathetic discharge and is therefore a benchmark that other drugs are compared against. Uses include:
      a. Management of acute allergic reactions.
      b. Management of bronchospasms via its potent dilation of the smooth muscles of the bronchioles.
      c. Treatment of cardiac arrest causing dilation of the coronary arteries.
      d. Vasoconstriction for hemostasis and vasoconstriction for local anesthetics to decrease absorption and increase duration; this occurs due to the initial predominance of alpha-receptor response in the peripheral tissue vasculature.
   2. Levonordefrin. A synthetic vasoconstrictor; similar to epinephrine only less potent and consequently less CNS and CVS stimulation.

L. Selection of a vasoconstrictor.
   1. Epinephrine and levonordefrin. Two most commonly used vasoconstrictors in the United States.
   2. Selection criteria.
      a. Length of procedure. Longer procedures require a longer duration of anesthesia; therefore, epinephrine is of benefit. Consequently, shorter procedures would not benefit with epinephrine present.
      b. Hemostasis needed during and after the procedure. Decreased blood loss during and after the procedure is a benefit to the operator to increase visibility and the overall safety of the patient.
      c. Postoperative pain control. The longer duration of anesthesia may be a benefit in those procedures that create postoperative pain.
      d. Patients with cardiovascular disease. Due to the effects on the coronary vessels, as well as the peripheral vasculature, it is *not* recommended to introduce epinephrine to a patient who already has a weakened heart or increased blood pressure.
      e. Patients with noncardiovascular disease, i.e., thyroid disorders, diabetes, or sulfite sensitivity. These conditions may already exhibit

increased adrenergic responses, which would be aggravated by more epinephrine.[9]

    f. Patients using certain drugs.[5]

      (1) Monoamine oxidase (MAO) inhibitors. Epinephrine may create a greater risk for dysrhythmias.

      (2) Tricyclic antidepressants. Epinephrine, if inadvertently administered intravascularly, can have a threefold effect; levonordefrin can have a six- to eightfold effect resulting in acute hypertension and dysrhythmias.

      (3) Beta blockers. Epinephrine, if inadvertently administered intravascularly, can decrease the heart rate to as low as 38 beats per minute ± 8 beats.

      (4) Cocaine may exaggerate the response to any vasoconstrictor, resulting in dysrhythmia, myocardial infarction, or stroke.

      (5) Thyroxin, when in elevated circulating amounts and exposed to a vasoconstrictor, may cause cardiac abnormalities as a result of overstimulation of myocardial metabolism.

      (6) Illicit drugs may induce a mild respiratory acidosis, decreasing protein binding of the local anesthetic agent, permitting more of the free drug to distribute to the CNS, hence decreasing the seizure threshold.

      (7) Medications for dyspepsia or ulcers, angina, or high blood pressure may slow the elimination of local anesthetic agents, possibly leading to toxic levels of the anesthetic agent in the blood stream, causing adverse reactions.

M. Specific local anesthetic agents. Many are available today; however, only a few are commonly used in dentistry. They meet most, if not all, of the desirable qualities previously mentioned and have been approved for use in dentistry.

    1. Duration is affected by:

      a. Individual variation. Different individuals may react to the same drug in different ways, due to variances in body chemistry.

      b. Accuracy in administration. Deposition of the agent closer to the nerve results in better anesthesia.

      c. Tissue status at deposition site. Infected or damaged tissue may react to the local anesthetic differently.

      d. Anatomical variation. Different individuals may have some normal variation in the anticipated location of a nerve.[10]

      e. Type of injection, i.e., supraperiosteal, nerve block. Different types of injections will have differing durations due to their relationship to different tissues.[11]

    2. Specific local agents.

      a. Procaine (Novocain). Most famous local anesthetic; however, it is no longer available.

      b. Lidocaine.

      (1) Most commonly used local anesthetic agent by dentists in the United States.[12]

      (2) Only available for dentistry with a vasoconstrictor because the duration without a vasoconstrictor is so short that it is of little practical application.

      (3) Onset. Rapid (2 to 3 minutes).

CLINICAL TIP:

Innervating Your Knowledge: Only one-third of the normal maximum dose of epinephrine should be administered if a patient is taking a tricyclic antidepressant. An additional, similar, dose may be administered 30 minutes later, if no problems are encountered.[5]

CLINICAL TIP:

Innervating Your Knowledge: Review of the social history with the patient using cocaine must include when the drug was last used, because a vasoconstrictor must be avoided for at least 24 hours after cocaine use.[5]

          (4) Duration.
              (a) Pulpal anesthesia, 60 minutes.
              (b) Soft tissues, 3 to 5 hours.

    c. Carbocaine 3% (Mepivacaine hydrochloride); Carbocaine 2% with Neo-cobefrin® 1:20,000 (Mepivacaine hydrochloride and levonordefrin).[13]
        (1) Onset. Rapid.
              (a) Maxilla, 30 seconds to 2 minutes.
              (b) Mandible, 1 to 4 minutes.
        (2) Duration.
              (a) Pulpal, without a vasoconstrictor, 20 minutes in maxilla; 40 minutes in mandible.
              (b) Pulpal, with a vasoconstrictor, 1 to 2.5 hours in maxilla; 2.5 to 5.5 hours in mandible.
              (c) Soft tissues, 2 to 3 hours without a vasoconstrictor; 3 to 5 hours with a vasoconstrictor.

    d. Articaine; 4% Articaine HCL with 1:100,000 epinephrine (Septocaine™).
        (1) It is believed to diffuse through soft and hard tissues more reliably than other anesthetics.[14]
        (2) Onset. Rapid (2 to 3 minutes).
        (3) Duration. Similar to lidocaine with epinephrine.[15]

    e. Bupivacaine 0.5% (Marcaine) with 1:200,000 epinephrine.
        (1) Onset. Slow (6 to 10 minutes).
         (2) Duration.
               (a) Pulpal, 90 to 120 minutes.
              (b) Soft tissues, 4 to 12 hours.

    f. Etidocaine. Similar to bupivacaine in all respects, but believed to be more effective for block anesthesia due to a somewhat faster onset caused by its lower pKa.

N. Topical anesthetics. Anesthetic agents that are applied directly to skin or mucous membranes rather than injected.
1. Useful for atraumatic, painless block, and infiltration injections.
2. Concentrations are usually higher than for injectible varieties.
3. Only affect superficial tissues.
4. Available as liquids, gels, or sprays.
5. Specific topical anesthetic agents include:
    a. Benzocaine (an ester).
    b. Lidocaine (an amide).
    c. Dyclonine (a ketone). No longer commercially available.
    d. Cocaine. Abuse potential is very high, therefore it is not used in dentistry.

O. Criteria for selection of a local anesthetic (vasoconstrictor combination). The selection of an anesthetic with or without a vasoconstrictor should be made based upon the specific needs of each patient and procedure.
1. Pain control duration, i.e., 30 minutes, 60 minutes, or several hours.
2. Postoperative pain control desired. Determine if the planned procedure is anticipated to create pain after the anesthesia has subsided.
3. Hemostasis. Determine if the procedure will cause significant bleeding that will decrease visibility during the procedure or cause greater risk to the health and safety of the patient.

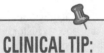

CLINICAL TIP:

Innervating Your Knowledge: There is such a wide range of concentrations and variations among topical anesthetic agents that comparison should be made on the specific tasks, requirements, and patient's health history.

    4. Absolute contraindications.
      a. Known allergy to any of the drugs included in the anesthetic/vaso-constrictor combination.
      b. Physical status of patient. Determine if the patient's general health can accept the type and amount of anesthetic to perform the planned procedure.

P. General practice stocking suggestions.
    1. Stock a minimum of two different agents on hand with no more than four available.
      a. Benefits.
        (1) Limiting the choices simplifies the preparation and allows the operator to be familiar with all the variables of a specific agent or agents.
        (2) Limited choices also allow for a reasonable usage rate of the agents without fear of an infrequently used item exceeding its shelf life and necessitating being discarded unused.
      b. Duration.
        (1) Short duration agent. 30 minutes of pulpal anesthesia.
        (2) Intermediate duration. 60 minutes of pulpal anesthesia.
        (3) Long duration. Up to 90 minutes of pulpal anesthesia.
      c. Availability of an ester if an amide fails or is contraindicated. This choice is not currently feasible as esters are not available in dental cartridges.
    2. A topical anesthetic for tissue/injection preparation.

III. Toxicity of Local Anesthetics

Local anesthetics do exhibit systemic effects. When adverse reactions occur due to toxicity, the effects are usually reversible and temporary in nature.[16] Serious complications are rare when the guidelines of administering agents are followed. However, local anesthetics are capable of reaching toxic and potentially fatal levels due to a variety of factors or combination of those factors discussed regarding the drug's uptake, breakdown, elimination, and effects on various end organs. In general, local anesthetics cause depression, which can eventually lead to seizures/convulsions at toxic levels. Local anesthetics do cross the blood–brain barrier as well as the placental barrier.[17]

A. Preconvulsive signs indicate that a minimal to moderate overdose has occurred.
    1. Each agent, or combination of agents, has a specific amount or dosage that will cause the signs and symptoms of an overdose.
    2. Specific signs and symptoms include slurred speech, shivering, muscle twitching, facial muscle and extremity tremors, numbness of tongue, warm flushed skin, pleasant dreamy state, lightheadedness, dizziness, inability to focus, tinnitus, drowsiness, disorientation, talkativeness, apprehension, increased blood pressure, increased heart rate, and increased respiratory rate.

B. Convulsive stage signs indicate a moderate to high overdose has occurred.
    1. Symptoms are a progression from the preconvulsive signs of the depressive effects on the various systemic organs.
    2. Signs and symptoms include tonic/clonic seizures, generalized CNS depression, and depressed blood pressure, heart rate, and respiratory rate.

IV. Overdoses/Complications of Local Anesthesia[5,8,18]

A. Causes of overdose are related to one or more factors.

1. Intravascular injection of the agent or combination of agents greatly increases the plasma levels to twice the expected amount absorbed into the bloodstream with an extravascular injection.

2. A metabolic disorder resulting in slowing of the metabolism of the agents. Decreased liver or renal function may slow the metabolism or elimination/excretion of the drug, causing more to remain in the bloodstream than is expected under normal conditions.

3. The operator may have injected more than the recommended dose of local anesthetic agent.

B. Overdose situations and emergent treatment.

1. Rapid, severe onset within 1 minute.
   a. Usually leads to loss of consciousness due to intravascular (IV) injection of local anesthesia.
   b. Emergent treatment involves:
      (1) Discontinuing injection and remove syringe.
      (2) Protecting patient from self.
      (3) Calling 911.
      (4) Providing basic life support (BLS), as needed.
      (5) Preparing to administer IV anticonvulsants, if qualified.
      (6) Administering vasopressors, if qualified.
      (7) Allowing the patient to recover.

2. Mild to slow onset, approximately 5 minutes.
   a. Usually caused by rapid absorption and too great a dose.
   b. Emergent treatment involves:
      (1) Reassuring patient.
      (2) Administering oxygen.
      (3) Monitoring vital signs.
      (4) Administering IV anticonvulsants, if qualified.
      (5) Allowing patient to recover.

3. More than 15 minutes to onset.
   a. Usually caused by abnormal biotransformation or renal dysfunction.
   b. Emergent treatment involves:
      (1) Reassuring patient.
      (2) Administering oxygen.
      (3) Monitoring vital signs.
      (4) Administering IV anticonvulsants, if qualified.
      (5) Calling 911.
      (6) Physician exam may be indicated after emergent phase has been controlled.
      (7) Determining cause of overdose for future treatment modifications.

4. Slow onset, between 5 and 15 minutes.
   a. Usually due to too large a dose, rapid absorption, abnormal biotransformation, and/or renal dysfunction.
   b. Emergent treatment involves:
      (1) Stopping treatment.
      (2) Providing basic life support, as needed.
      (3) Administering IV anticoagulants, if qualified.
      (4) Calling 911.
      (5) After seizure subsides, maintaining BLS and administering vasopressors, if qualified.

CLINICAL TIP:

Innervating Your Knowledge: A recent study shows that in 45 percent of the cases adverse reactions occurred at the time of the injection with another 29 percent occurring within the first 2 hours following the injection.[16]

CLINICAL TIP:

Innervating Your Knowledge: Each patient will react differently to an overdose. The operator must exhibit sensible clinical judgment. Monitoring of vital signs is required in all types of medical emergencies related to an overdose. A supine or Trendelenburg position is suggested to decrease peripheral pooling and to increase vascular circulation.[8]

CLINICAL TIP:

Innervating Your Knowledge: Fifty-five percent of medical emergencies occurring during dental treatment are due to psychogenic stress or excessive uptake of the anesthetic agent within the first 5 minutes of the injection.[19]

C. Vasoconstrictor overdoses.

 1. An overdose can result from the amount of vasoconstrictor administered as part of a local anesthetic combination independent of the amount of anesthetic delivered.

 2. Amount of anesthetic may be well below the recommended toxic levels, but the amount of vasoconstrictor can exceed the recommended dosage or, more commonly, the patient's response or tolerance of the vasoconstrictor.

 3. Signs, symptoms, and treatment to a vasoconstrictor overdose.

  a. Signs include fear, anxiety, tenseness, restlessness, throbbing headache, tremor, perspiration, weakness, dizziness, pallor, respiratory difficulty, palpitations, increased blood pressure, increased heart rate, and cardiac dysrhythmias.[9]

  b. Emergent treatment. Episode is usually so short in duration that no formal management is necessary; however, if it is not a short episode:

   (1) Stop treatment.

   (2) Reposition the patient, NOT SUPINE.

   (3) Reassure the patient.

   (4) Monitor blood pressure.

   (5) Administer oxygen.

   (6) Monitor vital signs every 5 minutes.

   (7) Allow the patient to recover.

 4. Best way to avoid an overdose, of any kind, is to be well versed in the recommended dosage of all agents administered, follow a safe protocol for administering the agent, as well as have a thorough knowledge of the patient's medical history.

D. Local complications of local anesthetics. Occur at or near to the site of injection, affecting only the immediate area where the injection was administered.

 1. Broken needle. Usually caused by a sudden unexpected movement by the patient; if this occurs, the protocol to follow is:

  a. Retrieve needle, if visible, using a hemostat or cotton forceps.

   (1) It may be more prudent to leave the needle where it is than to retrieve it; this may take a consultation with a specialist to determine how difficult or dangerous the surgery would be to retrieve the fragment.

   (2) Refer the patient to an oral surgeon for evaluation; the specialist should determine the course of action, including possible retrieval of the remaining needle.

  b. Inform the patient a complication has occurred.

  c. Document the incident so that all details are included just in case a medical–legal situation should arise.

  d. Save the remaining fragment; it will aid in determining the portion size that fractured and remained with the patient.

  e. Notify your liability insurance carrier so that in the event of a medical–legal challenge you can be advised how to proceed.

 2. Pain with injection. Commonly indicates pain from the needle penetration and/or the deposition of local anesthetic. This complication can best be avoided by following the technique for atraumatic injections; common causes include:

  a. Poor technique.

  b. Attitude that "this is going to hurt."

CLINICAL TIP:

Innervating Your Knowledge: Avoid adverse reactions by implementing the following safety protocols.[5]

1. Monitor the amount of anesthetic solution being administered. Always stay below the recommended maximum level.

2. Aspirate during the injection to ensure the solution is not being deposited intravascularly.

3. Slowly inject the anesthetic solution.

4. Review the medical history for possible contraindications, i.e., conditions and/or medications, to anesthetic agents.

CLINICAL TIP:

Innervating Your Knowledge: A dull needle may be produced after providing numerous injections. A barbed needle has a small extension of metal protruding from the tip, resulting in trauma to adjacent tissue during movement of the needle.

      c. Dull needle.

      d. Barbed needle.

      e. Expressing solution too rapidly.

3. Burning with injection. A burning sensation of the anesthetic solution in the area of the injection occurs quite often; reasons include:

      a. Injecting solution too quickly.[19] The rate of injection should be approximately one cartridge per minute.[5,8]

      b. Contaminated cartridge. Storing the cartridge in alcohol or other sterilizing solution can contaminate the solution. Preparing the syringe hours before use allows the copper from the needle cannula to be released, resulting in copper ion contamination of the solution.[20]

      c. Solution is too warm.

      d. pH is too low. Local anesthetics range from 3 to 5 pH.

4. Persistent anesthesia/paresthesia. Denotes a total loss of sensation or an altered sense of feeling. Fairly uncommon due to administration of a local anesthetic, but continues to be the most frequent cause for dental liability claims; possible causes include:[12,21,22,23,24]

      a. Neurovascular bundle is severed in spite of proper injection technique.

      b. Alcohol or another ingredient is in the cartridge rather than local anesthetic agent.

      c. Trauma to the tissues occurs from hemorrhage secondary to the injection.

5. Trismus—prolonged tetany or "lock jaw"—caused by physical or chemical trauma to a muscle of mastication, either along the lines of proper injection or a deviation from recommended technique.[23]

      a. Trauma to the musculature or vasculature in the infratemporal fossa.

      b. Local anesthetic is myotoxic, which causes a progressive necrosis of exposed muscle fibers.

      c. Treatment. Use heat, saltwater rinses, analgesics, muscle relaxants, and/or progressive physical therapy.

      d. Usually symptoms appear within 24 to 48 hours[20] and resolve in 48 to 72 hours.

      e. Schedule patient for a followup exam to verify resolution.

6. Hematoma, commonly referred to as a " bruise," or more correctly, bleeding into the tissue due to damaged blood vessels.[23] Usually not a serious problem because it is often resolved with no consequence or sequelae; mostly inconvenient and embarrassing to the patient.

      a. Causes.

        (1) Needle unavoidably lacerates a vessel as it passes to the site for deposition.

        (2) Deposition is immediately adjacent to the neurovascular bundle without first aspirating to establish needle location.

      b. Treatment.

        (1) Treat site with direct pressure as soon as possible.

        (2) Apply an ice pack, if feasible, for 20 to 30 minutes.

        (3) Apply heat after 24 hours has passed.

      c. Healing. Usually takes from 7 to 14 days for "tincture of time" healing to occur.

7. Infection. Soft tissue infection occurring along the tract where the needle coursed during the injection.[20]

      a. Causes.

(1) A contaminated needle used for two different patients, which is *never* recommended.

(2) Contact with a contaminated surface or object prior to injection.

b. Treatment. Antibiotics may be useful; administer orally for 7 to 10 days, as with most soft tissue, bacterial intraoral infections.

8. Edema. A swelling of tissues caused by many different means. This is a sign, not a syndrome; it can indicate a hemorrhage or hematoma formation or the injection of an irritating substance; cause can be a result of an allergic reaction to topical anesthetic or other agent applied to the mucosal surfaces.

9. Sloughing of tissues. Characterized by epithelial desquamation; should be an infrequent complication if judicious use of topical and local anesthetics, with high concentrations of vasoconstrictor, is followed.

    a. Causes.

    (1) Excessive application of a topical anesthetic agent.

    (2) Sterile abscess caused by excessive use of a vasoconstrictor in conjunction with a local anesthetic agent.

    b. May be painful.

    c. Treatment.

    (1) Analgesics should be prescribed, as needed.

    (2) Epithelial desquamation will resolve in a few days and the sterile abscess will disappear in 7 to 10 days.

10. Soft tissue injuries. Usually are self-inflicted and unintentional by the patient after dismissal from the office.[25]

    a. Most often occurs with children or disabled adults.

    b. Treat locally.

    (1) Apply pressure, if bleeding.

    (2) Suture, if necessary (rarely performed).

    (3) Instruct patient in postoperative home care to keep area clean.

    (4) Avoid irritating foods for 3 to 4 days.

    (5) Antibiotics may be necessary if the wound becomes secondarily infected; follow a course normally prescribed for intraoral, bacterial soft tissue infections.

11. Facial nerve paralysis (7th cranial nerve). Caused by local anesthetic injected into the deep lobe of the parotid gland; occurs most frequently when attempting to anesthetize the maxillary canine or administer an infraorbital block.

    a. Unilateral "drooping face" is observed.[23]

    b. Occurs infrequently.

    c. Is a transitory phenomenon, usually subsiding within a few hours.

    d. Treat with reassurance; may wear an eye patch, if necessary (due to paralysis of the eyelids); discontinue wearing contacts.

    e. Record the event in the patient's treatment record.

12. Postanesthetic intraoral lesion. Results in recurrent aphthous stomatitis or herpes simplex.

    a. Infections are aroused by the trauma from the injection of local anesthetic solutions, just as with their occurrence in other locations from other types of trauma.

    b. As is often the case with these types of lesions, they have occurred previously under these circumstances or in other areas common to herpetic infection.

    (1) Lesions tend to be painful, and analgesics may be necessary.

(2) Avoid applying Kenalog or similar agents, because the lesions may be virile and this steroid would cause the infection to worsen. However, some of the anti-virile topical medications may provide some relief.

c. Most often occur within approximately 2 days postoperatively.

d. Lesions resolve in 7 to 10 days with or without treatment in a healthy individual.

13. Record keeping for administration of local anesthetics. A record of the visit must be made in the patient's permanent dental treatment record and includes:

a. Type and amount of local anesthetic and vasoconstrictor administered.

b. Name and location of the injection(s) provided.

c. Description of how the patient tolerated the procedure and the anesthetic agent.

d. Condition of the patient when dismissed.

V. Armamentarium

A. **Syringe.** A device to which a needle is attached that allows an anesthetic solution to be injected; most popular type is the breech-loading, metallic, aspirating, syringe due to its ergonomic design and ease of obtaining needles and anesthetic carpules of the proper dimension.

1. Parts (Figure 1–1).

a. Thumb ring. Circular component where the thumb is placed.

b. Finger grip. Area of the syringe where fingers are placed to grip syringe.

c. Piston with harpoon. Rod with harpoon at end to engage in rubber stopper, allowing for aspiration and expelling solution from the carpule.

d. Syringe barrel. Houses the carpule; has one large and one smaller opening. It is important to position the larger opening toward the operator during an injection to watch for a positive aspiration.

e. Needle adapter. Area where needle is threaded on syringe.

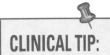

CLINICAL TIP:

Innervating Your Knowledge: A positive aspiration indicates the bevel of the needle is in a blood vessel during aspiration.

Figure 1–1   (A) Breech-loading Aspirating Syringe. (B) Parts of syringe: A. Thumb ring. B. Finger grip. C. Piston with harpoon. D. Syringe barrel. E. Needle adapter.

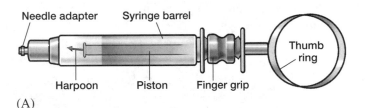

Needle adapter   Syringe barrel   Thumb ring

Harpoon   Piston   Finger grip

(A)

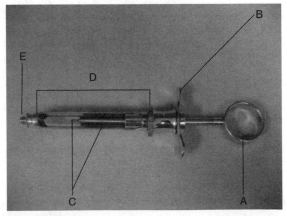

(B)

2. Care.
   a. After each use. Sterilize syringe in accordance with infection control guidelines for contaminated instruments.
   b. After every five autoclave cycles. Disassemble syringe and lubricate with a silicone lubricant; clean the harpoon with a brush.
   c. Replace the harpoon and piston when the harpoon no longer engages the stopper adequately.
3. Problems.
   a. Off-center needle penetration into the rubber diaphragm of the anesthetic carpule may cause the needle to bend or prevent the local anesthetic solution from being expressed.
   b. A broken cartridge, due to worn syringe, occurs when the metal of the cylinder wears, causing the cartridge to be held more loosely than ideal; creates torque on the carpule and leads to breakage.
   c. A bent harpoon from improper reassembly or damage prevents the harpoon from engaging the stopper of the local anesthetic carpule.
   d. Disengagement of harpoon during aspiration makes it impossible to properly **aspirate** prior to injecting the anesthetic solution; causes include:
      (1) Improper engagement of the harpoon into the stopper of the local anesthetic carpule.
      (2) Worn harpoon that cannot remain engaged.
   e. Surface deposits due to corrosion and/or oxidation deposits on the metal components of the syringe cause it to function improperly.
B. Needles.
   1. Types.
      a. Reusable. Seldom, if ever, used today; not advised for typical dental use.
      b. Nonreusable. May be reused for the same patient during the same appointment, then discarded at the end of treatment.
   2. Parts (Figure 1–2).
      a. Bevel. Angled insertion tip of the needle.
      b. Shank. Long straight portion of the needle.
      c. Hub. Portion of the needle assembly that attaches to the needle adaptor of the syringe; may be plastic or metal.
      d. Syringe-penetrating end. Extends out the opposite end of the hub from the shank and beveled end, but is much shorter; penetrates the rubber diaphragm of the local anesthetic carpule.

> **CLINICAL TIP:**
>
> **Innervating Your Knowledge:** If the harpoon disengages during aspiration, remove the needle from the tissue and re-engage the harpoon into the stopper.

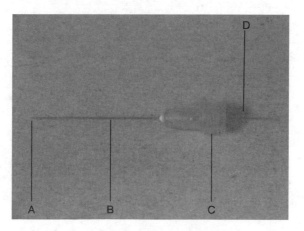

Figure 1–2   Needle. A. Bevel. B. Shank. C. Hub. D. Syringe penetrating end.

CLINICAL TIP:

Innervating Your Knowledge:
The gauge of a needle refers to the diameter of the needle lumen.

CLINICAL TIP:

Innervating Your Knowledge:
The scoop technique involves using only one hand to recap the needle. Place the cap of the needle on its side. While holding the syringe with one hand, insert the needle into the cap.

CLINICAL TIP:

Innervating Your Knowledge:
Careful visual inspection of the bevel prior to use can identify a barb. If a barb is observed, change the needle before use.

CLINICAL TIP:

Innervating Your Knowledge:
A hemostat in the local anesthetic setup can be used to retrieve a broken needle.

e. Gauge. The standard by which needle diameter, or bore or lumen, is measured; the larger the number or gauge, the smaller the diameter or bore/lumen of the needle.
   (1) Many different gauges are available including 23, 25, 27, and 30; most frequently used gauge is 27.
   (2) Bigger is better with regard to needle gauge; larger gauge needles are deflected less readily, break less often, and aspiration results are more reliable.[26] It is often mistakenly believed that a smaller diameter needle is less painful upon injection for the patient; however, it has been shown that there is little difference between needles commonly used in dentistry today as noted by the patient in regard to discomfort upon insertion.[26]

f. Lengths. The type of injection to be administered will determine the length of needle required (Figure 1–3).
   (1) Long: Approximately 32 millimeters from bevel tip to hub.
   (2) Short: Approximately 20 millimeters from bevel tip to hub.

g. Care. All needles are single-patient use.
   (1) Change after every three to four injections because the needle will become dull, making insertion more difficult and uncomfortable for the patient.
   (2) Cover when not in use; recap with scoop or other technique to avoid accidental injection of operator, assistant, or patient and potential risk of serious injury or infection.
   (3) Always be aware of needle position to eliminate possibility of injury or injection into an unintended area.
   (4) Use **sharps container.** A puncture-resistant container used to store sharp objects, like needles, after use, prior to their disposal, minimizing accidental injury and/or infection.

h. Problems.
   (1) Discomfort with insertion. The needle may have a "barb" or "burr" on its tip, from the manufacturer or from handling during assembly; this barb will make the needle drag and tear as it pierces the mucosa, causing discomfort.
   (2) Breakage. The needle is weakest where it joins the hub.
      (a) If the patient jumps or moves unexpectedly, it can break at the hub.
      (b) Avoid inserting the entire length of the needle into the tissue; if needle breakage occurs, enough of the needle will be protruding to be easily recovered.

Figure 1–3   Needle lengths. The top needle is short—approximately 20 millimeters from bevel tip to hub. The bottom needle is long—approximately 32 millimeters from bevel tip to hub.

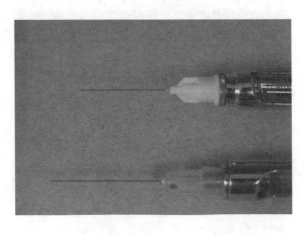

(c) Bending the needle prior to insertion, or changing direction, causes unnecessary and unintended stress on the needle, leading to potential breakage.

(3) Discomfort upon withdrawal. A barb can be created if the tip of the needle contacts bone, causing discomfort as the needle is withdrawn.

C. Cartridges (or carpule). Most common and easily obtainable means for delivering dental local anesthesia.

1. Components[18] (Figure 1–4).

   a. Cylinder. Glass tube containing 1.7 or 1.8 milliliters of solution.[3,7]

   b. Rubber stopper. Seals one end of the glass tube where harpoon on the syringe engages. It is pushed through the glass tube to express the local anesthetic solution through the needle.

   c. Aluminum cap. Attaches the diaphragm to the end of the glass tube; opposite the stopper.

   d. Rubber diaphragm. Semipermeable membrane held onto the cartridge by the aluminum cap. It is pierced by the syringe-penetrating end, allowing the anesthetic solution out of the cartridge and through the needle.

   e. Thin plastic label. Attached to the outside of the cartridge; contains the information regarding the contents of the cartridge as well as the manufacturer and the expiration date.

2. Contents.[18]

   a. Local anesthetic agent. Provides local anesthesia to the injected area or region.

   b. Vasopressor (Vasoconstrictor). Provides localized vasoconstriction to control bleeding and slows uptake and elimination of the anesthetic, thus prolonging its action.

   c. Vasopressor preservative. An antioxidant, typically sodium bisulfite; prolongs the shelf life of the vasoconstrictor.

   d. Sodium chloride. Adjusts the pH of the solution for ideal biocompatibility and anesthetic effectiveness.

   e. Distilled water. Acts as a diluting agent to adjust the solution to the ideal concentration in order to prevent toxicity to the tissues injected with the solution.

   f. Air bubble. 1 to 2 cc nitrogen bubble that verifies integrity of the carpule; incorporated into the cartridge to prevent oxygen from being trapped in the cartridge.

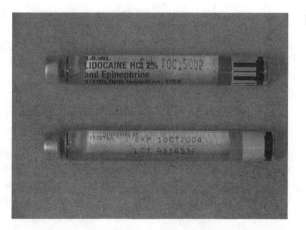

Figure 1–4   Anesthetic carpule.

3. Care.
   a. Store in original container to eliminate confusion as to which anesthetic to use; do not sterilize—autoclaving can cause accelerated degradation of the vasopressor and decrease the duration of anesthesia.
   b. Do not store in a disinfectant because alcohol and other cold sterilization solutions can penetrate the diaphragm and contaminate the solution.
   c. Do not heat because if the solution is warmer than body temperature, the patient may feel that it is too warm and may complain of a burning sensation.
4. Problems.
   a. Enlarged bubble can indicate that the solution has frozen; stopper may be extruded as well; integrity and sterility of the contents cannot be assured.
   b. Extruded stopper with a bubble suggests freezing as noted above; no bubble indicates prolonged storage in disinfection (sterilization) solution and diffusion of the solution into the cartridge.
   c. Burning injection can be attributed to:
      (1) Cartridge being too hot, affecting the pH; if the solution contains a vasopressor, the pH will be lowered, producing a burning sensation for some patients. Even normal temperatures can produce a burning sensation in some patients.
      (2) Sterilization solution leaking into the cartridge.
   d. Corroded cap indicates that the cartridge has been soaked in a sterilization agent and diaphragm penetration has likely occurred, resulting in possible contamination of the solution.
   e. Rust on cap may be caused from a broken, leaky cartridge in the dispensing tin; the entire tin should be examined and possibly discarded.
   f. Leakage. The diaphragm may have been punctured and thus does not seal tightly around the needle; most often caused by improper syringe and needle assembly or a damaged syringe.
   g. Broken cartridge. Most often, broken cartridges are delivered as such from the manufacturer, but breakage can also be caused by excessive force applied upon injection against a plugged needle or excessive force applied with a blow to the thumb ring to engage the harpoon.

VI. Anatomy

Prior to administering the anesthetic agent, it is critical for the operator to have a full and complete understanding of the surrounding neuroanatomy, i.e., blood supply, nerve supply, muscles, osteology, as well as the local anesthetic agent, to ensure the anesthetic agent is deposited in the correct location. Different injections have different results. Providing block anesthesia produces an interruption of the flow of impulses along a nerve trunk;[16] whereas, infiltration anesthesia is more site specific as numbness is attained in the immediate area where the agent is administered.

A. Trigeminal nerve (5th cranial nerve)[27] (Figure 1–5).
   1. Predominantly sensory.
   2. Forms the semilunar (Gasserian) ganglion, which lies in Meckel's cavity in the middle cranial fossa.
   3. Composed of three large trunks/divisions; ophthalmic nerve (V_1), maxillary nerve (V_2), and the mandibular nerve (V_3); only the maxillary and mandibular divisions will be discussed because they relate to local anesthesia of the oral cavity.

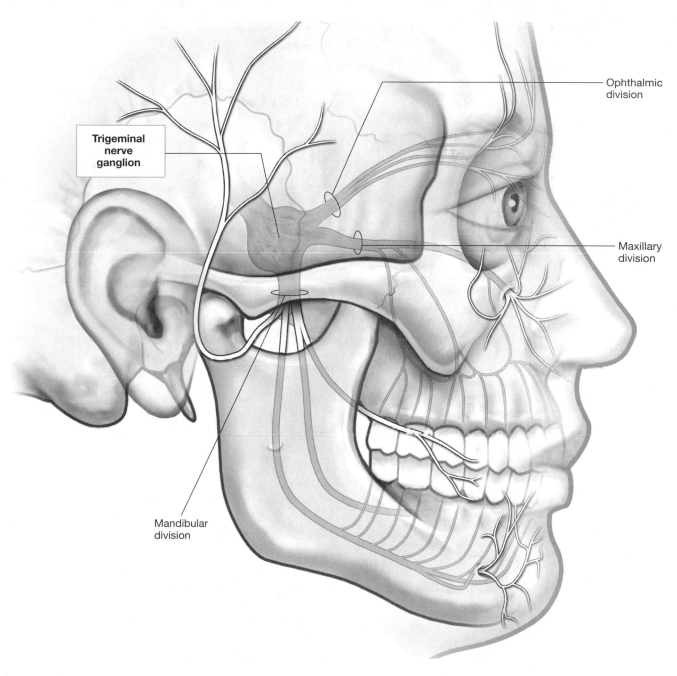

Figure 1–5   Trigeminal nerve.

B. Divisions.
    1. Maxillary division (V$_2$)[20,28,29] (Figure 1–6).
        a. Pathway. Exits the cranial fossa via the foramen rotundum and pro-
           ceeds to the superior portion of the pterygopalatine fossa within the
           infratemporal fossa, giving off numerous branches within the fossa.
           It continues in an anterior direction, passing through the inferior or-
           bital fissure, traversing the infraorbital groove and canal (there the
           nerve becomes the infraorbital nerve) where two branches are given
           off, exits via the infraorbital foramen, and concludes on the face in
           several terminal branches.

Figure 1–6   Maxillary division (V$_2$) of the trigeminal nerve.

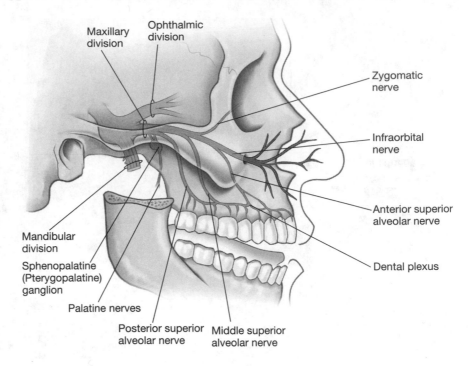

Maxillary division

Ophthalmic division

Zygomatic nerve

Infraorbital nerve

Anterior superior alveolar nerve

Dental plexus

Mandibular division

Sphenopalatine (Pterygopalatine) ganglion

Palatine nerves

Posterior superior alveolar nerve

Middle superior alveolar nerve

b. Branches in the pterygopalatine fossa.
   (1) Zygomatic nerve.
       (a) Enters the orbit via the inferior orbital fissure and divides into two branches:
           i. Zygomaticofacial nerve. Sensory nerve.
           • Pathway: Travels along the inferior and lateral portion of the orbit and penetrates a foramen in the zygomatic bone, perforates the orbicularis oculi muscle.
           • Innervation: Supplies the skin on the cheek.
           ii. Zygomaticotemporal nerve. Sensory nerve.
           • Pathway: Travels along the lateral portion of the orbit and penetrates a foramen in the zygomatic bone, continues in a posterior direction to the temporal fossa, terminates within the temporalis muscle superior to the zygomatic arch.
           • Innervation: Supplies the skin on the side of the forehead and anterior temporal areas of the skull.
   (2) Sphenopalatine ganglion. Located deep in the pterygopalatine fossa.
       (a) Nasopalatine nerve[1] (Figure 1–7). Sensory nerve.
           i. Pathway: Leaves the sphenopalatine ganglion through the sphenopalatine foramen, passing forward and downward on the nasal septum through the incisive canal to the incisive foramen; runs in a posterior direction.
           ii. Innervation: Nasal septum, mucous membrane, and gingiva of the anterior hard palate.
       (b) Greater palatine nerve (see Figure 1–7). Sensory nerve.
           i. Pathway: Leaves the sphenopalatine ganglion and descends through the greater palatine canal to the greater palatine foramen; continues in an anterior direction.
           ii. Innervation: Mucous membrane, glands, and gingiva of the posterior hard palate.

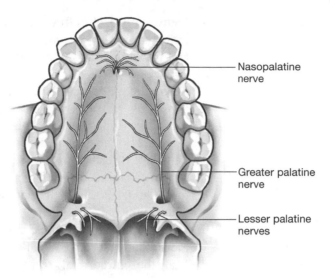

Figure 1–7   Nasopalatine nerve and greater palatine nerve.

(3) Posterior superior alveolar nerve (Figure 1–8). Sensory nerve.
    (a) Pathway. Given off immediately prior to the nerve entering the infraorbital groove; penetrates posterior of maxillary tuberosity via posterior superior alveolar foramen, travels forward under the mucosa of the maxillary sinus.
    (b) Innervation: Supplies the maxillary third and second molars, and the first molar with the exception of the mesiobuccal root, the respective facial gingiva, periosteum, and mucous membranes of the buccal mucosa.
c. Branches in the infraorbital groove.
(1) Middle superior alveolar nerve (see Figure 1–8). Presence is irregular; if it is not present, the posterior superior alveolar and anterior superior alveolar branches converge and provide innervation to the structures[1]; sensory nerve.

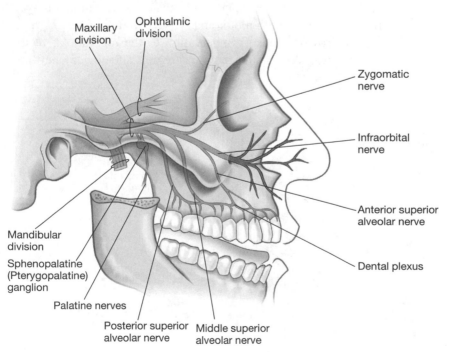

Figure 1–8   Divisions of the maxillary nerve (V_2).

(a) Pathway: Branches from the infraorbital nerve near the posterior portion of the infraorbital canal and runs downward and forward along the maxillary sinus, to apices of respective teeth.

(b) Innervation: Supplies the maxillary first and second premolars along with the mesiobuccal root of the maxillary first molar, the respective facial gingiva, and periosteum.

(2) Anterior superior alveolar nerve (see Figure 1–8). Sensory nerve.

(a) Pathway: Branches from the infraorbital nerve in the infraorbital canal just before the nerve exits the infraorbital foramen; descends down the anterior portion of the maxillary sinus to the apices of the respective teeth.

(b) Innervation: Supplies the canine, lateral incisor, and central incisor and respective facial gingiva and periosteum.

d. Branches at the infraorbital foramen. Originating on the face (Figure 1–9).

(1) Inferior palpebral. Sensory nerve.

(a) Pathway: Ascends behind the orbicularis oculi.

(b) Innervation: Supplies skin and conjunctiva of the lower eyelid, joining at the lateral angle of the orbit with the facial and zygomaticofacial nerves.

(2) External nasal. Sensory nerve.

(a) Pathway: Skin of nose.

(b) Innervation: Supplies the skin of the side of the nose and the movable portion of the septum; joins with the terminal endings of the nasociliary nerve.

(3) Superior labial. Sensory nerve.

(a) Pathway: Descends behind the labii superioris.

(b) Innervation: Supplies the skin of the upper lip, labial mucous glands, and mucous membrane of the upper lip and labial vestibule.

2. Mandibular division (V_3)[20,29,30] (Figure 1–10).

a. Largest of the three major divisions of the trigeminal nerve.

b. Mixed nerve, both motor and sensory in function.

(1) Provides sensory innervation to the mandibular teeth and gingiva; skin of the temporal region and lower one-third of face,

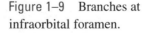

Figure 1–9   Branches at infraorbital foramen.

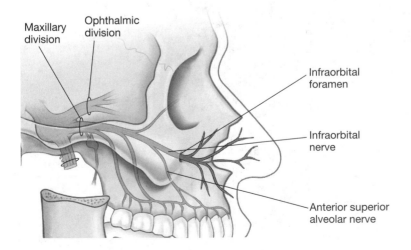

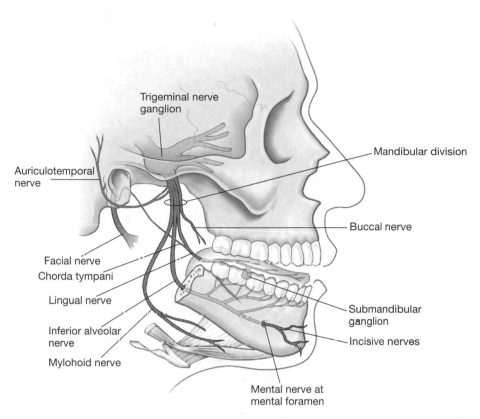

Figure 1–10   Branches of the mandibular division (V$_3$).

ear, and lower lip; and mucous membrane of the anterior two-thirds of the tongue and floor of mouth.

(2) Provides motor to muscles of mastication, tensors veli palatini and tympani, mylohyoid muscle, and anterior belly of the digastric muscle.

(3) Pathway: Exits the middle cranial fossa via the foramen ovale; descends into the infratemporal fossa where branches are given off.

(4) Branches.

    (a) Buccal nerve, also called long buccal nerve or buccinator nerve (Figure 1–11). Sensory nerve.

        i. Pathway: Travels laterally in the infratemporal fossa between the two heads of the lateral pterygoid muscle, passes superiorly to the medial pterygoid muscle, pierces the buccinator muscle and gives off branches. One branch of interest to local anesthesia is that it travels along the medial side of the ramus of the mandible, crosses the ramus near the anterior border, and sends terminal branches to the buccal mucosa and gingiva up to the mental foramen.

        ii. Innervation: Supplies the buccal gingiva and mucosa from the mental foramen posteriorly.

    (b) Inferior alveolar nerve (Figure 1–12). The largest branch of the mandibular division; sensory nerve.

        i. Pathway: Passes downward from the infratemporal fossa below the inferior head of the lateral pterygoid muscle, lateral to the sphenomandibular ligament and medial to the ramus entering the mandibular foramen; travels in

Figure 1–11 Buccal nerve (long buccal nerve or buccinator nerve).

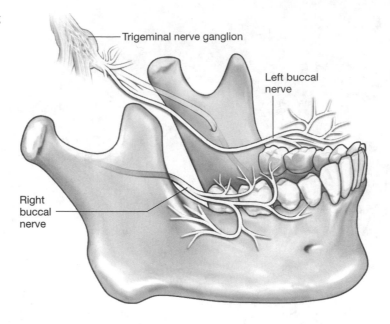

the mandibular canal giving off branches to the teeth; near the mental foramen it divides into the mental nerve and the incisive nerve.

  ii. Innervation: Supplies all anterior and posterior teeth and the respective periosteum along with the facial gingiva of the teeth anterior to the mental foramen.

  iii. Branches: Include mental and incisive nerves.

(c) Mental nerve (see Figures 1–12, 1–13, and 1–14). Sensory nerve.

  i. Pathway: Branches from the inferior alveolar nerve passing through the mental foramen proceeding toward the midline of the mandible.

Figure 1–12 Mandibular division.

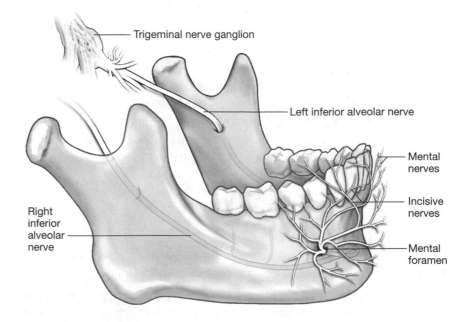

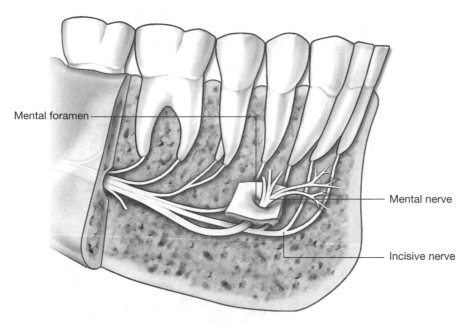

Figure 1–13   Mental nerve and incisive nerve.

ii. Innervation: Supplies the facial gingiva from the mental foramen to the midline of the mandible and skin and mucosa of the lower lip.
(d) Incisive nerve (see Figures 1–12 and 1–13). Sensory nerve.
   i. Pathway: Continuation of the inferior alveolar nerve within the incisive canal, at the mental foramen, to the midline of the mandible.
   ii. Innervation: Supplies the teeth anterior to the mental foramen, and the respective periosteum.
(e) Lingual nerve (Figure 1–15). Sensory nerve.
   i. Pathway: Passes downward with the inferior alveolar nerve, communicating with the chorda tympani of the

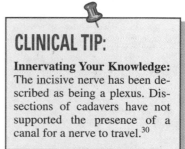

CLINICAL TIP:

Innervating Your Knowledge: The incisive nerve has been described as being a plexus. Dissections of cadavers have not supported the presence of a canal for a nerve to travel.[30]

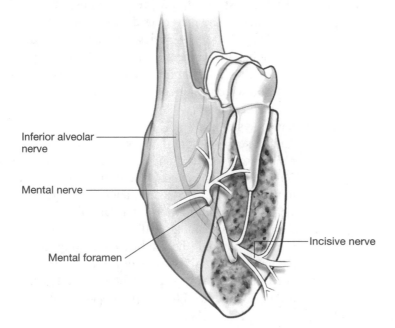

Figure 1–14   Mental nerve.

Figure 1–15 Mandibular division.

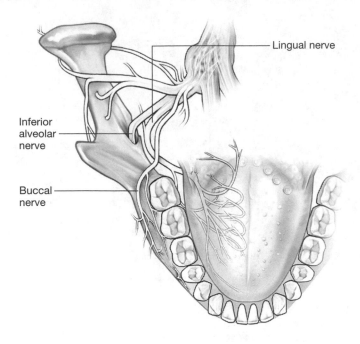

facial nerve; crosses obliquely to the side of the tongue running in an anterior direction across the submandibular salivary gland and along the tongue to its tip, lying beneath the mucous membrane.

ii. Innervation: Supplies the mucous membrane of the anterior two-thirds of the tongue and the lingual gingiva up to the midline of the mandible.

VII. Review of the Medical and Dental Histories

A thorough review of the patient's medical and dental histories is essential because some information may alter the anesthetic plan or, if left unacknowledged, could create a serious, even life-threatening complication.

A. Ascertain the patient's chief complaint. Ask yourself, "Why is the patient in the chair?" "What is his or her greatest need?"

B. Determine the history of the present illness. Detail the specifics of the problem that brings the patient to the office that day.

C. Review of dental history. A review of the patient's dental history may suggest some induced complications. Examples of these include intravascular injection, hematoma formation, and lacerations; it may also suggest unusual anatomic form, which resulted in inadequate anesthesia in past experiences.

D. Review of medical history.

1. Review of systems.

   a. Cardiovascular system. This may affect the decision on the type of anesthetic, vasoconstrictor, and/or both that can be safely administered.

   b. Central nervous system. There are potential body chemistry variations that would make one anesthetic agent preferable to another, such as pH, solubility, or other variables.

   c. Liver and renal function. If function is impaired, metabolism, excretion, or both could be inhibited, resulting in increased plasma levels and more potential for an overdose.

   d. Heart murmur. May suggest the relative strength of the heart as well as the possible need for prophylactic antibiotic coverage.

e. Psychiatric treatments and drugs. Life-threatening drug–drug interactions exist between many common drugs and those present in anesthetic solutions.

2. Dialogue history. Discussion between the operator and the patient should follow review of the systems and any positive responses.
   a. Pre-existing contraindications to local anesthesia may be identified. Examples of these would include malignant hyperthermia, atypical plasma cholinesterase, and methemoglobinemia.
   b. Recent hospitalizations. May indicate the patient's overall health is compromised.
   c. Current medications, including over-the-counter and homeopathic drugs. Must be identified to determine any possible drug–drug interactions with the local anesthetic agent and/or vasoconstrictor.
      (1) Provider must be aware of the potential for drug–drug interactions as well.
      (2) Some examples of these include sulfonamides and esters, beta-blockers and epinephrine, tricyclic antidepressants and epinephrine, and MAOs and epinephrine.
      (3) While it is ultimately the responsibility of the provider to recognize the potential for these incompatible relationships, a pharmacist can be a great resource in this rapidly growing area of concern.
   d. All known allergies. Avoid limiting this to "drug" allergies. A cosmetics allergy or reaction could indicate an allergy to para amino benzoic acid (PABA), a common ingredient in many cosmetics that has been used as a preservative in some anesthetic solutions in the past; reaction to some jewelry items could suggest a nickel or other metal allergy, which may affect the dental treatment plan.[31]

VIII. Local Anesthetic Injections

Developing a routine helps the operator provide safe injections focusing on safety for the patient, and both anatomical and anesthetic considerations.[1]

A. Preparation of patient. Keeping the patient calm is essential.[23]
   1. Positioning of patient. Proper supine positioning allows for comfort of the patient while allowing the operator to ensure proper positioning for maximum direct vision, fulcrum placement and access to the target site.
   2. Preparing armamentarium.
      a. Review health history, obtain blood pressure, and select appropriate preinjection analgesia and local anesthetic agent.[23]
      b. Determine gauge and length of needle to be used.
      c. Prepare the syringe.
         (1) Review the type of agent written on cartridge.
         (2) Ensure agent has not reached expiration date (Figure 1–16).
         (3) Check the rubber stopper and diaphragm to ensure integrity of cartridge.
         (4) Load cartridge in syringe by inserting rubber stopper end first, retract thumb ring to seat rest of cartridge, and engage harpoon in rubber stopper by applying gentle pressure to thumb ring (Figure 1–17).
         (5) Thread needle onto syringe, being careful not to bend the syringe-penetrating end inserting into the diaphragm (Figure 1–18).

CLINICAL TIP:

Innervating Your Knowledge: Malignant hyperthermia is a genetically transferred defect, believed to affect the distribution of myoplasmic calcium. It is characterized by tachycardia, cardiac arrhythmias, muscle rigidity, cyanosis, and death. The response occurs when the patient is exposed to a triggering agent, most often a general anesthetic agent. However, amide local anesthetics have been implicated as a triggering agent.[3] **Atypical plasma cholinesterase** is a variation of the normal choline-ester substrates (substances), such as ester local anesthetic agents, which are hydrolyzed in the blood by this enzyme produced in the liver.[8] **Methemoglobinemia** is a condition of a cyanosis-like state with or without cardiac or respiratory changes. It is caused by an inborn error in metabolism, or it can be induced by certain drugs. When severe, the blood appears chocolate brown and can lead to respiratory depression, syncope, and even death.[6]

CLINICAL TIP:

Innervating Your Knowledge: Positioning the anxious patient in a supine position may help prevent syncope.[26]

Figure 1–16   Anesthetic cartridge. Confirm anesthetic agent and expiration date.

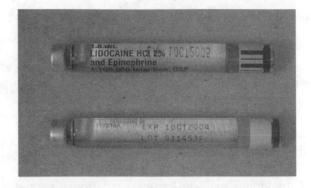

Figure 1–17   Loading syringe. Insert rubber stopper end first.

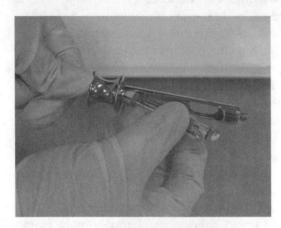

Figure 1–18   Threading needle onto syringe.

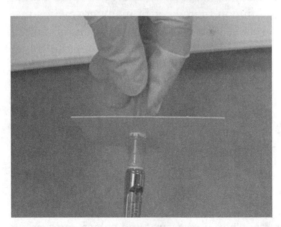

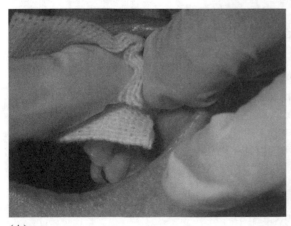

(A)

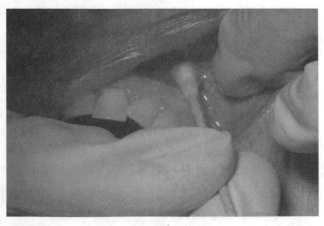

(B)

Figure 1–19   Topical anesthesia. (A) Drying area. (B) Applying topical ointment.

(6) Remove cap of needle and ensure flow of solution through the lumen of needle by expressing a small amount of agent and check for a barb; replace the needle cap.

d. Topical antiseptic (e.g., betadine). Swab the area to be injected with the antiseptic agent on a cotton-tipped applicator to reduce the chance of infection from the injection. Note: This step is commonly omitted.

e. Preinjection analgesia.

(1) Topical anesthetic ointment (Figure 1–19).
(a) Purpose. Mucosal anesthesia at injection site.
(b) Procedure. Apply a small amount to the injection site with a cotton-tipped applicator after drying the area with a gauze square. The topical anesthetic should be allowed to remain on the area 1 to 2 minutes prior to administering the injection to be effective. Wipe off excess.
(c) Concern. Tissue sloughing in immediate area.

(2) Topical anesthetic spray.
(a) Purpose. Mucosal anesthesia at injection site.
(b) Procedure. Spray solution on mucosal tissue at injection site.
(c) Concerns. Bad taste, increase in salivation, and difficult to restrict spray to injection site area.

(3) Distraction anesthesia (Figure 1–20).
(a) Purpose. Implemented in lieu of topical anesthetic, reducing the amount of drug introduced to system.
(b) Procedure. Apply gentle tension to vestibular area of injection site, allowing the needle to insert with ease; apply gentle pressure away from the injection site or lightly compress (squeeze) lip.
(c) Concerns. The patient may be apprehensive without having topical anesthetic at injection site.

(4) Pressure anesthesia (Figure 1–21).
(a) Purpose. Produces anoxia of the area, reducing sensation to the palatal mucosa.
(b) Procedure. Apply firm, constant pressure with the cotton-tipped end of an applicator to the injection site.
(c) Concerns. Pressure should result in the patient feeling uncomfortable, with the intent of reducing the discomfort associated with the insertion of the needle.

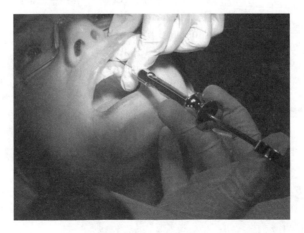

Figure 1–20 Distraction anesthesia.

Figure 1–21   Pressure anesthesia. (A) Nasopalatine. (B) Greater palatine.

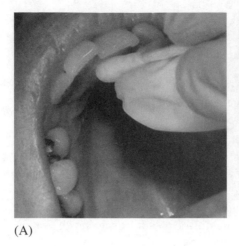

(A)

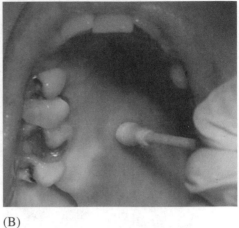

(B)

CLINICAL TIP:

Innervating Your Knowledge: Aspiration is recommended to ensure the end of the needle is not in a blood vessel. A positive aspiration will produce blood in the cartridge, confirming the needle is in a blood vessel. A negative aspiration will not produce blood in the cartridge, confirming the needle is in an area safe to deposit the local anesthetic agent.

f. Cotton-tipped applicator. Used to apply topical antiseptic and topical anesthetic.

g. Gauze squares or cotton rolls. Used to dry the soft tissue area prior to applying topical anesthetic and wiping off excess topical anesthetic immediately prior to needle insertion.

h. Hemostat. Used to retrieve separated (broken) needle if it occurs.

3. Determination of injection site. Review anatomy of area to determine any variation that may affect the injection technique.

4. Injection technique (see CD for photos).

a. Gently retract tissue so injection site is clearly visible and mucosa is taut. This allows the needle to pierce the tissue easily with minimal trauma.[26]

b. Establish a fulcrum to provide a constant and stable reference and rest for syringe.

c. Insert needle at injection site.

d. Proceed to target site maintaining a direct, continuous movement.

e. Aspirate by gently retracting the thumb ring; turn the syringe one-quarter turn, aspirate again. Confirm a double negative aspiration has occurred prior to depositing any solution. If a positive aspiration has occurred, the needle should be removed from the tissue and the cartridge should be replaced.

f. Slowly deposit anesthetic solution at an approximate rate of 1 cartridge per minute.[5,8]

g. Withdraw the needle maintaining a direct, continuous movement.

h. Recap the needle.

i. Rinse the patient's mouth.

j. Document the injection.

5. Post-injection protocol.

a. Remain with the patient and be alert for allergic or other adverse reactions.

b. Confirm spread of analgesia.

6. Specific local anesthetic injections.

a. Maxillary injections.

(1) Anterior superior alveolar nerve block (Figure 1–22).

(a) Landmark: Canine eminence.

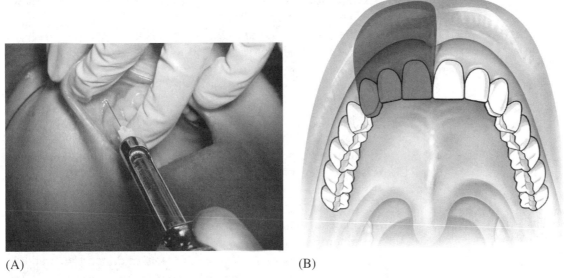

(A)   (B)

Figure 1–22   Anterior superior alveolar. (A) Injection technique. (B) Spread of analgesia.

        (b) Injection site: Height of vestibule on mesial side of canine eminence.
        (c) Insertion angle: Approximately 5 degrees to long axis of tooth.
        (d) Penetration depth: 5 to 6 millimeters to apex of root.
        (e) Amount of solution deposited: One-fourth to one-half cartridge; 0.45 to 0.9 milliliters.
        (f) Tissues innervated: Maxillary canine, lateral incisor, central incisor, and the respective facial gingiva and periosteum.
   (2) Middle superior alveolar nerve block (Figure 1–23).
        (a) Landmark: Apex of second premolar and buccal frenum.

> **CLINICAL TIP:**
>
> **Innervating Your Knowledge:** Modification to the middle superior alveolar nerve block may be indicated due to anatomical features such as an extensive bony prominence, the zygomaticoalveolar crest, preventing the needle's approach to the target site.[1]

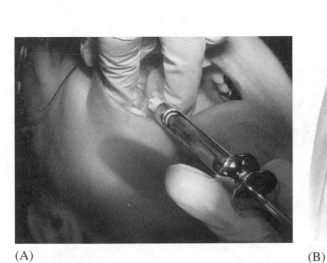

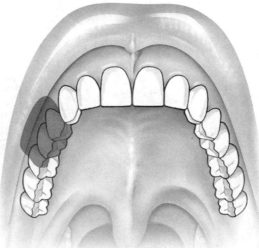

(A)   (B)

Figure 1–23   Middle superior alveolar. (A) Injection technique. (B) Spreading of analgesia.

(b) Injection site: Height of vestibule at apex of second premolar; avoid inserting into frenum.
(c) Insertion angle: Parallel to long axis of second premolar.
(d) Penetration depth: Approximately 5 millimeters to apex of root.
(e) Amount of solution deposited: One-fourth to one-half cartridge; 0.45 to 0.9 milliliters.
(f) Tissues innervated: Maxillary first and second premolars, along with the mesiobuccal root of the maxillary first molar, and the respective facial gingiva and periosteum.
(3) Posterior superior alveolar nerve block (Figure 1–24).
(a) Landmarks: Maxillary tuberosity and posterior superior alveolar foramen.
(b) Injection site: Height of vestibule posterior to maxillary tuberosity.
(c) Insertion angle: 45 degrees out from midline of arch and 45 degrees down from maxillary occlusal plane.
(d) Penetration depth: Approximately 15 millimeters; 1.5 centimeters.
(e) Amount of solution deposited: One-half cartridge; 0.9 milliliters.
(f) Tissues innervated: Maxillary third and second molars, first molar with the exception of the mesiobuccal root, and the respective facial gingiva, periosteum, and mucous membranes of the buccal mucosa.
(4) Greater palatine nerve block (Figure 1–25).
(a) Landmark: Greater palatine foramen.
(b) Insertion site: Greater palatine foramen.
(c) Insertion angle: Approximately 45 degrees from hard palate.
(d) Penetration depth: 2 to 3 millimeters; cover the bevel of the needle.

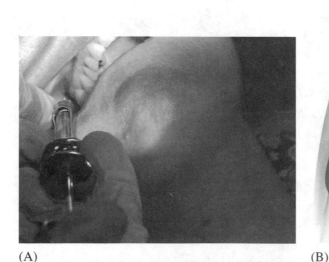
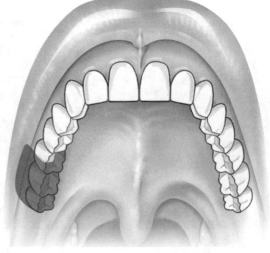

(A)　　　　　(B)

Figure 1–24   Posterior superior alveolar. (A) Injection technique. (B) Spread of analgesia.

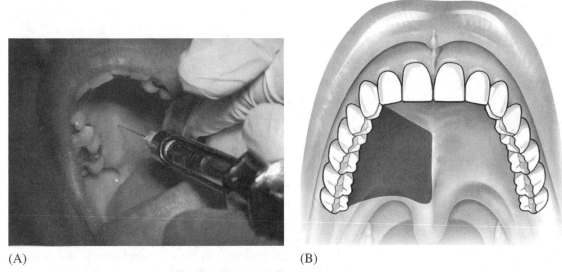

(A)   (B)

Figure 1–25   Greater palatine. (A) Injection technique. (B) Spread of analgesia.

(e) Amount of solution deposited: One-eighth cartridge; stopper full or until tissue blanches in immediate area; 0.1 milliliters.
(f) Tissues innervated: Mucous membrane and glands and gingiva of the posterior hard palate.
(5) Nasopalatine nerve block (Figure 1–26).
(a) Landmark: Incisive papilla.
(b) Injection site: Lateral to the incisive papilla.
(c) Insertion angle: Direct the needle upward, backward, and slightly medially.[1]
(d) Penetration depth: 2 to 3 millimeters, covering the bevel of the needle.

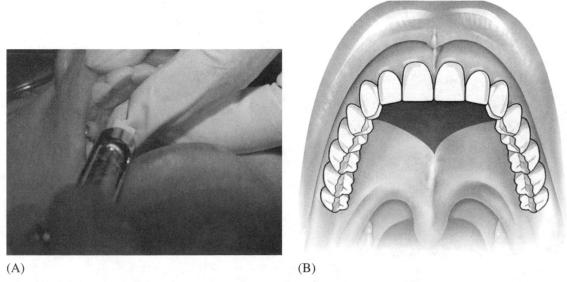

(A)   (B)

Figure 1–26   Nasopalatine. (A) Injection technique. (B) Spread of analgesia.

CLINICAL TIPS:

Innervating Your Knowledge:
Permanent paresthesia, anesthesia, or dysesthesia of both the inferior alveolar and lingual nerves, rarely occurs with an incidence ranging from 1 in 26,000 to 1 in 800,000.[32]

CLINICAL TIP:

Innervating Your Knowledge:
Operators must be fully aware of the anatomical structures in the vicinity of the inferior alveolar nerve and along the pathway to reach the deposition site.

CLINICAL TIP:

Innervating Your Knowledge:
Moving or angling the needle higher along the ramus may result in penetration of arterial supply.[1]

(e) Amount of solution deposited: One-third cartridge; stopper full or until tissue blanches in immediate area; 0.1 milliliters.
(f) Tissues innervated: Nasal septum, mucous membrane, and gingiva of the anterior hard palate.
b. Mandibular injections. Block anesthesia is most effective on the mandibular structures due to the dense buccal cortical plate preventing infiltration of the agent to the nerve.[1]
(1) Inferior alveolar nerve block (Figure 1–27).
(a) Landmarks: Pterygomandibular raphe (Figure 1–28); coronoid notch have the patient open wide to see the pterygomandibular raphe; palpate the anterior border of the ramus of the mandible to locate the coronoid notch.
(b) Injection site: Approximately 10 millimeters, 1 centimeter, coronal to the occlusal plane of the mandibular molars, just medial to the digit locating the coronoid notch, and just lateral to the pterygomandibular raphe.
(c) Insertion angle: Barrel of syringe is placed over the opposite premolars; pathway of insertion should stay in same plane, not at an angle.
(d) Penetration depth: Approximately 26 to 28 millimeters into the pterygomandibular space.[1]
(e) Amount of solution deposited: Three-fourths cartridge; 1.3 to 1.4 milliliters.
(f) Tissues innervated: All anterior and posterior teeth, the respective periosteum, along with the facial gingiva of the teeth anterior to the mental foramen.
(2) Lingual nerve block (see Figure 1–27).
(a) Landmarks: Pterygomandibular raphe and coronoid notch; have the patient open wide to view the pterygomandibular

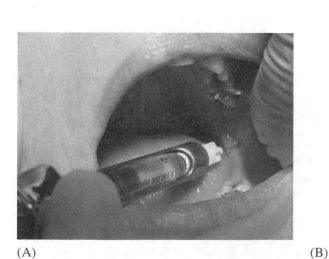

(A)

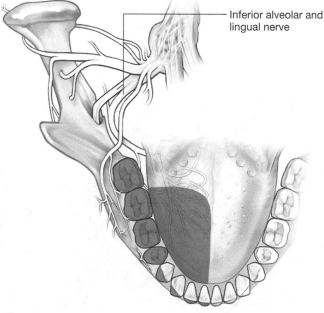

Inferior alveolar and lingual nerve

(B)

Figure 1–27   Inferior alveolar and lingual. (A) Injection technique. (B) Spread of analgesia.

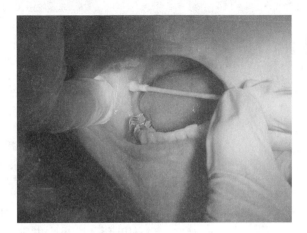

Figure 1–28   Pterygomandibular raphe. Application of the cotton-tipped applicator lateral to landmark.

raphe; palpate the anterior border of the ramus of the mandible to locate the coronoid notch.

(b) Injection site: Approximately 10 millimeters, 1 centimeter, coronal to the occlusal plane of the mandibular molars, just medial to the digit locating the coronoid notch, and lateral to the pterygomandibular raphe.

(c) Insertion angle: Barrel of syringe is placed over the opposite premolars; pathway of insertion should stay in same plane, not at an angle.

(d) Penetration depth: Approximately 13 to 14 millimeters.

(e) Amount of solution deposited: One-fourth cartridge; 0.4 to 0.5 millimeters.

(f) Tissues innervated: Mucous membrane of the anterior two-thirds of the tongue and the lingual gingiva up to the midline of the mandible.

(3) Long buccal nerve block (also known as buccal nerve block) (Figure 1–29).

(a) Landmarks: Anterior border of ramus of mandible.

(b) Injection site: Anterior border of ramus of mandible, approximately 1 millimeter coronal to the occlusal plane of the mandibular molars.

(c) Insertion angle: Barrel of syringe is placed parallel to the central groove of the mandibular molars.

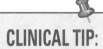

CLINICAL TIP:

Innervating Your Knowledge: Attaining anesthesia for the lingual nerve is commonly done in unison with the inferior alveolar nerve block. The anesthetic solution can be deposited at the target site for the lingual nerve prior to advancing to the penetration depth for the inferior alveolar nerve block or upon retrieval from that injection.

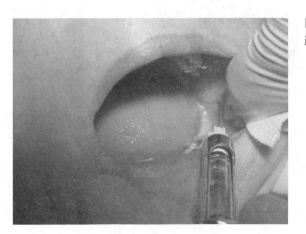

Figure 1–29   Long buccal nerve injection technique.

CLINICAL TIP:

Innervating Your Knowledge:
Radiographs aid in locating the mental foramen, especially with the edentulous patient.

CLINICAL TIP:

Innervating Your Knowledge:
Other injection techniques may be used to achieve anesthesia, such as intraligamentary, intraosseous, intrapulpal, the Gow-Gates block, and Vazirani-Akinosi. These techniques are not discussed in this book but may be learned from an advanced anesthesia course.

    (d) Penetration depth: 2 to 3 millimeters, covering the bevel of the needle.
    (e) Amount of solution deposited: One-eighth cartridge; stopper full; 0.1 milliliters.
    (f) Tissues innervated: Buccal gingiva and mucosa from the mental foramen posteriorly.
  (4) Mental nerve block (Figure 1–30).
    (a) Landmark: Mental foramen.
    (b) Injection site: Depth of vestibule at mental foramen.
    (c) Insertion angle: Slightly toward bone of mandible.
    (d) Penetration depth: To depth of mental foramen; to the area, but not entering the foramen.
    (e) Amount of solution deposited: One-half cartridge; 0.9 milliliters.
    (f) Tissues innervated: Facial gingiva from the mental foramen to the midline of the mandible and the skin and mucosa of the lower lip.
  (5) Incisive nerve block. The incisive nerve can be innervated by displacing the anesthetic solution from the mental injection into the mental foramen; this can easily be accomplished by placing the index finger in the area posterior to the foramen and moving it in an anterior direction.
B. Summary. Providing local anesthesia requires the operator to conduct a thorough review of the medical and dental histories, choose the appropriate local anesthetic agent, utilize proper local anesthetic technique keeping in mind anatomical considerations and areas to be innervated, and observing the patient for possible complications of the injection.

IX. Nitrous Oxide

Nitrous oxide combined with oxygen is a colorless, almost odorless to sweet-smelling gas; it is the only inorganic inhalation agent.[33] It is neither explosive or flammable, however it supports combustion, just like oxygen.[26] It is a supplemental component, commonly used in conjunction with local anesthesia, in

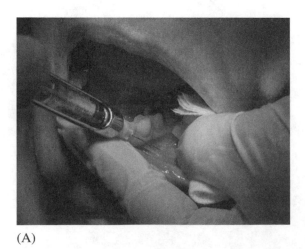
(A)

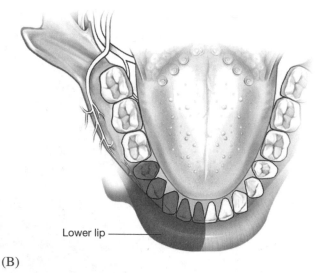
Lower lip
(B)

Figure 1–30   Mental nerve/incisive nerve. (A) Injection technique. (B) Spread of analgesia.

achieving pain control. It is estimated that approximately 50 percent of the dentists in the United States have the equipment to deliver this mixture to help patients deal with their anxiety.[34]

A. History of nitrous oxide. Joseph Priestly discovered oxygen in 1771 and nitrous oxide a year later.[33] In 1798, Sir Humphrey Davy first speculated that nitrous oxide may diminish the pain of surgery. Dr. Horace Wells is the first dentist credited with utilizing nitrous oxide in his dental practice in 1844.[33] Dr. Wells and Dr. William T.G. Morton advanced its use in medicine and dentistry. Dr. Edmund Andrews suggested the addition of oxygen to the nitrous oxide in the mid-1800s, and in 1887 Sir Fredrick Hewitt invented a machine to administer fixed proportions of nitrous oxide and oxygen. Since that time, the mixture, apparatus, and technique have been refined to provide nitrous oxide sedation safely and easily as we do today.[21]

B. Pharmacology of nitrous oxide.
  1. Pharmacological effects.
    a. Nitrous oxide is the weakest of all inhalation and sedation agents.[35]
      (1) Its effect is primarily through the displacement of nitrogen in the bloodstream.
      (2) Its action is purely physical because it does not combine with hemoglobin, other tissues, or undergo biotransformation.[36]
    b. Its pharmacological effect is extremely mild when administered with adequate oxygen.
  2. Physiologic effects.
    a. Central nervous system (CNS). Primary site of action.
      (1) Signs and symptoms include:
        (a) Low nitrous oxide/high oxygen levels. Relaxation, reduced sense of anxiety/fear, glazed eyes, tingling in parts of the body, and flushed cheeks.
        (b) Increased nitrous oxide/moderate oxygen levels. Previous signs and symptoms listed may intensify or disappear; uncontrolled laughing, disassociation from the environment, too warm or hot, slurred words, fidgety, dizziness, and restlessness.
        (c) High nitrous oxide/low oxygen levels (not recommended and usually not necessary). Previous signs and symptoms listed may intensify or disappear; hallucinations, sexual fantasizing, nausea, vomiting, incoherent vocabulary with possibly no response to verbal commands, and fluctuation between consciousness and unconsciousness.
      (2) Somnolence, or the production of sleep, can begin at very low levels.
      (3) The lowest level of nitrous oxide–oxygen that can produce unconsciousness or light general anesthesia is 45 percent; the optimal, or most common level for dental procedural relaxation and sedation is 35 percent.
    b. Cardiovascular system. Response is similar to that produced by 100 percent oxygen administration, namely an insignificant rise in mean arterial pressure and cardiac output decreases slightly. Nitrous oxide has a very low solubility in the bloodstream; therefore, its effects are rapid, and the termination of its effects are equally rapid, usually within 3 to 5 minutes.

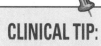

CLINICAL TIP:

Innervating Your Knowledge: If the patient reaches a state of sedation where uncontrolled laughing occurs, he or she may experience nausea as the level of nitrous oxide–oxygen is fluctuating. Encourage the patient to continue to breathe through the nose to maintain consistent levels of the agent in the body.

CLINICAL TIPS:

Innervating Your Knowledge: If the patient begins to exhibit unwanted signs/symptoms, the operator must immediately increase the amount of oxygen and decrease the amount of nitrous oxide being delivered.

    c. Respiratory system. Effects of nitrous oxide are negligible when administered with adequate oxygen.

      (1) Nitrous oxide increases the respiratory minute volume without depressing the response to carbon dioxide.

      (2) Gas is transported across the pulmonary epithelium, which accounts for the uptake and excretion of most of the nitrous oxide in the body.

      (3) It is eliminated unchanged through the lungs, with a very small amount excreted through the skin.

    d. Other organ systems. When administered with adequate oxygen, nitrous oxide can almost be considered inert and nontoxic.

      (1) Produces little to no effects on any body system, except on the CNS.

      (2) Any tissue damage in other organs can usually be attributed to a hypoxia caused by inadequate oxygen, not as a direct result of the nitrous oxide.

      (3) Chronic exposure, even at low levels, may lead to some hematopoietic changes that can affect reproduction.

      (4) Chronic, higher-than-therapeutic levels have been shown to cause some neurological changes, as well as death, from hypoxia in abuse situations.[37]

C. Patient evaluation and preparation.

  1. Review of the health history. Physical and psychological aspects of the patient must be considered prior to nitrous oxide sedation.

    a. Generally, the poorer the health of the patient, the greater the need for conscious sedation. Patients in poor health are less able to cope with the physical stresses of a long dental experience.

    b. Some specific physical or health conditions that need to be considered in the evaluation for sedation are respiratory conditions and pregnancy.

  2. Nitrous oxide is the indicated sedation method for most medically compromised patients. It is considered useful for those patients determined to be mildly apprehensive; patients who are moderately to very apprehensive will need to receive other more potent sedative agents.

  3. Classifications and stages. American Society of Anesthesiologists Physical Status Classification System is a standardized set of physical status classifications to provide a general measure of the patient's severity of illness, allowing for the uniform interpretation of data. Prior to administering nitrous oxide–oxygen, the operator must determine the patient's ability to withstand the procedure and use of the sedative agent.

    a. ASA I: Patient without systemic disease; a normal, healthy patient.

    b. ASA II: Patient with mild systemic disease.

    c. ASA III: Patient with severe systemic disease that limits activity but is not incapacitating.

    d. ASA IV: Patient with incapacitating systemic disease that is a constant threat to life.

    e. ASA V: A moribund patient not expected to survive 24 hours with or without operation.

    f. ASA E: Emergency operation of any variety; "E" precedes the number indicating the patient's physical status (e.g., ASAE-III).

  4. Preoperative preparation. Since the goal of nitrous oxide–oxygen sedation is to provide the patient with a feeling of pleasant relaxation, anal-

CLINICAL TIP:

Innervating Your Knowledge: Pregnancy is not considered an absolute contraindication. However, any treatment that can be deferred until after the conclusion of the first trimester, including the sedation, is advisable.

gesia and amnesia should not be sought as objectives; the patient should be prepared as follows:

a. Assure patient that he or she will be fully aware and in control of his or her faculties, yet will be calm and indifferent to the dental treatment.

b. Operator should suggest a positive experience and use appropriate descriptions of the subjective symptoms to enhance the psychosedative component of the procedure.

c. Provide patient with a minimal amount of physical preparation; instruct patient to wear loose, comfortable clothing because it is easier to get into a relaxed mode when restrictive clothing is not an issue.

d. Suggest that patient have light liquids, such as broth, 2 to 3 hours before the appointment. Food in the stomach should not pose a serious threat. However, since the patient is awake with all protective reflexes intact, it is best to avoid the possibility of nausea and vomiting.[26]

   (1) Because one of the signs of overdose/over sedation is nausea, try to avoid the unpleasant experience of vomiting, if possible.

   (2) Discourage fasting prior to the scheduled appointment because a mild hypoglycemia can occur and increase the potential for nausea and, consequently, vomiting.

5. Indications for nitrous oxide–oxygen sedation. This sedation is considered for nearly all dental procedures where the patient exhibits mild anxiety and apprehension. The procedure may be as minimally invasive as an initial examination or as extensive as endodontics or tooth extraction.

6. Contraindications for nitrous oxide–oxygen sedation.

a. Absolute contraindications include:[26]

   (1) Inability to use nasal hood due to anatomical or disease-induced obstructions.

   (2) Upper respiratory infection or blocked sinus due to deviated septum, nasal polyps, or severe sinusitis.

   (3) Recent history of ear surgery may lead to an increase in pressure of the tympanic membrane or eustachian tube.

b. Relative contraindications.[26,36]

   (1) Compulsive personality: Patient does not like to lose control.

   (2) Claustrophobic patients: The breathing apparatus may increase their fears of claustrophobia.

   (3) Children with severe behavior disorders.

   (4) Adults with severe personality disorders, especially those using mood-elevating antidepressant medications: The use of nitrous oxide–oxygen may increase the negative effects of the condition.

   (5) Acute respiratory conditions that may include the common cold, mild acute or chronic sinusitis, chronic mouth breathing, mild allergies, tuberculosis, bronchitis, or cough: These conditions may compromise the patient's ability to breathe through the nose, resulting in insufficient amounts of nitrous oxide–oxygen entering the respiratory system.

   (6) Chronic obstructive pulmonary disease (COPD): Supplemental oxygen within the nitrous oxide–oxygen mixture may increase the oxygen blood saturation level to a point where breathing could cease.

   (7) A patient who does not want nitrous oxide–oxygen (forcing a patient to use nitrous oxide) during treatment could result in a

compromised patient/operator trust situation and could lead to legal problems.

(8) Pregnancy: While it is considered safe for the pregnant patient, it is best to avoid any elective treatment during the first trimester because nitrous interferes with the metabolism of vitamin B_{12} that is necessary for DNA production and cellular reproduction.[36]

7. Current and contemporary issues surrounding nitrous oxide–oxygen sedation.

a. Potential biohazard from long-term exposure.

(1) Nitrous oxide has historically been considered to be physiologically harmless.

(2) Studies on record suggest long-term exposures, even at low levels, can cause some health risks.

(a) Female employees who are of childbearing age and exposed to nitrous oxide–oxygen in the work environment need to evaluate possible exposure to the agent.

(b) This has not been proven conclusively.[17]

(3) It has been well documented that long-term exposure to high levels of nitrous oxide, higher than is therapeutically utilized, can cause **leukopenia** and a pernicious anemia–like condition as well as some neurological disorders; these hazards are minimized by appropriate concentrations, using scavenging systems, and monitoring dental personnel for trace exposures.

(4) Recreational abuse.[35,36] As may be expected, due to the euphoria produced by nitrous oxide, it has been used and abused for recreational purposes to the point of addiction and death.

(5) Chronic abuse can lead to neuropathies and eventually hypoxia and death; counseling, peer groups, and other support groups are available for those who are addicted; however, state licensing boards and others often become involved.

b. Sexual awareness regarding nitrous oxide.[35,36] It has been documented that nitrous oxide produces a euphoria, but at higher concentrations, it can lead to dreaming hallucinations, specifically increased feelings of sexuality, or, as Sir Humphrey Davy described it in 1798, "voluptuous sensations."

(1) In many cases, where the patient has misinterpreted these hallucinations as reality, the operator of the nitrous oxide consistently allowed the following circumstances to occur.

(a) Patient was treated alone, without the benefit of a witness in the room.

(b) High concentrations of nitrous oxide were delivered, with failure to titrate to the patient's range of therapeutic sedation.

(2) Following simple guidelines to avoid these situations should ensure that the administrator of nitrous oxide has no difficulties with any sexual issues.[38]

8. Maintenance and monitoring of nitrous oxide and equipment.[36] A properly installed delivery system should include scavenging equipment, readily visible and accurate flowmeter, a vacuum system capable of 45L per minute per workstation, and a variety of masks.

a. Vacuum and ventilation exhausts should vent to the outside.

b. Room air should be well ventilated.

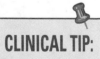

CLINICAL TIP:

Innervating Your Knowledge: Titration is the administration of small incremental doses of a drug until a desired clinical action is observed.

c. Each time the machine is turned on and every time the gas cylinders are changed, the connections should be checked for leaks; other high-pressure connections should be checked routinely. A simple solution of soapy water may be used to check for leaks.

d. All equipment, including the reservoir bag, tubing, masks, and connectors should be checked for cracks, holes, or tears each day before the machine is used.

e. Connect the mask to the tubing with the vacuum pump to verify flow rates.

f. Each patient should be fitted with an appropriately comfortable mask, and the reservoir bag should be checked for proper inflation prior to administering nitrous oxide.

g. The patient should be encouraged to minimize talking and mouth breathing, as much as possible, to minimize the amount of nitrous oxide–oxygen contaminating the office air.[35]

h. The reservoir bag should be checked frequently for changes in tidal volume and the vacuum flow rate verified.

i. Upon completion of all procedures, the patient should breath 100 percent oxygen for 3 to 5 minutes; this purges both the patient and the system of nitrous oxide.

j. Dental personnel should be checked semiannually for trace nitrous exposures with a dosimeter.

9. Equipment
a. Types of inhalation sedation apparatus. In the United States, the most commonly used machine in dentistry is the continuous flow unit; there are three types of delivery systems for nitrous oxide–oxygen administration, which include:

(1) Portable. The entire system, including the gas cylinders, regulating and monitor devices, can be transported from operatory to operatory. It is a self-contained, stand-alone system.

(2) Central storage system. The large nitrous oxide and oxygen cylinders are maintained in a central storage area with the gases piped into each operatory; each operatory is equipped with the regulating and monitoring devices; the patient simply needs to be "plugged in" via the delivery hoses.

(3) Central storage system with mobile heads. This is a hybrid of the other two systems. The large gas cylinders are stored in a central area and the gases are piped into each operatory; the regulating, delivery, and monitoring devices are moved from operatory to operatory and attached to the gas sources via a quick connect arrangement.

b. Compressed gas cylinders. Nitrous oxide and oxygen gas are supplied in steel cylinders under high pressure (Figure 1–31). Cylinders are color-coded and the valve/coupling system is pin-indexed specifically for each type of gas.

(1) These two features prevent accidental crossing or confusion of the gases.

(2) American Society of Anesthesiologists, the American Hospital Association, and the medical gas industry have established a uniform color code and pin-indexing configuration.

(a) Oxygen is supplied in a green cylinder.

📌
CLINICAL TIP:

Innervating Your Knowledge: The colors of gas cylinders are uniform in the United States: blue = nitrous oxide, green = oxygen. These colors are not consistent internationally.[36]

Figure 1–31   Compressed gas cylinders. Color coding helps prevent accidental crossing of the gases to the gas lines. The oxygen cylinders are green. The nitrous oxide cylinders are blue.

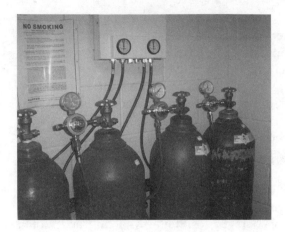

(b) Nitrous oxide comes in a blue cylinder.
(c) Cylinders are available in a wide variety of sizes ranging from approximately 3 pounds to more than 125 pounds, depending on the specific needs of the practice.
c. Regulators, also known as reducing valves, are located between the compressed gas cylinders and the flowmeter.
(1) The regulator reduces the high-pressure gas coming from the cylinder to a pressure that is safe for the patient and the sedation unit.
(2) A manifold is used in central systems to join multiple gas cylinders.
(3) Yokes are used only in portable systems; they hold the cylinder of gas tightly in contact with the nipples of the portable sedation unit.
(4) Metal pins below the collar of the nipple area (where the pin index safety system is found) are incorporated to prevent attachment of the wrong gas cylinder.
d. Flowmeters. The gases flow from the reducing valves to the back of the unit and then into the flowmeter, which permits the precise delivery of either gas to the patient; they measure the actual flow of the gas, not the pressure (Figure 1–32).
(1) A float, either a ball or a rotameter, measures the volume of the gas flow. The gauge is read from the middle of the ball, and the rotameter is read from the top of the bobbin.
(2) Calibrated markings on the flowmeter tubes indicate gas flow in liters per minute.

Figure 1–32   Flowmeter. Permits precise delivery of either gas to the patient.

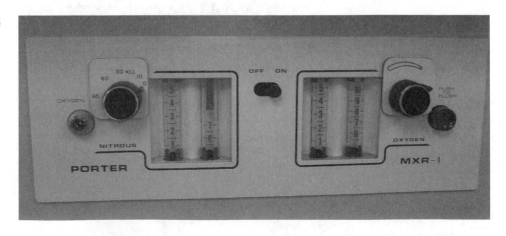

(3) Gas flow is adjusted by a fine needle valve for each flowmeter. As the gases leave each flowmeter, they are combined in a mixing chamber in the head of the sedation unit. The combined gases exit the sedation unit through the outflow tube or bag/tee—tee because it is T-shaped—a component of the system that mixes the metered gases prior to delivery to the patient. The oxygen is combined with the nitrous oxide and then passes to the patient for inhalation.

e. Emergency air intake valve. Located on the bag/tee above the reservoir bag, it provides a supply of atmospheric air to the patient in the event the sedation unit malfunctions or gas flow is interrupted.

f. Rubber goods. These include the reservoir bag, conducting tubing, facemasks, nasal hoods, and nasal canula. The gases flow from the outlet tube to the patient.

(1) The reservoir bag is a bladder-type bag that attaches to the base of the bag/tee immediately below the emergency air inlet valve. A small amount of gas is diverted into the bag and may be used for several purposes (Figure 1–33).

(a) Primary function: To provide a reservoir for additional gas should the patient's respiratory demands exceed the gas flow of the sedation machine.

(b) May be used to monitor respirations and is a means for providing oxygen during assisted ventilation, if needed.

(2) Conducting tubes (breathing tubes) connect the bag/tee to the breathing apparatus. Large diameter corrugated tubing is attached to a smaller diameter tube that connects to the breathing apparatus.

(3) Breathing apparatus can be a full-face mask, nasal cannula, or, most commonly, a rubber or silicon nasal hood with four tubes attached.

(a) Two tubes carry fresh gas to the patient, and two tubes carry the exhausted gases to a safe repository. This is called a scavenging nasal hood; the hood may also contain some other valves to help regulate the gas flow as needed.

(b) A scavenger hood is two hoods in one—an inner and an outer hood. The inner hood delivers fresh nitrous oxide–oxygen to the nose of the patient and is disposable or may be autoclavable. The outer hood connects with the vacuum system and may be cold disinfected[35] (Figure 1–34).

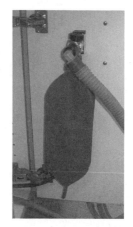

Figure 1–33   Reservoir bag.

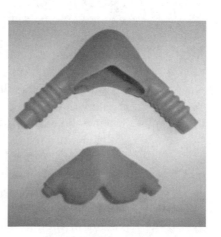

Figure 1–34   Scavenger hoods.

10. Listing of safety features.
    a. Pin index safety system. Metal pins protruding from the attachment apparatus to which the gas cylinders attach; prevents gas cylinder from being attachment to a wrong portal.
    b. Diameter index safety system. Each hose is gas specific and has a unique, standardized diameter of the coupling attaching to the cylinder.
    c. Minimum oxygen liter flow. The minimum amount of oxygen, in liters, that flows through the unit.
    d. Minimum oxygen percentage. The minimum amount of oxygen, in percentage, that flows through the unit. Units manufactured today require a 30 percent oxygen level.[36]
    e. Oxygen fail-safe mechanism. Prevents the delivery of 100 percent nitrous; oxygen must be flowing to the machine for nitrous to be delivered.
    f. Emergency air inlet. Provides additional source of atmospheric air if the reservoir bag is not efficient or there is a decrease in the flow of the gas.
    g. Alarm. Visual or auditory alert indicating a depleting oxygen supply.
    h. Oxygen flush button. Delivers oxygen to the reservoir bag in a rapid manner.
    i. Reservoir bag. Bladder-type bag that holds a reserve of oxygen.
    j. Color-coding of cylinders. Allows for immediate identification of gaseous agent.
    k. Lock. Prevents unauthorized use and abuse.
    l. Quick connect. Allows for positive pressure oxygen delivery.
11. Complications.
    a. Inadequate or incomplete sedation is usually due to poor patient selection.
    b. Poor patient experience is usually attributable to oversedation; this can be avoided by titrating the concentration to the desired clinical relaxation endpoint.
    c. Equipment performance can also complicate the experience. This can be prevented by routine examination, inspection, and maintenance.
    d. Oversedation (rare). Nitrous oxide concentration is greater than 50 percent or the duration is longer than an hour.
    e. Potential list includes nausea and vomiting, tooth pain associated with sinus pressure, vertigo, bowel discomfort, claustrophobia, contact lens drying out, and anatomic obstructions.
    f. Management of these complications can best be achieved by avoiding them through judicious titration and delivering the minimal concentration to achieve the clinical level of sedation; also closely monitor the patient during sedation.
12. Techniques of administration.[36] It is important for the operator to develop a routine when administering nitrous oxide–oxygen to ensure patient safety during the procedure.
    a. Review the health history and obtain vital signs for any possible contraindications for use.
       (1) Obtain informed consent before each use.
       (2) Evaluate equipment ensuring proper working conditions.
       (3) Select the appropriate breathing apparatus, making sure it fits snugly around the nose to eliminate unnecessary gas into the room air.

CLINICAL TIP:

Innervating Your Knowledge: It is important to continuously monitor the patient using nitrous oxide–oxygen for possible complications.

(4) Activate the scavenger system, adjusting the suction so it does not pull the gas away from the patient prior to inhalation.

(5) Fill the reservoir bag approximately two-thirds full with oxygen using the oxygen flush button; turn off the oxygen flush button.

(6) Establish a flow rate with 100 percent oxygen and position the nasal hood.

(7) Establish appropriate flow rate while the patient is still breathing 100 percent oxygen. The reservoir bag is neither expanding nor collapsing, but remains uniform.

(8) Encourage the patient to close mouth and breath through the nose.

(9) Start the flow of nitrous oxide, usually beginning at 10 percent to 20 percent and titrating at 5 percent to 10 percent increments every 60 seconds.

(10) Question the patient to determine level of sedation; ideal level of clinical sedation is reached when the patient claims feeling a pleasant, relaxed, and comfortable state.

b. Treatment phase.
   (1) Perform the planned procedure(s).
   (2) Monitor the patient's responses and the reservoir bag to make sure adequate titration level and flow is continued.

c. Recovery phase.
   (1) Terminate the nitrous oxide flow and administer 100 percent oxygen at the flow rate already determined for the patient for 3 to 5 minutes or until the signs of the sedation have subsided.
   (2) Obtain vital signs.
   (3) Dismiss the patient only after it is determined that all signs of the agent are exhausted from the body.

d. Record keeping. Enter information into the treatment record including the date, reason for use of nitrous oxide–oxygen sedation, treatment completed, vital signs (before and after sedation), patient's tidal volume, peak percentage of nitrous oxide–oxygen administered, amount of time in recovery phase breathing 100 percent oxygen, and any negative experiences/conditions.

CLINICAL TIP:

Innervating Your Knowledge: Nasal hoods come in a variety of colors and scents.

CLINICAL TIP:

Innervating Your Knowledge: Evaluate each patient individually when titrating nitrous oxide–oxygen. Avoid developing the "cookie cutter" mentality that all patients require the same concentration.

CLINICAL TIP:

Innervating Your Knowledge: The exact configuration of delivery mechanisms varies by manufacturer. Prior to administering nitrous oxide–oxygen, the operator must become familiar with the oxygen and nitrous controls.

Using nitrous oxide–oxygen may alleviate nervousness in the dental hygiene patient. While it is a safe drug for most people, it is essential to carefully review the patient's health history and monitor the agent delivered, as well as the patient's response to the drug.

QUESTIONS

1. A loss of sensation in a circumscribed area of the body, caused by depression of excitation in nerve endings or an inhibition of the conduction process in peripheral nerves, is
   a. nitrous oxide–oxygen sedation.
   b. general anesthesia.
   c. local anesthesia.
   d. no anesthesia.

2. All of the following are methods of inducing local anesthesia EXCEPT one. Which one is the EXCEPTION?
   a. Anoxia
   b. Chemical agents
   c. Lowering the temperature
   d. Hypnosis

3. Which of the following statements identifies the property of an "ideal" local anesthetic agent?
   a. Permanently alters the nerve ending.
   b. Does not produce an allergic reaction.
   c. Effective when introduced into the gastrointestinal system.
   d. Shows high systemic toxicity.

4. Local anesthetic agents, delivered in recommended amounts, generally produce
   a. vasodilatation.
   b. vasoconstriction.
   c. significant respiratory difficulty.
   d. immunoglobulin E-mediated allergic reactions.

5. All of the following are recommended methods of administering local anesthetic agents for dental procedures EXCEPT one. Which one is the EXCEPTION?
   a. Topical
   b. Injection
   c. Subcutaneous
   d. Oral

6. Which two organs are the major targets for local anesthetic toxicity?
   a. Brain and liver
   b. Liver and kidneys
   c. Kidneys and heart
   d. Heart and brain

7. Plasma pseudocholinesterase is responsible for initiation of hydrolysis for which anesthetic agent?
   a. Procaine
   b. Articaine
   c. Bupivacaine
   d. Lidocaine

8. Renal impairment may result in a problem with the
   a. metabolism of the drug.
   b. administration of the drug.
   c. excretion of the drug.
   d. uptake of the drug.

9. Mild signs of central nervous system (CNS) stimulation include all of the following EXCEPT one. Which one is the EXCEPTION?
   a. Localized muscle twitching
   b. Convulsions
   c. Inability to focus
   d. Disorientation

10. All of the following are benefits of the addition of vasoconstrictors to local anesthetic agents EXCEPT one. Which one is the EXCEPTION?
    a. Increased blood flow to the site.
    b. Slower rate of absorption.
    c. Decrease in the risk of overdose.
    d. Less amount of anesthetic solution needed to achieve anesthesia.

11. Which percentage of vasoconstrictor would produce more of a hemostasis effect?
    a. 1:200,000
    b. 1:100,000
    c. 1:50,000
    d. They all produce an equal state of hemostasis.

12. Epinephrine is acceptable for patients with cardiovascular disease. The preferred concentration would be 1:50,000 to minimize stress on the heart.
    a. Both statements are TRUE.
    b. Both statements are FALSE.
    c. The first statement is TRUE. The second statement is FALSE.
    d. The first statement is FALSE. The second statement is TRUE.

13. Which class of drugs may be a contraindication for use with epinephrine?
    a. Beta blockers
    b. Calcium channel blockers
    c. Oral contraceptives
    d. Antibiotics

14. All of the following are forms of topical anesthetics EXCEPT one. Which one is the EXCEPTION?
    a. Liquid
    b. Gel
    c. Spray
    d. Foam

15. It is important to select an anesthetic agent that will provide an appropriate length of anesthesia. An anesthetic of intermediate duration provides approximately 90 minutes of pulpal anesthesia.
    a. Both statements are TRUE.
    b. Both statements are FALSE.
    c. The first statement is TRUE. The second statement is FALSE.
    d. The first statement is FALSE. The second statement is TRUE.

16. Adverse reactions occurring due to toxicity of a local anesthetic agent are usually irreversible and permanent in nature. Toxicity may be minimized when guidelines for administration are followed.
    a. Both statements are TRUE.
    b. Both statements are FALSE.
    c. The first statement is TRUE. The second statement is FALSE.
    d. The first statement is FALSE. The second statement is TRUE.

17. Intravascular injection of the anesthetic agent may result in
    a. increased amount of excretion of the drug.
    b. increase in the plasma level of the drug.
    c. decreased toxicity to the drug.
    d. decreased amount absorbed into the bloodstream.

18. An overdose of a local anesthetic agent that presents itself more than 15 minutes from when the agent was administered is most likely caused from
    a. an intravascular injection.
    b. rapid absorption of the drug.
    c. too great a dose of the drug.
    d. abnormal biotransformation.

19. Common causes of pain with an injection may be associated with all of the following EXCEPT one. Which one is the EXCEPTION?
    a. Injecting the solution too slowly.
    b. Poor technique during administration.
    c. Expressing solution too rapidly.
    d. Using a dull needle.

20. Persistent anesthesia may occur as a result of administration of local anesthesia. One possible cause is the needle severed the neurovascular bundle.
    a. Both statements are TRUE.
    b. Both statements are FALSE.
    c. The first statement is TRUE. The second statement is FALSE.
    d. The first statement is FALSE. The second statement is TRUE.

21. What is the first step in treating a hematoma that is a result of a local anesthetic injection?
    a. Apply heat
    b. Apply ice
    c. Apply direct pressure
    d. Elevate the feet

22. Off-center penetration of the needle into the rubber diaphragm may
    a. increase the amount of solution expressed during the injection.
    b. prevent anesthetic solution from being expressed.
    c. prevent aspiration.
    d. lead to a broken cartridge.

23. A positive aspiration indicates that the
    a. operator has retracted the thumb ring during the injection.
    b. tip of the needle has reached the target site for the injection.
    c. bevel of the needle is in a blood vessel.
    d. patient is having an allergic reaction to the anesthetic agent.

24. Which injection (nerve block) provides innervation to the maxillary first and second premolar, along with the mesiobuccal root of the maxillary first molar?
    a. Anterior superior alveolar
    b. Middle superior alveolar
    c. Posterior superior alveolar
    d. Greater palatine

25. The incisive papilla is the landmark for which of the following injections (nerve blocks)?
    a. Nasopalatine
    b. Anterior superior alveolar
    c. Greater palatine
    d. Middle superior alveolar

26. Which injection (nerve block) requires a penetration depth of approximately 26 to 28 millimeters?
    a. Middle superior alveolar
    b. Posterior superior alveolar
    c. Inferior alveolar
    d. Lingual

27. Nitrous oxide–oxygen sedation levels must be carefully monitored. The amount of agent administered should be the same for all patients.
    a. Both statements are TRUE.
    b. Both statements are FALSE.
    c. The first statement is TRUE. The second statement is FALSE.
    d. The first statement is FALSE. The second statement is TRUE.

28. Nitrous oxide–oxygen sedation is contraindicated for patients with respiratory conditions because the patient's ability to inhale and exhale efficiently may be compromised.
    a. Both the statement and reason are correct and related.
    b. Both the statement and reason are correct but not related.
    c. The statement is correct. The reason is not.
    d. The statement is not correct. The reason is correct.

29. Oxygen is supplied in a blue tank. Nitrous oxide is supplied in a green tank.
    a. Both statements are TRUE.
    b. Both statements are FALSE.
    c. The first statement is TRUE. The second statement is FALSE.
    d. The first statement is FALSE. The second statement is TRUE.

30. The component of the nitrous oxide–oxygen sedation delivery mechanism that delivers fresh nitrous oxide–oxygen to the nosepiece, while eliminating exhausted gas via a vacuum system, is(are) the
    a. conducting tubes.
    b. reservoir bag.
    c. scavenger hood.
    d. oxygen flush button.

REFERENCES

1. Blanton P, Jeske A. The key to profound local anesthesia: Neuroanatomy. *Journal of the American Dental Association,* Vol. 134, June 2003, 753–60.

2. States where dental hygienists may administer local anesthesia, http://www.adha.org/downloads/LocalAnthsiamap.pdf, April 4, 2004.

3. Malamed SF. *Handbook of Local Anesthesia.* St. Louis: Mosby, 1997.

4. Allen GD. *Dental Anesthesia and Analgesia (local and general),* 2nd ed. Baltimore: Williams & Wilkins, 1979.

5. Koerner K, Taylor S. Emergencies associated with local anesthetics. *Dentistry Today,* October 2002, 72–79.

6. Haas, DA. An update on local anesthesia in dentistry. *Journal of the Canadian Dental Association,* Vol. 68, Number 9, October 2002, 546–51.

7. Dentsply Pharmaceutical. Product brochure 3% Polocaine® Dental; 2% Polocaine® Dental. http://www.dentsplypharma.com/Prescribing%20Information/Polocaine%20Pl.pdf, May 22, 2004.

8. Chen A. Toxicity and allergy to local anesthesia. *Journal of the California Dental Association,* September 1998, http://www.cda.org/member/pubs/jounral/jour998/allergy.html, May 22, 2004.

9. Germishuys PJ. Hyperresponders and adrenaline in local anaesthetic solutions. *Journal of the South African Dental Association,* Vol. 56, Number 4, April 2001, 175–77.

10. Anil AT, Peker HB, Turgut IN, Gulekon FL. Variations in the anatomy of the inferior alveolar nerve. *British Journal of Oral and Maxillofacial Surgery* Vol. 41, 2003, 236–39.

11. Meechan JG. Supplementary routes to local anaesthesia. *International Endodontic Journal,* Vol. 35, 2002, 885–96.

12. Pogrel MA, Thamby S. Permanent nerve involvement resulting from inferior alveolar nerve blocks. *Journal of American Dental Association,* Vol. 131, July 2000, 901–7.

13. Cook-Waite. Product brochure—Carbocaine 3% injection; Carbocaine 2% with Neo-cobefrin 1:20,000 injection. http://www.kodak.com/global/plugins/acrobat/en/health/pdf/prod/dental/intra/carbocaine.pdf, May 25, 2004.

14. Malamed SF, Gagnon S, LeBlanc D. Efficacy of articaine: A new amide local anesthetic. *Journal of the American Dental Association,* Vol. 131, May 2000, 635–42.

15. VISN 21 Drug Use Criteria for Septocaine™ (4% Articaine HCl with 1:100,000 epinephrine), June 2003. Product brochure. http://www.visn21.med.va.gov/resources/docs/pharmacy/druginfo/duc/articaine.doc, May 25, 2004.

16. Kaufman E, Goharian S, Katz Y. Adverse reactions triggered by dental local anesthetics: A clinical survey. *Anesthesia Progress,* Vol. 47, Number 4, Winter 2000, 134–38.

17. Turner M, Shahid RA. Management of the pregnant oral and maxillofacial surgery patient. *Journal of Oral and Maxillofacial Surgery,* Vol. 60, Number 12, December 2002, 1479–88.

18. Malamed S. Allergy and toxic reactions to local anesthetics. *Dentistry Today,* April 2003. http://www.dentistrytoday.com/mod/forum/discuss.php?d=48, May 28, 2004.

19. Nicholson J, Berry T, Summitt J, Yuan C, Witten T. Pain perception and utility: A comparison of the syringe and computerized local injection techniques. *General Dentistry,* Vol. 49, Number 2, March-April 2001, 167–73.

20. Evers H, Haegerstam G. *Introduction to Local Anaesthesia,* Switzerland: Mediglobe SA, 1990.

21. Bennett C. *Conscious Sedation in Dental Practice.* St. Louis: Mosby, 1974.

22. Lydiatt DD. Litigation and the lingual nerve. *Journal of Oral Maxillofacial Surgery,* Vol. 61, 2003, 197–200.

23. Blanton PL, Jeske AH. Avoiding complications in local anesthesia inductions: Anatomical considerations. *Journal of the American Dental Association,* Vol. 134, July 2003, 888–93.

24. Dower JS Jr. A review of paresthesia in association with the administration of local anesthesia. *Dentistry Today,* February 2003, http://www.dentistrytoday.com/mod/forum/discuss.php?d=40, April 30, 2004.

25. College C, Feigal R, Wandera A, Strange M. Bilateral versus unilateral block anesthesia in a pediatric population. *Pediatric Dentistry,* Vol. 22, 2000, p. 6.

26. Dionne RA, Phero JC, Becker DE. *Management of Pain and Anxiety.* Philadelphia: W.B. Saunders, 2002.

27. Shankland WE. The trigeminal nerve. Part I: An over-view. *The Journal of Craniomandibular Practice,* Vol. 18, Number 4, October 2000, 238–48.

28. Shankland WE. The trigeminal nerve. Part III: The maxillary division. *The Journal of Craniomandibular Practice,* Vol. 19, Number 2, April 2001, 78–83.

29. *Gray's Anatomy,* The trigeminal nerve, http://education.yahoo.com/reference/gray/200.html#49, April 3, 2004.

30. Shankland WE. The trigeminal nerve. Part IV: The mandibular division. *The Journal of Craniomandibular Practice,* Vol. 19, Number 3, July 2001, 153–61.

31. Requa-Clark B. *Applied Pharmacology for the Dental Hygienist,* 4th ed. St. Louis: Mosby, 2000.

32. Pogrel MA, Schmidt BL, Sambajon V, Jordan RCK. Lingual nerve damage due to inferior alveolar nerve blocks, a possible explanation. *Journal of the American Dental Association,* Vol. 134, February 2003, 195–99.

33. Cameron E, May P. *Nitrous Oxide–Laughing Gas,* http://www.chm.bris.ac.uk/motm/n2o/n2oh.html, May 31, 2004.

34. Quarnstrom F. Comparison of time to anesthesia for block, infiltration, and intraosseous local anesthetic injections: A clinical study. *Dentistry Today,* Vol. 20, Number 2, February 2001, 114–19.

35. Malamed S, Clark M. Nitrous oxide-oxygen: A new look at a very old technique. *Dentistry Today,* May 2003, http://www.cda.org/member/pubs/journal/jour0503/malamed.html, May 28, 2004.

36. Clark M, Brunick A. *Handbook of Nitrous Oxide and Oxygen Sedation.* St. Louis: Mosby, 1999.

37. Malamed SF. *Sedation, A Guide to Patient Management,* 4th edition. St. Louis: Mosby, 2003.

38. Holroyd I, Roberts GJ. Inhalation sedation with nitrous oxide: A review. *Dental Update,* Vol. 27, Number 3, April 2000, 141–2, 144, 146.

Chapter 2

Advanced Instrumentation

Nancy K. Mann, RDH, MSEd

MediaLink

A companion CD-ROM, included free with each new copy of this book, supplements the procedures presented in each chapter. Insert the CD-ROM to watch video clips and view a large collection of color images that is also included. This multimedia library is designed to help you add a new dimension to your learning.

KEY TERMS

alternate fulcrum
  cross arch
  extraoral
  finger on finger
  opposite arch
  reinforced
area-specific curette

debridement
endoscopy
extended terminal shank
file
fulcrum
mechanical therapy

nonsurgical periodontal therapy
periodontal debridement
root planing
scaling
shortened blade curette
universal curette

LEARNING OBJECTIVES

After reading this chapter, the student will be able to:

- compare and contrast area-specific curettes;
- discuss instruments used for advanced root instrumentation;
- compare and contrast universal curettes and area-specific curettes;
- identify intraoral sites of use when utilizing the following area-specific curettes:
  - a. 1/2
  - b. 3/4
  - c. 5/6
  - d. 7/8
  - e. 9/10
  - f. 11/12
  - g. 13/14
  - h. 15/16
  - i. 17/18
- name the characteristics of an area-specific curette;
- differentiate between regular- and extended-length curettes;
- list the advantages of shortened-bladed curettes;
- list the characteristics of Langer universal curettes;
- state the surface areas used for the posterior area-specific curettes;
- list and describe the four grades of furcation involvement;

- define periodontal debridement;
- differentiate between scaling, root planing, and periodontal debridement;
- define nonsurgical periodontal therapy;
- state the goal of periodontal debridement;
- discuss what determines the end point of root planing;
- demonstrate alternate seating positions used to accomplish greater access to specific areas of the mouth;
- demonstrate alternate fulcrums:
  - a. extra oral
  - b. cross arch
  - c. opposite arch
  - d. reinforced
  - e. finger on finger
- discuss the challenges of furcation debridement;
- name the benefits of magnification provided by eye loupes;
- discuss new technologies to detect subgingival calculus;
- demonstrate proper instrument sharpening technique;
- discuss new technologies in instrument sharpening.

I. Introduction

Advanced **scaling** and root instrumentation are challenging, yet rewarding tasks in dentistry, requiring meticulous clinical skills to achieve a successful response from the patient. A thorough knowledge of root anatomy is essential to properly adapt various instruments strategically. A thorough assessment, dental hygiene diagnosis, and treatment planning are prerequisites for root instrumentation. Ongoing evaluation during and after treatment is integral to a successful case. Following is a discussion of hand instrumentation that will be used for **nonsurgical periodontal therapy.** For skills relating to calculus detection and assessing the periodontal pocket, refer to *Essentials of Dental Hygiene: Preclinical Skills.*[1]

II. Hand Instruments Used in Advanced Root Instrumentation

A. Area-Specific Curette

1. Definition. A periodontal instrument with one useful cutting edge and rounded back per working end that is easily adapted subgingivally because of its design; ends are designed for use on specific surfaces and areas; blade curves toward the tooth.
2. Purpose. To access root surfaces for effective **periodontal debridement** and **root planing.**
3. Characteristics.
   a. Internal angle. Angled between 70 and 80 degrees between face and lateral sides; this provides optimal cutting edge for calculus removal (Figure 2–1).
   b. Blade. Angled 60 to 70 degrees from terminal shank and curved in two planes for offset angulation.
   c. Lower cutting edge. Located at each end and positioned next to tooth/root surface with paired mirror image working ends.
   d. Cross section. Half-moon shape.
   e. Rounded back. Located where the lower portion of the lateral surfaces meet; always remains next to the soft tissue.
   f. Curved face. Tilted at a 60 to 70 degree angle to the lower shank; when in use, face tilts toward tooth surface (Figure 2–2).

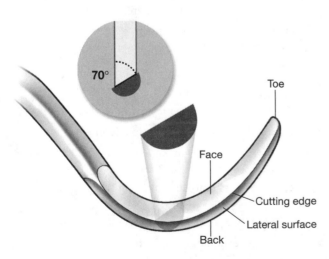

Figure 2–1   Characteristics of an area-specific curette, including internal angle.

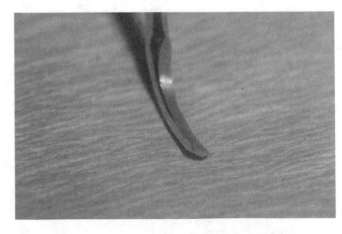

Figure 2–2   Curved face tilts toward tooth surface.

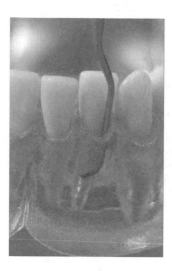

Figure 2–3 Anterior area-specific curette. Note straight shank. *Photo courtesy of Hu-Friedy Manufacturing Co., Inc.*

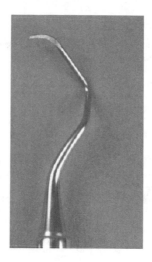

Figure 2–4 Posterior area-specific curette. Note curved shank. *Photo courtesy of Hu-Friedy Manufacturing Co., Inc.*

CLINICAL TIP:

Adapting Your Knowledge: An example of a set of Gracey curettes used to complete the entire dentition includes the 5/6, 11/14, and 12/13.

g. Long functional shank. Designed with straight or multiple bends to allow adaptation throughout the mouth.
   (1) Straight shank: Usually indicates more anterior use.
   (2) Longer, more angled shank: Generally used in the posterior area(s) (Figures 2–3 and 2–4).
h. Terminal (lower) shank. Placed parallel to the tooth surface being instrumented; also known as self-angulating.
i. Rounded toe. Facilitates adaptation to root concavities (Figure 2–5).
j. Numbering system. Lower numbers identify anterior instruments (e.g., 1/2); higher numbers indicate posterior instruments (e.g., 17/18, used on the most posterior distal surface) (Table 2–1).
4. Types of area-specific curettes (Figure 2–8).[2] All of the following designs are available with a rigid shank, which is preferred for removal of heavy calculus. Although the shank is wider, the blade width is the same as a standard Gracey.
   a. Standard series. Original area-specific curette designed by Dr. Clayton Gracey in the 1930s; permits greater accessibility; numbered from 1 to 18 (Figure 2–9).
   b. Extended shank length. Designed with 3 additional millimeters in the terminal shank for increased accessibility in periodontal pockets

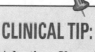

CLINICAL TIP:

Adapting Your Knowledge: The terms *terminal shank* and *lower shank* mean the same and can be used interchangeably.

CLINICAL TIP:

Adapting Your Knowledge:
Area-specific curette *mesial* ends include 11, 12, 15, or 16. (Figure 2–6)
Area-specific curette *distal* ends include 13, 14, 17, or 18. (Figure 2–7)

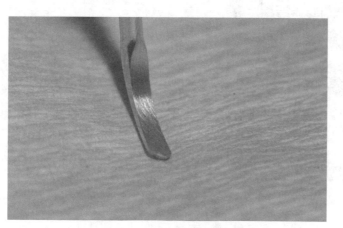

Figure 2–5 Rounded toe of an area-specific curette.

Table 2–1   Area of Use for Gracey Curettes

Instrument	Area of Use for Anterior Teeth	Area of Use for Posterior Teeth
Gracey 1–2	Maxillary and Mandibular Anteriors	
Gracey 3–4	Maxillary and Mandibular Anteriors	
Gracey 5–6	Maxillary and Mandibular Anteriors	All surfaces of premolars; buccal and linguals of molars
Gracey 7–8	Maxillary and Mandibular Anteriors	Posterior proximals and facial and lingual surfaces
Gracey 9–10		Facial and lingual surfaces of all molars
Gracey 11–12		Mesial, facial, and lingual surfaces of maxillary and mandibular teeth
Gracey 13–14		Distal surfaces of maxillary and mandibular posterior teeth
Gracey 15–16		Mesial surfaces of maxillary and mandibular posterior teeth
Gracey 17–18		Distal surfaces of maxillary and mandibular posterior teeth

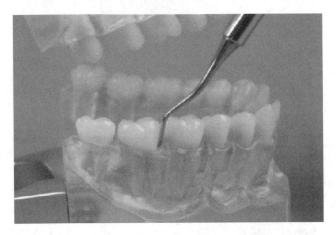

Figure 2–6   Gracey 15/16. Used for mesial surfaces only. *Photo courtesy of Hu-Friedy Manufacturing Co., Inc.*

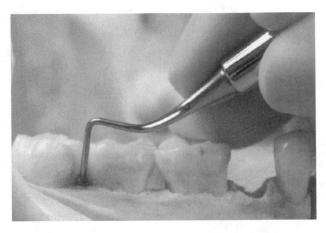

Figure 2–7   Gracey 17/18. Used for distal surfaces only. *Photo courtesy of Hu-Friedy Manufacturing Co., Inc.*

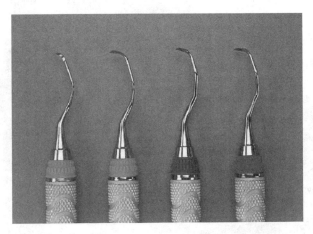

Figure 2–8   Types of area-specific curettes: Mini, After Five, Rigid, and Standard. *Photo courtesy of Hu-Friedy Manufacturing Co., Inc.*

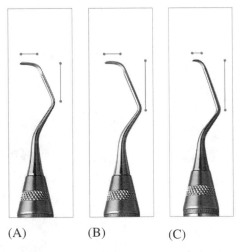

(A)   (B)   (C)

Figure 2–9   (A) Standard Gracey curette. (B) After Five curette. (C) Mini Five curette. *Photo courtesy of Hu-Friedy Manufacturing Co., Inc.*

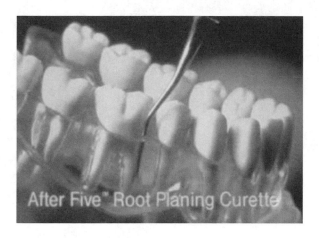

Figure 2–10 After Five root planing curette. *Photo courtesy of Hu-Friedy Manufacturing Co., Inc.*

of 5 millimeters and greater; thinner blade permits easier subgingival insertion[2] (Figures 2–10 and 2–11).

  c. **Shortened blade.** Half the blade length of regularly designed blades; blades are also thinner; available in regular or extended shank length; excellent for application on line angles and maxillary and mandibular anterior teeth, as well as narrow pockets, furcations, and developmental grooves.

    (1) Curvettes. Design includes:

      (a) Blade: Reduced length and width by 50 percent.

      (b) Toe: Turned up.

      (c) Blade identification marking at junction of handle and shank, as well as raised 5 and 10 millimeter markings on the terminal shank, allowing the operator a point of reference for the depth of insertion.

    (2) Mini-bladed Gracey curettes. Design includes:

      (a) Blade: Reduced and thinned by 50 percent.

      (b) **Extended terminal shank** (3 millimeters) to allow for access in deeper pockets (5 millimeters and beyond), furcations, line angles, and root concavities (Figure 2–12).

5. Correct working end. To determine correct working end use either:

  a. Option I.

    (1) Place the sharp cutting edge towards the tooth/root surface with the rounded back next to the soft tissue.

CLINICAL TIP:

Adapting Your Knowledge: If the face of the blade can be seen when **scaling,** the *wrong end* of the instrument has been selected.

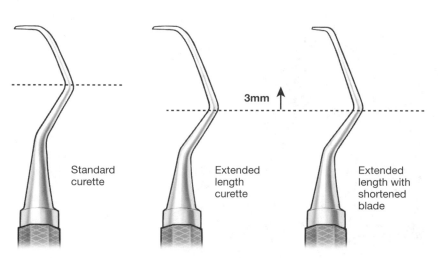

Standard curette

3mm

Extended length curette

Extended length with shortened blade

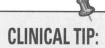

Figure 2–11 Comparison of shanks.

Figure 2–12   Standard blade vs. shortened blade. *Photo courtesy of Hu-Friedy Manufacturing Co., Inc.*

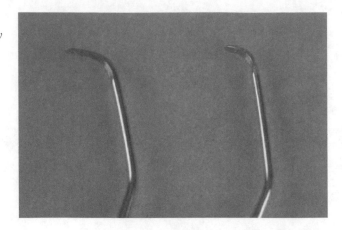

(2) Position the lowest tilted edge against the tooth surface.
(3) Place the terminal shank parallel to the surface being instrumented (Figure 2–13).
  b. Option II
    (1) Hold instrument with terminal shank perpendicular to the floor.
    (2) View the working end and determine which side is lower (this is the cutting edge).
6. Grasp. Use modified pen grasp.
7. **Fulcrum.** A variety of fulcrums are available for maximum adaptation and angulation. (Please see section IV for a complete explanation with photos.)

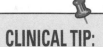

CLINICAL TIP:

Adapting Your Knowledge: Strokes are completed with vertical, horizontal, and oblique motions.

8. Insertion. Insert at or as near 0 degrees as possible; close and tilt blade toward the tooth as the rounded back is slipped under the free margin of the gingiva (Figure 2–14).
9. Adaptation.
  a. Place 1 to 2 millimeters of side of toe flush against tooth.
  b. Roll instrument with thumb and index finger around line angles to keep toe adapted to tooth at all times.
10. Angulation. Open blade between 60 and 80 degrees by pivoting on fulcrum to accomplish working and planing strokes. To open blade, tilt instrument away from the tooth by pivoting on fulcrum.[3,4]
11. Custom working end configuration available. To scale both the mesial and distal surfaces with one instrument, instrument manufacturing com-

Figure 2–13   Shank parallel to long axis of tooth. *Photo courtesy of Hu-Friedy Manufacturing Co., Inc.*

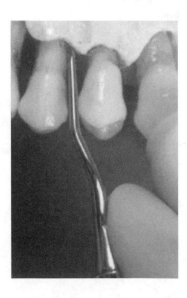

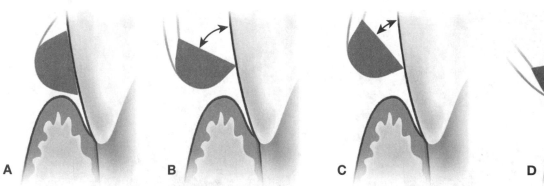

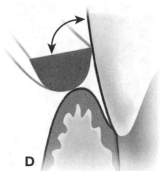

Figure 2–14   Blade angulation. (A) Correct angulation for blade insertion—zero. (B) Correct angulation for scaling—45 degrees to 90 degrees. (C) Blade too closed for scaling—less than 45 degrees. (D) Blade too open for scaling—more than 90 degrees.

panies can pair the 11/14 or the 12/13 ends together upon request, normally, the 11/12 and 13/14 are paired together for scaling mesial and distal surfaces respectively

B. Review of **Universal Curettes.** Initially introduced and discussed in *Essentials of Dental Hygiene: Preclinical Skills;*[1] available for periodontal instrumentation.

1. Definition. A rounded, curved, scaling instrument used on any tooth for periodontal debridement.
2. Purpose. To deplaque and remove hard deposits anywhere in the mouth with the convenience of using one instrument.
3. Characteristics (Figure 2–15).
   a. Internal angle. Face of the blade and cutting edges meet at an internal angle of 70 to 80 degrees.
   b. Blade. Angled 90 degrees (perpendicular) to the shank.
   c. Cutting edges. Curve and meet at the round toe with both parallel cutting edges utilized; formed at the junction of the lateral surfaces and facial surface on either side.
   d. Cross section. Half-moon shape.
   e. Rounded back. Lower portions of the lateral surfaces meet toward the toe third and remain next to the soft tissue.
   f. Curved face. Perpendicular to the lower shank and curves upward.
   g. Working ends. Paired mirror images.

> **CLINICAL TIP:**
>
> **Adapting Your Knowledge:** The 11/14–12/13 instrument combination is convenient for students.

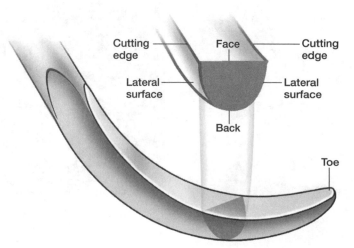

Cutting edge — Face — Cutting edge

Lateral surface — Lateral surface

Back

Toe

Figure 2–15   Characteristics of a universal curette.

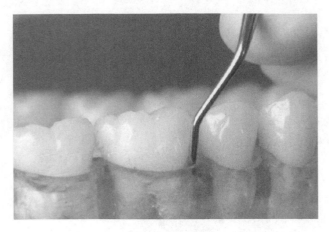

Figure 2–16   Langer 1/2. *Photo courtesy of Hu-Friedy Manufacturing Co., Inc.*

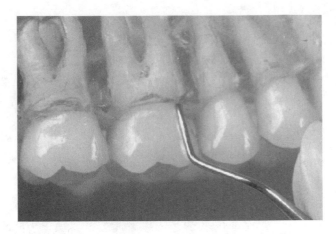

Figure 2–17   Langer 3/4. *Photo courtesy of Hu-Friedy Manufacturing Co., Inc.*

CLINICAL TIP:

Adapting Your Knowledge: When using a Langer curette, both the mesial and distal surfaces can be scaled with the same instrument since it is a universal blade.

4. Types of universal curettes. All universal instruments are designed to use throughout the entire dentition, which is convenient. The "anterior" and "posterior" designation actually refers to variations in shank length and design. Examples of advanced periodontal universal curettes include the Langer curettes. Their unique design features terminal shanks that mimic area-specific curettes, yet with universal blades. They are available in both shortened blade length and extended shank length varieties and are used in the following areas.

   a. Langer 1/2. Used to instrument mesial and distal mandibular posterior surfaces (Figure 2–16).
   b. Langer 3/4. Used to instrument mesial and distal maxillary posterior surfaces (Figure 2–17).
   c. Langer 5/6. Used to instrument mesial and distal maxillary and mandibular anterior surfaces (Figure 2–18).
   d. Langer 17/18. Used to instrument maxillary and mandibular second and third molars (Figure 2–19).

5. Determination of correct working end.

   a. Place toe of instrument into interproximal area. Align terminal shank parallel to surface so handle extends out of mouth, not toward patient's

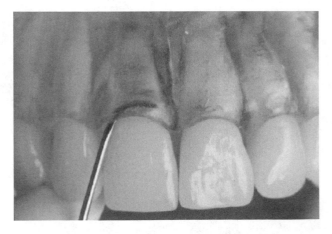

Figure 2–18   Langer 5/6. *Photo courtesy of Hu-Friedy Manufacturing Co., Inc.*

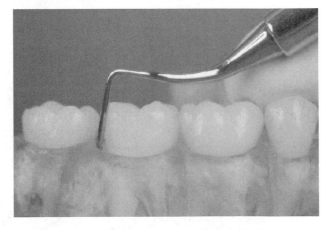

Figure 2–19   Langer 17/18. *Photo courtesy of Hu-Friedy Manufacturing Co., Inc.*

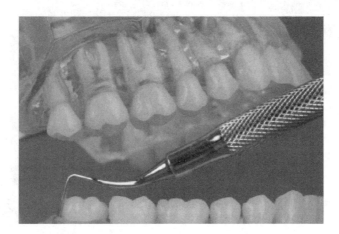

Figure 2–20 Determination of correct working end. Align terminal shank parallel to the tooth surface so handle extends out of mouth. *Photo courtesy of Hu-Friedy Manufacturing Co., Inc.*

throat (Figure 2–20). When the correct end is adapted, most of the instrument face cannot be seen. If the face can be seen, the wrong end is being adapted; to correct, switch ends.

   b. Blade will curve toward the tooth.

6. Grasp. Use modified pen grasp.
7. Fulcrum. Use traditional intraoral finger rests, or **alternate fulcrums,** which are helpful and enhance blade placement to base of pocket (see section IV for a discussion and explanation of alternate fulcrums).
8. Insertion. Insert at or as near 0 degrees as possible; blade is closed, and tilted toward the tooth as the rounded back is slipped under the free margin of the gingiva.
9. Adaptation.
   a. Place 1 to 2 millimeters of toe flush against tooth.
   b. Roll instrument with thumb and index finger around line angles to keep toe adapted to tooth at all times.
10. Angulation. Open blade between 45 and 90 degrees by pivoting on fulcrum to accomplish working and planing strokes; to open blade, tilt instrument away from the tooth.
11. Stroke. Apply lateral pressure against the tooth and pull upward while maintaining contact with the tooth[2] (Figure 2–21).

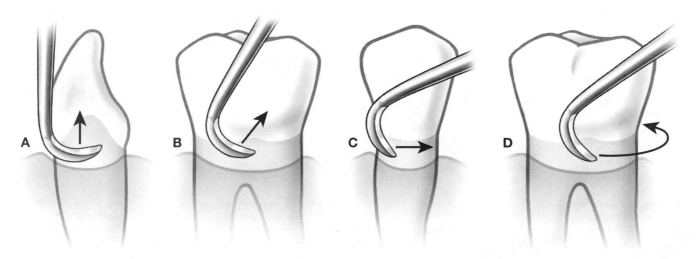

Figure 2–21 Basic stroke directions. (A) Vertical (B) Oblique (C) Horizontal. (D) Circumferential.

Figure 2–22   Horizontal stroke. Place toe toward gingiva, then pull horizontally.

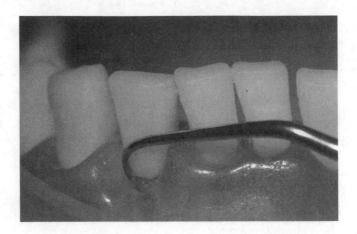

a. Vertical. Begin at the base of the pocket and activate instrument in a straight direction using short, overlapping strokes (see Figure 2–21a).
b. Oblique. Appropriate for direct facial and lingual surfaces since range of motion for the operator is increased on these surfaces. Begin strokes at the base of the pocket and proceed with short, over-lapping, oblique strokes (see Figure 2–21b).
c. Horizontal. Best accomplished with the instrument toe directed toward the gingiva; beginning at the base of the pocket, complete strokes sideways, methodically in sections (see Figure 2–21c).
d. Circumferential. Extension of horizontal strokes by continuing around the line angles from facial or lingual aspect of tooth (see Figure 2–21d) (Figure 2–22).

III. Alternate Seating Positions

In preparing for advanced root instrumentation, the student will build on the fundamental principles introduced in *Essentials of Dental Hygiene: Preclinical Skills.*[1] After proficiency is gained in the basic skills, variations can be implemented in many avenues, including seating positions. These variations enhance accessibility to move beyond the seating positions learned in the preclinical laboratory, advancing into alternate seating positions. For example, when the right-handed operator is instrumenting the maxillary right lingual, it is helpful yet untraditional to sit between 1:30 o'clock to 2:00 o'clock with the patient's chin up and turned slightly away. Excellent adaptation can be obtained in this position, with maximum root-blade contact. Likewise, access can also be obtained when the right-handed operator sits between 12:30 o'clock to 1:00 o'clock, fulcrums on the maxillary arch, while reaching down with an extended

Table 2–2   Alternate Seating Positions for the Right-Handed Operator to Accomplish Power Strokes

Area of Mouth	Seating Position (o'clock)	Fulcrum	Grasp	Patient Head
Mandibular Right Lingual	1:00	Occlusals of Mandibular Right Lingual	Extended	Slightly right or straight
Maxillary Right Lingual	1:30–2:00	Occlusals of Maxillary Right	Slightly extended	Chin up; head turned to right
Mandibular Right Buccal Mesial Surfaces	12:00	Maxillary Right Premolars	Extended	Straight

Table 2–3 Alternate Seating Positions for the Left-Handed Operator to Accomplish Power Strokes

Area of Mouth	Seating Position (o'clock)	Fulcrum	Grasp	Patient Head
Mandibular Left Lingual	11:00	Occlusals of Mandibular Left Lingual	Extended	Slightly left or straight
Maxillary Left Lingual	10:00–11:30	Occlusals of Maxillary Left	Slightly extended	Chin up; head to left
Mandibular Left Buccal Mesial Surfaces	12:00	Maxillary Left Premolars	Extended	Straight

grasp to instrument the mesial-facial or lingual surfaces of the mandibular right quadrant. This becomes a power stroke for the operator with excellent root-blade contact. Continue to follow ergonomic principles, always keeping the wrist and back in the neutral position to decrease stress and strain. (See Tables 2–2 and 2–3.)

IV. Alternate Fulcrums

Point of stabilization achieved other than on the adjacent incisal or occlusal tooth surface; used to enhance instrumentation; examples include:

A. **Cross arch** (same arch). Place fulcrum in the opposite quadrant of the same arch (Figure 2–23).

B. **Extraoral.** Place fulcrum on a point outside the mouth, such as on the border of the mandible, cheek, or chin; helpful when working on the maxillary molars where traditional fulcrums are often split, resulting in a loss of strength of lateral pressure and parallelism of terminal shank; position palm either up or down, depending on side being instrumented (Figure 2–24).

C. **Finger on finger.** Place fulcrum on index finger of nondominant hand to increase access in deeper pockets; especially effective in the vestibule of the mandible to access a variety of mandibular areas or provide a rest for a fulcrum when teeth are missing (Figure 2–25).

D. **Opposite arch.** Place fulcrum on the arch opposite the one being instrumented (Figure 2–26).

E. **Reinforced.** Supplemental fulcrum applied with index finger of nondominant hand to dominant hand to gain additional force in a stroke when needed (Figure 2–27).

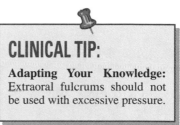

CLINICAL TIP:

Adapting Your Knowledge: Extraoral fulcrums should not be used with excessive pressure.

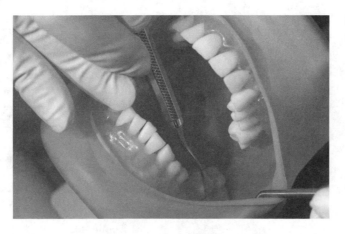

Figure 2–23 Alternate fulcrum. Crossing same arch.

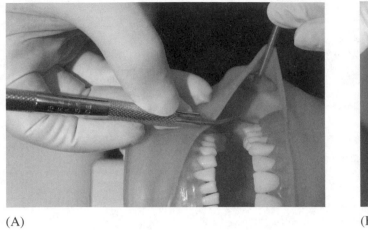

(A)

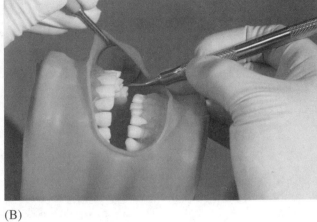

(B)

Figure 2–24   Extraoral fulcrum. (A) Palm up. (B) Palm down.

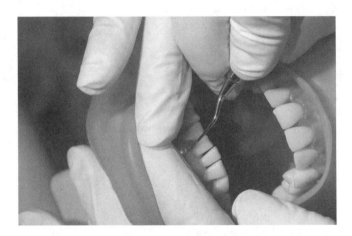

Figure 2–25   Alternate fulcrum. Finger on finger.

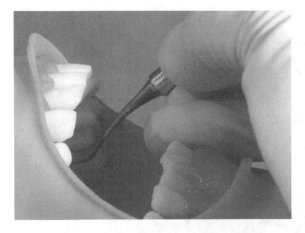

Figure 2–26   Alternate fulcrum. Opposite arch.

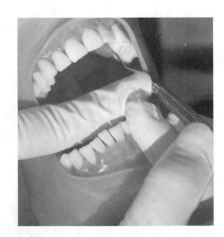

Figure 2–27   Alternate fulcrum. Reinforced.

V. Periodontal Debridement

In some areas of the country, the terms root planing and periodontal debridement are interchangeable, although any differences seem to be in the matter of degree.[5,6] Periodontal debridement is more of an all-encompassing term that includes all types of **mechanical therapy**—hand and power-assisted instrumentation—to deplaque, scale, and/or root plane tooth surfaces. The evaluation of successful periodontal debridement depends on the soft tissue response following therapy. While Oberholzer and Rateitschak concluded that it is unnecessary to strive for total root smoothness, the value of a clean tooth surface cannot be minimized in periodontal tissue healing response.[7]

A. Periodontal debridement. Encompasses:
1. Deplaquing the roots. Use lighter pressure to remove nonattached, free-floating plaque biofilm and toxic by-products of bacterial metabolism from the sulcus or pocket; recommended at maintenance and reevaluation appointments.
2. Scaling. Use short, overlapping strokes with firmer pressure for deliberate plaque, calculus, and stain removal from crown and root surfaces.
3. Root planing (extension of scaling). In the beginning, use smooth, multidirectional strokes with medium pressure to remove residual calculus that harbors biofilm and its toxic by-products; complete procedure with longer strokes, while applying lighter lateral pressure.

B. Goals of periodontal debridement (also called nonsurgical periodontal therapy by some).
1. Managing oral infection.
2. Establishing gingival health.
3. Gaining periodontal attachment.
4. Maintaining an oral environment conducive to periodontal health.[4]

C. Post-instrumentation instructions for patient following periodontal debridement include:
1. Isotonic salt rinse (one teaspoon salt mixed in 8 ounces of warm water). Use three times daily for three days to reduce swelling, if indicated.
2. Chlorhexidine gluconate antimicrobial (.12 percent) oral rinse. Use as needed and prescribed.
3. Over-the-counter (OTC) analgesic (i.e., ibuprofen). Use for discomfort, if necessary.
4. Prescribed plaque control home care regimen. Instruct according to patient's needs.
5. Desensitizing dentifrice. Use as needed for sensitivity.

VI. Technique for Traditional Root Planing

During root planing, the goal is to produce a biologically compatible root surface with surrounding tissues in a state of health. The end result is not a glassy, smooth root surface, but complete calculus removal.[8] Review the periodontal chart and radiographs before beginning treatment and refer to them often during instrumentation. The use of topical or, preferably, local anesthetic enhances patient comfort during the procedure.

A. Insert the instrument at the proximal area at or as near to 0 degrees as possible at the base of the pocket until the junctional epithelium is felt (Figures 2–28a and b).
B. Open blade 45 degrees to 90 degrees; this is accomplished by pivoting on fulcrum.

CLINICAL TIP:

Adapting Your Knowledge: When deplaquing the roots, use light pressure.

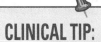

CLINICAL TIP:

Adapting Your Knowledge: During beginning root planing strokes, pressure is applied against the handle with the operator's thumb.

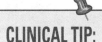

CLINICAL TIP:

Adapting Your Knowledge: "The endpoint of all periodontal debridement is to produce a root that is biologically acceptable for a healthy attachment."[5]

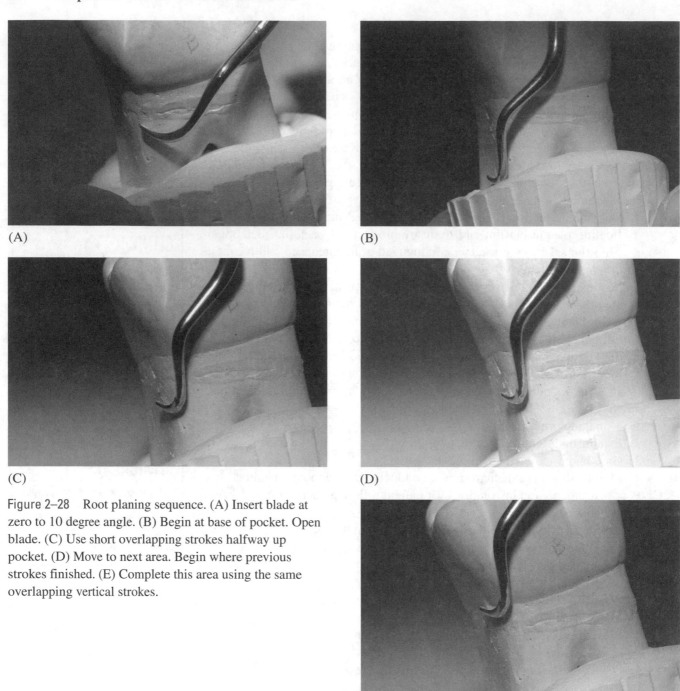

Figure 2–28 Root planing sequence. (A) Insert blade at zero to 10 degree angle. (B) Begin at base of pocket. Open blade. (C) Use short overlapping strokes halfway up pocket. (D) Move to next area. Begin where previous strokes finished. (E) Complete this area using the same overlapping vertical strokes.

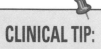

CLINICAL TIP:

Adapting Your Knowledge: Begin initial strokes at the base of the pocket.

C. Use short, overlapping vertical strokes, with moderate pressure, halfway up the pocket, which will depend on the amount of clinical attachment loss (Figure 2–28c).

D. Continue from the halfway point of pocket toward the cementoenamel junction (CEJ) (Figure 2–28d); complete this section using the same moderate pressure and short, overlapping vertical strokes (Figure 2–28e).

E. Again, reinsert to the base of the pocket and use light pressure, sweeping the entire length of the root surface in longer strokes; re-explore intermittently.

F. Move to the middle third section and use a combination of oblique and horizontal strokes, always beginning with firmer pressure and short strokes, and ending with longer, lighter strokes.

G. Re-explore, using a calculus-detecting explorer to check for complete deposit removal.

VII. Furcations and Root Anatomy

The complexity of root anatomy adds to the difficulty of periodontal instrumentation and requires skill. A thorough knowledge of dental anatomy is required for a complete understanding of advanced periodontal instrumentation. The morphology of each tooth, as well as irregular and fused roots, makes working subgingivally a challenge.

A. Naber's furcation probe. Curved, blunted, mirror-image assessment instrument with paired working ends used to detect bone loss in furcations; lower shank is parallel to the long axis of tooth when properly positioned; varieties include (Figure 2–29):
   1. With markings. Has millimeter markings at the 3-6-9 junctions, although there is no actual measurement—it is a guide to note the distance the probe can be inserted.
   2. Without markings. No markings are indicated since its purpose is to note how far the probe enters the furcation—none, partially, or completely through.

B. Teeth with furcations include:
   1. Maxillary molars (trifurcation).
   2. Maxillary first premolar (bifurcation).
   3. Mandibular molars (bifurcation).

C. Teeth with depressions that can harbor subgingival deposit include[9] (Figure 2–30):
   1. Maxillary first premolars.
   2. Mandibular canines.
   3. Maxillary molars.
   4. Mandibular molars.

D. Types of furcations include (Figure 2–31):
   1. Grade or Class I. Fluted depression is detectable.
   2. Grade or Class II. Open either at the facial or lingual side, but not both.

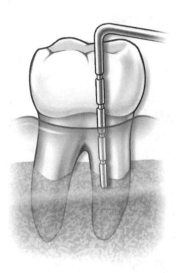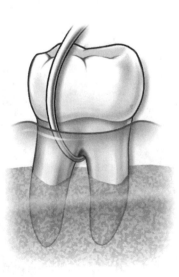

Figure 2–29   Comparison of standard vs. furcation probe.

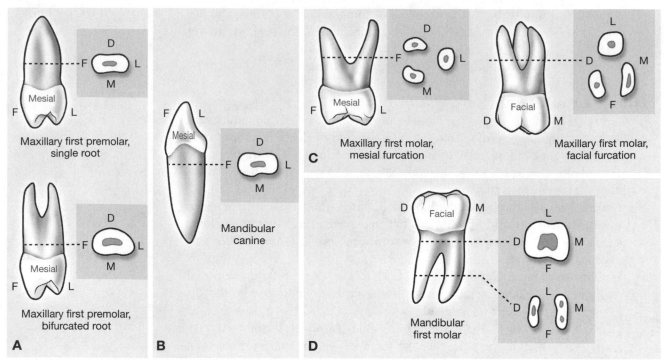

Figure 2–30   (A) Maxillary first premolar. (B) Mandibular canine. (C) Maxillary first molar. (D) Mandibular first molar.

3. Grade or Class III. Through and through furcation with no bone present interradicularly; gingival tissue covers the crotch.
4. Grade or Class IV. Through and through furcation with no soft tissue obstructing opening; can be accessed with interdental brush or other auxiliary aids.

E. Accessing furcations. Since molars have mesial, distal, and/or lingual roots, these areas must be instrumented the same as tooth surfaces.

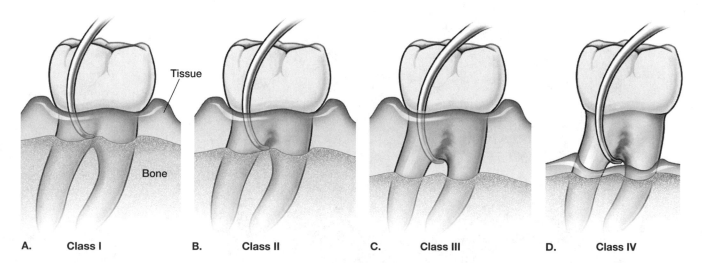

Figure 2–31   Classification of furcation involvement.

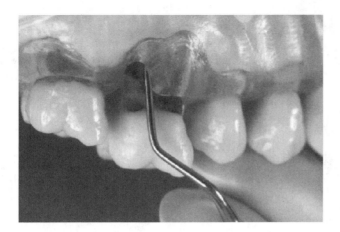

Figure 2–32 Accessing the mesial aspect of the distal root of tooth #3. An 11/12 or 15/16 area-specific curette can be used, preferably with a shortened blade with extended length shank. *Photo courtesy of Hu-Friedy Manufacturing Co., Inc.*

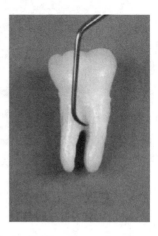

Figure 2–33 Accessing the crotch of the furcation with the toe of a curette. *Photo courtesy of Hu-Friedy Manufacturing Co., Inc.*

1. Surfaces.
   a. Mesial surfaces. Use the Gracey 11-12 or 15-16 (Figure 2–32).
   b. Distal surfaces. Use the Gracey 13-14 or 17-18.
2. Proper adaptation. Place the cutting edge toward the tooth or root surface and the terminal shank parallel to the long axis of the tooth; this enables the instrument to self-angulate or be at the correct angle.
   a. Assess crotch or roof of furcations with the toe of the curette (Figure 2–33).
   b. Available in many blade lengths and widths to assist in accessing these challenging surfaces.
   c. Use a calculus-detecting explorer to help determine the end point for periodontal debridement and develop increased tactile sensitivity.
3. Furcation **files.**
   a. Consist of a 360 degree medical-grade diamond coating with thin tips and unique bends to access furcations, small narrow pockets, line angles, root depressions, and deep developmental grooves.
   b. Extended shank and pronounced curvature enhance crown clearance for scaling.
   c. Use light pressure, multidirectional in and out strokes to effectively clean and polish the root surface while conserving root structure[10] (Figures 2–34 and 2–35).

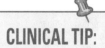

CLINICAL TIP:

Adapting Your Knowledge: When using **shortened blade curettes,** a variety of strokes adapt well to root anatomy.[10]

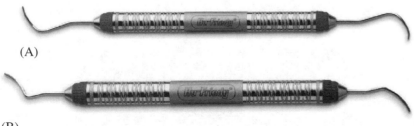

(A)

(B)

Figure 2–34 (A–B) Diamond-coated files for furcations. *Photos courtesy of Hu-Friedy Manufacturing Co., Inc.*

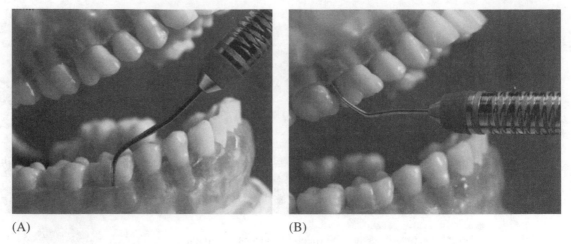

(A)   (B)

Figure 2–35   (A) Accessing furcation and root depression with diamond-coated file. (B) Accessing line angle and developmental groove with diamond-coated file. *Photos courtesy of Hu-Friedy Manufacturing Co., Inc.*

VIII. Adjuncts in Assessing and Detecting Subgingival Deposits

    A. Rationale. Failure of periodontal therapy is most often due to incomplete scaling—leaving residual toxins to cause irritation. **Endoscopy** makes it possible to view into pockets to determine reasons for lack of tissue resolution. Most often it is unresolved due to residual calculus remaining on the tooth. Whether using hand or power-assisted scalers, mechanical debridement is essential for pocket resolution. While instrumentation and anatomic limitations exist, efficacy of periodontal therapy is directly related to the ability to treat lower levels of pathogenic bacteria.[11] Meticulous hand instrumentation, with a combination of strokes, is utilized to accomplish complete root **debridement** and is crucial in pocket resolution. The use of dental endoscopy has proved this (see www.dentalview.com for more information).[12]

    B. Endoscopic periodontal viewing. Periodontal applications include (Figure 2–36):

Figure 2–36   Endoscope for subgingival calculus detection.

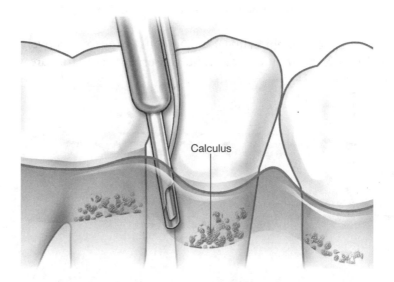

Calculus

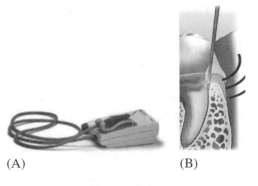

Figure 2–37   (A) DetecTar electronic calculus detecting device. (B) Low intensity light detects calculus. *Photos courtesy of Ultradent Products, Inc.*

(A)   (B)

1. Visualizing root surfaces, tooth structures, and other areas.
2. Locating and removing residual/missed areas of calculus.
3. Allowing for more complete healing to be achieved due to more thorough debridement.
4. Diagnosing other subgingival problems.

C. Electronic calculus detection. DetecTar, by Ultradent Products, Inc., is a device that emits a safe red and low infra-red wavelength of moderate intensity (no heat generated) with a high energy light emitting diode (L.E.D.) to identify calculus, regardless of blood, saliva, suppuration, or water (Figure 2–37). In the presence of subgingival calculus, this unit beeps and flashes a small green light.[13] (For further information, go to www.ultradent .com.)

D. Magnification with eye loupes.
1. Physical benefits from having an enlarged image include:
   a. Reduce eyestrain.
   b. Enhance visual acuity.
   c. Promote ergonomic posture (Figure 2–38).
   d. Relieve neck and back strain.
2. Clinical Benefits. Increase the operator's ability to:
   a. Read periodontal probe and radiographs.
   b. Detect supragingival deposits.
   c. Identify early pathology.[14]

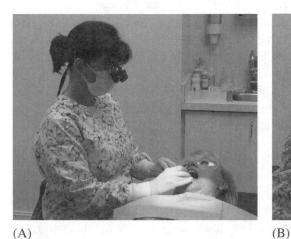
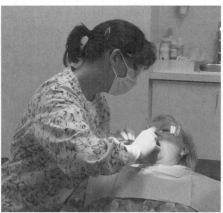

Figure 2–38   (A) Proper posture enhanced with eye loupes. (B) Improper posture which could be corrected with magnification. *Photos courtesy of SheerVision Optical Loupes.*

(A)   (B)

IX. Instrument Sharpening

Sharpening is an important maintenance step for scaling instruments, which will assist the dental hygienist in achieving the best performance possible. Ideally, instruments should be sharpened after sterilization.

A. Objective of sharpening. Produce a sharp cutting edge without changing the original design of the instrument.[15,16,17]

B. Rationale for sharpening.

1. Keeps instruments sharp and true to their original design by preserving the correct angulation between the instrument face and the lateral surface.[18]

2. Enhances job efficiency and quality of care to patient since sharp instruments reduce appointment time and lateral pressure.

3. Improves tactile sensitivity because a sharp instrument allows the use of a relaxed grasp and a controlled stroke.

4. Reduces operator fatigue since fewer strokes are needed; dull instruments must be used with excessive pressure to achieve results.

5. Increases comfort to patient due to fewer strokes needed.

6. Reduces incidence of trauma to patient and operator.

C. Armamentarium.

1. Sharpening stones. Sharpening stones are abrasive devices used to restore the cutting edge on a dull instrument without changing its original design. They are made of gritty, abrasive particles compressed into a solid piece that is harder than the metal of the instrument. Coarse stones have large particles that cut rapidly. Fine stones have smaller particles that cut more slowly.

a. Types of sharpening stones.

(1) Fine-to-medium stones.

(a) Arkansas oil stone. Fine-grained natural stone quarried from natural mineral deposits and used for routine sharpening.

i. Available in flat, rectangular, wedge, cylindrical, or round shapes.

ii. Flat, rectangular, or wedge-shaped stones may have grooves for the special adaptation of curved blades.

iii. Edges may be rounded or square.

(b) I stone (formally called India stone). Synthetic (man-made) medium-textured stone used to sharpen dull cutting edges.

(c) Ceramic stone. Fine-grained synthetic stone.

(2) Coarse stones. Synthetic coarse-grained stone used for extensive sharpening and reshaping of working ends that have dull or worn cutting edges; especially good for blades that have been improperly sharpened.

b. Stone design. Sharpening stones are available in varying sizes, shapes, and textures. Many come with guides and manufacturer's instructions that should be followed for best results.

(1) Unmounted stones (Figure 2–39).

(a) Rectangular or flat. Used to sharpen the blade of the instrument in three sections.

(b) Cylindrical or cone-shaped. Useful when sharpening the face of curettes or curved sickle scalers; most often used to remove wire edges (minute metal projections) that can form when the lateral sides are sharpened.

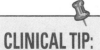

CLINICAL TIP:

Adapting Your Knowledge: Samples of sharpening stones are available for viewing at professional meetings, as well as advertisements in professional journals where manufacturers feature new designs and products frequently.

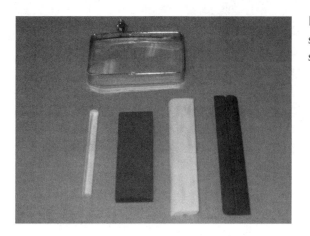

Figure 2–39 Unmounted sharpening stones, plastic testing stick, and magnifying glass.

      (c) Grooved. Designed to help cutting edge stay in proper angulation.

      (d) Wedge. Contains a rounded side that can be used like the cylindrical stone to accomplish the removal of the wire edge, or to sharpen the face of the blade; flat side is used to sharpen the lateral borders of the blade or cutting edges.

2. Lubricant (mineral oil or water).
  a. Application. Apply with cotton-tipped applicator or gauze square.
  b. Purpose.
    (1) Facilitates movement of the instrument over the stone.
    (2) Reduces frictional heat.
    (3) Prevents clogging of metal shavings into the surface of the stone. Use gauze square to remove the residue called "sludge" created by metal shavings and oil/water.

3. Light source. Use a good light source, such as the dental unit or a lab bench, since a sharp cutting edge does not reflect light. A dull cutting edge appears as a white area at the junction of the face and lateral surfaces.

4. Magnification. Can be helpful in identifying cutting edges and detecting dull edges; magnifying glass or magnification loupes are useful for this task.

5. Plastic testing stick. Process to determine instrument sharpness.
  a. Grasp stick with nondominant hand.
  b. Fulcrum on the top of the stick with dominant hand.
  c. Adapt the cutting edge against the stick at the same angle used to scale a tooth.
  d. Position the lower shank of the instrument parallel to the long axis of the stick.
  e. Cut into the stick with blade of instrument.
    (1) Sharp instrument will "bite" into the stick, and a pinging metallic noise can be heard.
    (2) Dull instrument will glide over the stick and not catch plastic.[15,16]
  f. Apply all three areas of the cutting edge (heel third, middle third, and lower one-third of blade) to test for sharpness; re-sharpen any portion of the blade that does not "bite" or grab into the stick.

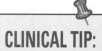

CLINICAL TIP:

Adapting Your Knowledge: Sharpening can also be done with a dry stone.

CLINICAL TIP:

Adapting Your Knowledge: Light reflects from a dull surface. The cutting edge of a sharp instrument has length but no width since it is a narrow line.[1,15]

g. Autoclave plastic testing sticks with sharpening stones.
6. Personal protective equipment (PPE). Operator should wear:
   a. Protective eyewear to prevent metal shavings from becoming lodged in eye.
   b. Gloves for protection.
   c. Mask, if instruments are contaminated.
7. Use clock positions as a reference to determine the proper positioning of the instrument and stone.[19]

D. Signs of instrument dullness. Repeated use of a dental instrument wears away minute particles of metal from the blade, causing the cutting edge to take on a rounded shape, resulting in a dull, ineffective blade. Instruments should be sharpened at the first sign of dullness, which may include one of the following:
1. Blade of instrument is not "biting" into plastic test stick but, instead, gliding over it.
2. White line is evident, due to the reflection of the light, along the cutting edge when examined under a light; best viewed under lighted magnification (Figure 2–40).
3. Cutting edge shows thickness and more depth. When an instrument is sharp, the cutting edge is only a line.
4. Scaling procedures take longer, due to inefficient cutting edge; deposit is "skipped" over, burnished, or may be only partially removed.

E. Technique.
1. Grasp instrument in nondominant hand.
2. To prevent slipping, stabilize back of fingers and instrument against a hard surface such as a tabletop or a lab bench.
3. Use clock positions (1:00 o'clock and 11:00 o'clock). Provide a guide to visualize the 110 degree angulation necessary between the blade and stone for sharpening to occur (Figure 2–41).

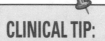

CLINICAL TIP:

Adapting Your Knowledge: Stabilize hand holding the instrument against a hard surface such as a table, desk, or lab bench in order to prevent slipping.

Figure 2–40   (A) Line of light showing a dull edge. (B) Line of light showing a sharp edge.

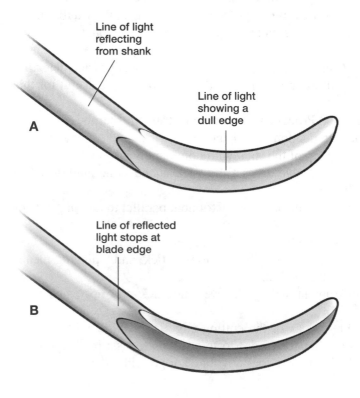

Line of light reflecting from shank

Line of light showing a dull edge

A

Line of reflected light stops at blade edge

B

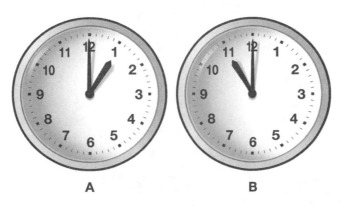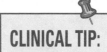

Figure 2–41   Clock positions used during instrument sharpening. (A) One o'clock (B) Eleven o'clock.

A   B

4. Identify cutting edge(s). Formed at the junction of the lateral sides and face of blade; lateral surfaces and face of universal and area-specific curettes meet at an internal angle between 70 and 80 degrees.
5. Position face of instrument parallel to floor.
6. Face toe toward operator.
7. Divide the blade into thirds—heel, middle, and toe.
8. At 12:00 o'clock position, apply stone to heel of blade at 90 degree angle; then open stone to 1:00 o'clock position, or 110 degree angle; using light pressure, move stone up and down with strokes that are 1/4″–1/2″ in length (Figure 2–42).
9. Continue moving stone to middle third of instrument (Figure 2–43).
10. Follow to toe third of instrument, finishing with down stroke to avoid creating a wire edge.[15]
11. Apply stone to *opposite* side of blade (*only applies to universal curettes*) at 11:00 o'clock position and sharpen entire blade in thirds (Figure 2–44).

CLINICAL TIP:

Adapting Your Knowledge: Remember the area-specific curette only has one cutting edge per working end.

CLINICAL TIP:

Adapting Your Knowledge: An excellent way to sharpen the toe is to use a grooved stone at a 45 degree angle.

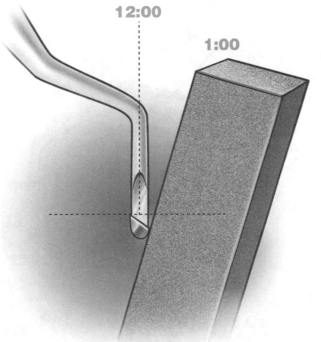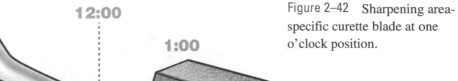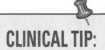

12:00   1:00

Figure 2–42   Sharpening area-specific curette blade at one o'clock position.

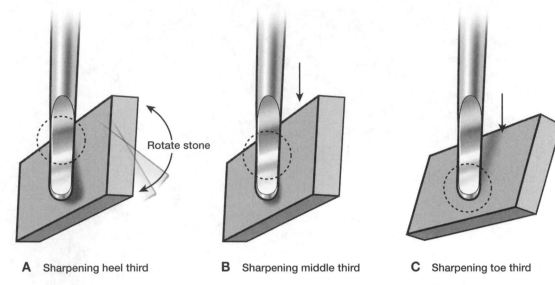

A Sharpening heel third   **B** Sharpening middle third   **C** Sharpening toe third

Figure 2–43   Sharpening curette. (A) Apply stone to heel third of blade.
(B) Continue moving stone to middle third of blade. (C) Follow to toe third of blade
and finish with a down stroke.

12. Continue the stroke around the toe to preserve its rounded contour by
    decreasing the stone angle to 45 degree (Figure 2–45). Only sharpening
    the lateral borders will result in the toe losing its roundness and taking
    on a pointed shape.
13. Sharpen the face. Use round or conical stone (Figure 2–46); roll the
    conical or round stone using light, even pressure toward the operator,
    beginning at the intersection of the shank and working end.

Figure 2–44   Sharpening
opposite side of universal curette
blade at eleven o'clock position.

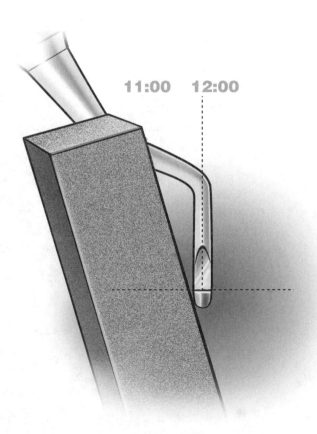

11:00   12:00

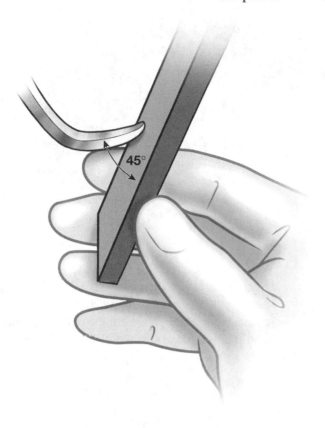

Figure 2–45   Rounding toe at forty-five degrees with sharpening stone.

a. Move stone toward the toe so both cutting edges are contacted at the same time.

b. Perform only periodically to avoid weakening the blade and shortening the life of the instrument.

c. Test for sharpness as previously described.

F. Care of Sharpening Stones.

1. Handle stones with care because they can break when dropped.

2. After use, clean stones in the ultrasonic cleaner to remove metal particles that become embedded into its surface during use; this also removes the oily layer that might have been applied prior to sharpening.

3. Wrap sharpening stone in gauze for protection and autoclave.

4. Follow lubrication recommendation for the particular stone used according to manufacturer's instructions.

5. Rotate area of use on stone to prevent grooving.

CLINICAL TIP:

Adapting Your Knowledge: Suggested sequence for sharpening instruments includes:

1. Sterilize.
2. Test cutting edges.
3. Sharpen.
4. Resterilize.

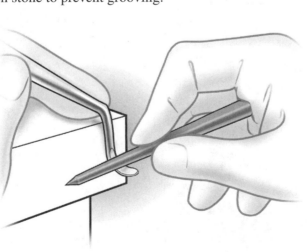

Figure 2–46   Sharpening the face of the curette with a conical stone.

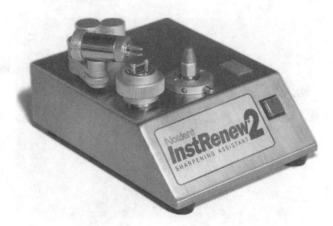

With proper care, sharpening stones will last for many years. Regular cleaning to remove metal particles will prevent stones from developing a smooth glaze. If glazing occurs due to imbedding of metal particles, roughen the stone with emery paper. In addition, proper packaging and handling will prevent stone breakage.

G. Innovations in sharpening with newer technology.
   1. Automated sharpening.
      a. InstRenew Sharpening System, by Nordent Manufacturing, Inc. (Figure 2–47). This compact stainless steel unit operates on standard 110v current. It features a blade positioner and a sharpening cone that provides a simple, accurate sharpening process that automatically locks each instrument to the correct angle. Sharpening cone is cut at a 75 degree angle for all sickle scalers and universal and area-specific curette blades[17] (for more information go to www.nordent.com).
      b. PerioStar 3000, by Kerr-Sybron (Figure 2–48). The instrument is inserted into a fixation device where it is stabilized and secured prior to sharpening with a magnetic orange beam that confirms the correct blade position. The sharpening stone is set mechanically at a consistent angle in relation to the blade, and a test stick confirms sharpness before the instrument is released.[17]
      c. Sidekick, by Hu-Friedy (Figure 2–49). This portable power (cordless) device has a small flat removable stone that is activated with a reciprocating motion. An instrument toe guide allows for easy positioning of universal and area-specific curettes, and a guide plate on top allows for easy access and accurate instrument positioning.[17]

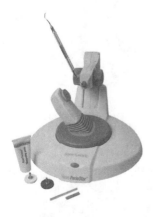

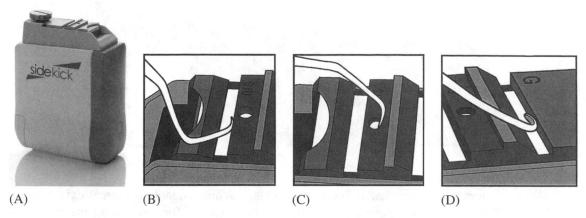

(A)   (B)   (C)   (D)

Figure 2–49 (A) Hu-Friedy Side Kick. (B) S/U Channel: For sickle scalers and universal curette. (C) Toe Guide: For Gracey curettes and universal curettes. (D) G Channel: For Gracey curettes. *Photos courtesy of Hu-Friedy Manufacturing Co., Inc.*

2. Nonautomated
   a. Remi Grip (www.rcmidental.com) (Figure 2–50). This design is a combination mouth mirror/sharpening stone; available in two styles. Interchangeable stones connect to a mouth mirror handle, autoclave as one, and provide a sterile stone for each patient. Stone shapes are triangular or circular.
   b. Ultimate Edge Kit, by Paradise Dental Technologies, has a flat stainless steel plate with angled bars to promote proper blade positioning for sharpening and includes an ultra fine grit ceramic stone and tester for cutting edges[17] (Figures 2–51).

Scaling and root planing are among the most challenging tasks to perfect in dentistry. A thorough knowledge of root anatomy, instrument design, and skill are required. It is the responsibility of the dental hygienist to perform periodontal debridement for patients requiring nonsurgical periodontal therapy. Excellent skills require time and experience to develop. The beginning operator should not be discouraged but rather accept the challenge to develop outstanding skills in advanced instrumentation. Fundamental principles acquired in the preclinical setting will be built upon with new information from continuing educational seminars and professional journals. Since the American Dental Hygienists' Association (ADHA) advocates evidence-based, patient-centered dental hygiene practice, operators are encouraged to stay current through courses offered by dental hygiene programs, state and local dental hygiene associations, distance education, private

Figure 2–50 Remi Grip. *Photo courtesy of Remi Dental Products, Inc.*

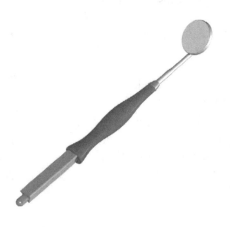

Figure 2–51 Ultimate Edge handheld sharpener. *Photos courtesy of Paradise Dental Technologies.*

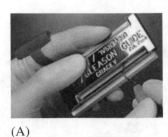

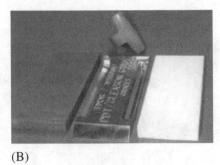

(A)   (B)

companies, and dental hygiene journals.[20] While valuable resources exist beyond the classroom, experience is still the best teacher for developing the more advanced skills to achieve a satisfying and rewarding dental hygiene career.

QUESTIONS

1. When a furcation probe can completely pass between the roots, with no recession present, the furcation is classified as Class
   a. I.
   b. II.
   c. III.
   d. IV.

2. The ultimate goal of nonsurgical periodontal therapy is to
   a. teach patient education.
   b. restore gingival health.
   c. save the patient from surgery.
   d. motivate the patient to value oral health.

3. The angulation, in degrees, for inserting an area-specific curette for periodontal debridement is
   a. 0.
   b. 45.
   c. 90.
   d. 110.

4. Utilizing eye loupes for magnification during periodontal debridement offers clinical as well as ergonomic benefits. Which of the following is NOT a benefit of wearing an eye loupe during advanced instrumentation?
   a. Assists in reading the periodontal probe.
   b. Enhances visual acuity.
   c. Relieves neck and back strain.
   d. Aids in supragingival calculus removal.
   e. Aids in subgingival calculus detection.

5. Your patient has a very small mouth and cannot open wide. However, there is a 7 millimeter periodontal pocket on the distal of tooth #17. Which is the best Gracey instrument to use in this area for thorough debridement?
   a. 11–12

   b. 13–14
   c. 15–16
   d. 17–18

6. The cross-section of a universal curette is a
   a. triangle.
   b. half moon.
   c. circle.
   d. nib.

7. The internal angle, in degrees, of a Gracey curette is
   a. 60 to 70.
   b. 45 to 60.
   c. 45 to 90.
   d. 70 to 80.

8. Where would a 15–16 Gracey be used?
   a. Mesial of molars
   b. Distal of molars
   c. Extruded premolars
   d. Anterior teeth

9. Tooth #31 has a Class III furcation involvement. Which Gracey instrument is best to use in order to scale the mesiobuccal aspect of the distal root?
   a. 11–12
   b. 13–14
   c. 1–2
   d. 9–10

10. When sharpening an area-specific curette, all of the following areas of the blade are sharpened EXCEPT one. Which one is the EXCEPTION?
    a. Toe
    b. Face
    c. One lateral side
    d. Both lateral sides

REFERENCES

1. Cooper M & Wiechmann L. In: *Essentials of Dental Hygiene: Preclinical Skills.* Upper Saddle River, NJ: Prentice Hall, 2004.

2. Hu-Friedy Manufacturing Company, Chicago, IL. Scaler/Curette brochure.

3. White DJ, Cox ER, et al. Instruments and methods for the quantitative measurement of factors affecting hygienist/dentist efforts during scaling and root planing of the teeth. *The Journal of Clinical Dentistry,* Vol. VII, Number 2, 1996, 32–40.

4. Schmidt CR. Task analysis of the Nevi 1 and Nevi 2 periodontal instruments. *The Journal of Practical Hygiene,* Vol. 11, Number 3, 2002, May/June, 15–19.

5. Drisko CH. Nonsurgical periodontal therapy. *Periodontology 2000,* Vol. 25, 2001, 77–88.

6. Cobb CM. Clinical significance of nonsurgical periodontal therapy: An evidence-based perspective of scaling and root planing. *Journal of Clinical Periodontology,* Supplement 2, Vol. 29, Number 5, 2002, 22–33.

7. Oberholzer R, Rateitschak, KH. Root cleaning or root smoothing: An in vivo study. *Journal of Clinical Periodontology,* Vol. 23, 1996, 326–330.

8. Schmidt CR, Mann GB, Mauriello SM. Task analysis of the Gracey 15/16 curette. *The Journal of Practical Hygiene,* Vol. 7, Number 4, 1998, July/August, 21–26.

9. McKechnie LB. Root morphology in periodontal therapy. *Dental Hygienist News.* Vol. 6, Number 1, 1993, 3–6.

10. Pattison AM, Matsuda S. Making the right choice. *Dimensions of Dental Hygiene.* Perio Focus Vol. 1, Number 7, 2004, 4–10.

11. Cobb CM. Non-surgical pocket therapy: mechanical. *Annals of Periodontology,* Vol. 1, 1996, 443–490.

12. Pattison AM, Pattison GL. Periodontal instrumentation transformed. *Dimensions of Dental Hygiene,* Vol. 1, Number 2, 2003, April/May, 18–22.

13. Benhamou V. Calculus detection goes high tech. *Dimensions of Dental Hygiene,* Vol. 1, Number 3, 2003, June/July, 16–18, 40.

14. Goldie MP. "Maximizing the value of the dental hygienist in the treatment of periodontal therapy." June 28, 2003, ADHA Annual Session, New York, NY.

15. Ellingson P. Instrument sharpening: How to solve your sharpening problems. *Journal of Practical Hygiene,* Vol. 2, Number 6, 1993, 23–25.

16. Hodges K. On the cutting edge. *Dimensions of Dental Hygiene,* Vol. 2, Number 4, 2004, April, 16–20, 36.

17. Burns S. Get the edge on instrument sharpening. *Journal of Practical Hygiene,* Vol. 13, Number 2, 2004, March/April, 43–44.

18. Cooper MD. Keeping the sharper edge. *RDH,* Vol. 19, Number 4, 1999, 46, 49–50.

19. Burns S. *It's about time.* Chicago. Hu-Friedy, 1995.

20. American Dental Hygienists' Association. Policy statements. Chicago, IL: Author. 1997. Accessed Oct 10, 2003 at www.adha.org.

GRACEY CURETTE/POCKET DEBRIDEMENT PERFORMANCE EVALUATION

Re-evaluation

Student ____________ Date ____________ Instructor ____________ Patient ____________

Instrument ____________

1 2 3 4 5 6 7 8 9 10 11 12 13 14 15 16

Date ____ Instr: ____ S–U S–U Date ____ Instr: ____

Date ____ Instr: ____ S–U S–U Date ____ Instr: ____

32 31 30 29 28 27 26 25 24 23 22 21 20 19 18 17

Instr: ____ Date ____ Patient ____ #'s ____

Instr: ____ Date ____ Patient ____ #'s ____

	S	U	Comments	S	U	Comments	S	U	Comments
1. Pocket debridement authorized by instructor.									
2. Gross removal of calculus on the root surfaces has been approved by dental hygiene instructor.									
3. Utilizes periodontal chart and radiographs.									
4. Provides anesthesia, when necessary.									
5. Confirms sharpening stone on tray.									
GRASP									
6. Stacks fingers together.									
7. Bends fingers slightly.									
8. Bends thumb tip out.									
9. Rests instrument on side of fat pad.									
FULCRUM									
10. Keeps finger straight.									
11. Stabilizes fulcrum.									
12. Utilizes alternative finger rests correctly.									
HAND									
13. Keeps wrist and forearm straight.									
14. Places palm toward occlusal plane, when applicable.									
ADAPTATION-ANGULATION									
15. Utilizes correct end of instrument.									
16. Inserts blade at closed angle (0–10°).									
17. Opens blade (60°–80°) at base of pocket.									
18. Maintains 1–2 mm of blade on tooth.									

STROKES						
19. Utilizes wrist/forearm action to move instrument.						
20. Keeps initial working strokes short, overlapping, and firm.						
21. Utilizes strokes with the same lateral pressure from beginning to end.						
22. Utilizes oblique/horizontal/vertical strokes.						
23. Completes with longer strokes and lighter pressure.						
24. Re-explores to check for thoroughness.						
25. Induces as little trauma as possible.						
DENTAL MIRROR; utilizes proper						
26. Grasp/fulcrum.						
27. Retraction.						
28. Reflection/illumination/transillumination.						
ERGONOMICS; utilizes proper						
29. Patient/operator positioning.						
30. Lighting						

Courtesy of Indiana University Purdue University Fort Wayne Dental Hygiene Program.

Chapter 3

Power-Driven Scaling

Anne N. Guignon, RDH, MPH and Harold A. Henson, RDH, MEd

 MediaLink

A companion CD-ROM, included free with each new copy of this book, supplements the procedures presented in each chapter. Insert the CD-ROM to watch video clips and view a large collection of color images that is also included. This multimedia library is designed to help you add a new dimension to your learning.

KEY TERMS

acoustics	in phase	root planing
active tip area	magnetostrictive ultrasonic scaler	scaling
amplitude	manually-tuned scaling unit	sonic scaler
automatically-tuned scaling unit	out of phase	stroke
biofilm	periodontal debridement	tip
cavitation	piezoelectric scaling tip	transducer
cycle	piezoelectric ultrasonic scaler	ultrasonic scaling insert
deplaquing	plaque	ultrasonics
frequency	power	

LEARNING OBJECTIVES

After reading this chapter, the student will be able to:

- determine the origins of power-driven scaling technology;
- determine the importance for incorporating power-driven scaling into clinical practice;
- identify the different types of power-driven scalers;
- identify the anatomy of an ultrasonic insert and tip;
- identify different types of ultrasonic tip designs;
- state the advantages and disadvantages of ultrasonic scaling devices;
- prepare the clinical workstation for ultrasonic scaling procedures;
- recall ultrasonic instrumentation techniques;
- identify the ergonomics of ultrasonic scaling;
- recall how to maintain the ultrasonic unit, inserts, and tips;
- understand the future of power driven technology.

I. Introduction

Ultrasonics devices were primarily used in the 1950s to cut tooth structure and remove dental caries. This application fell out of favor when the high-speed, air-driven handpieces were introduced. In 1955, Zinner introduced **ultrasonics** to the field of periodontics, which resulted in widespread acceptance in today's dental therapy.[1]

The first ultrasonic scalers were **magnetostrictive ultrasonic scalers,** which proved to be helpful in removing supragingival deposits; however, the size and diameter of the tips presented significant challenges for complex subgingival instrumentation. In the late 1960s a periodontist named Thomas Holbrook began to recontour and rebend the thick tips, creating tips that were much slimmer. His original design modifications, now universally accepted, have led to the development of many unique tip designs used in all types of ultrasonic scalers.[2]

Piezoelectric (Piezo) ultrasonic scalers were developed in the early 1970s. These scalers have a linear stroke in contrast to the elliptical stroke found in magnetostrictive ultrasonic units. Magnetostrictive ultrasonic units still remain the most widely used ultrasonic scalers in North America; however, piezoelectric ultrasonic scalers dominate the international market. Athough there are some differences between magnetostrictive and piezoelectric ultrasonics, a remarkable similarity is found in the actual clinical application of either type of device. Numerous reports in the literature indicate that if ultrasonic scalers are properly used, a superior clinical outcome can be obtained in contrast to other types of debridement, regardless of whether a magnetostrictive or piezoelectric ultrasonic scaler is used.

CLINICAL TIP:

Tuning Your Knowledge: A **cycle** is one complete linear or elliptical stroke path.

II. Types of Power-Driven Scalers
A. Sonic scalers.
1. Characteristics.
   a. Operate in an audible range by using compressed air to create vibrations that vary from 3,000 to 8,000 cycles per second (cps) (Figure 3–1).

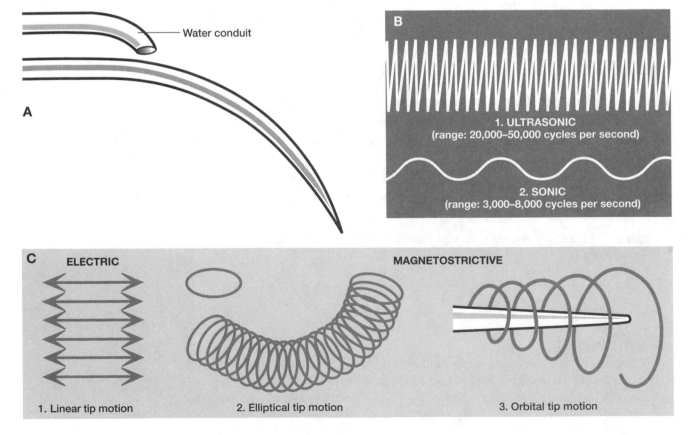

Figure 3–1   Audible ranges of power-driven scalers.

b. Compressed air passes over a series of metal plates, creating vibrations that are transferred to the sonic tip.

c. Both the **frequency** and **amplitude** are preset and cannot be adjusted by the operator.

2. Design.

   a. Handpiece attaches directly to the dental unit[3] slow speed handpiece air hose—portable and relatively inexpensive.

   b. Removes light-to-moderate or newly formed supragingival deposits, with limited application for subgingival deposit removal.

   c. Tips.

      (1) Available only in standard diameter **tips,** which limit access considerably, especially in areas that are clinically challenging.

      (2) Are threaded directly into handpiece.

      (3) **Stroke** is orbital in nature.

      (4) All sides of the insert are active.

      (5) Do not move rapidly enough to develop cavitational properties as the water flows over the moving tip.[4]

   d. Purpose of water.

      (1) Lubricates the active working tip.

      (2) Flushes debris from working area.

      (3) Flows through the working end of the tip.

B. Ultrasonic scalers, including magnetostrictive and piezoelectric scalers, create vibrations that are not audible to the human ear.

1. Characteristics.

   a. Both use electrical energy to create rapid movements, resulting in intense vibrations in the scaling tips.

   b. When fluid flows over an activated ultrasonic tip, ultrasonic sound wave energy (**acoustics**) creates fluid **cavitation,** which enhances the disruption of hard and soft deposits on teeth.

   c. Recent research has shown that cavitation is capable of disrupting plaque **biofilm** deposits.[5]

2. Types.

   a. Magnetostrictive ultrasonic scaler.

      (1) Characteristics.

         (a) Most use vibrations from magnetic strips that are passed through a **transducer** to the ultrasonic tip.

         (b) Creates a rapidly oscillating **active tip area** that removes deposits using an elliptical stroke operating at 25,000 to 30,000 cycles per second (cps) (see Figure 3–1).

         (c) One type of magnetostrictive unit uses a ferrite ceramic rod; this unit's transducer creates an orbital tip motion operating at 42,000 cps.

      (2) Operational mechanism.

         (a) An alternating electrical current, applied to a wire coil in the handpiece, creates a magnetic field.

         (b) A magnetic field forms as the metal strips or rod in the insert constrict and expand.

         (c) These rapid constrictions result in vibrations that are transferred to the active tip area via a transducer that is placed between the metal strips or the ferrite ceramic rod and the tip of the ultrasonic insert.

         (d) Stroke is elliptical or orbital (see Figure 3–1).

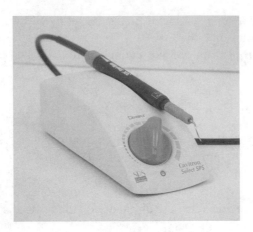

(e) Length and shape of the tip affect the stroke, as well as amplitude and frequency settings.

(f) Movement allows for simultaneous activation on all tip surfaces (360 degrees), allowing the operator the option of using the lateral surfaces, the convex, or concave surfaces on the tooth surface.

(3) Types.

   (a) **Automatically-tuned scaling units.** Designed with a preset frequency control within the unit (Figure 3–2).

     i. Scaler tunes each ultrasonic insert automatically, which creates a frequency/amplitude relationship.[4]

     ii. Single-stage units control amplitude settings from low-to-high ranges with a single power (amplitude) knob.

     iii. Dual-stage units feature an amplitude control knob on the unit. Footswitch has a boost mechanism that allows an increase in the scaler amplitude when the unit is set at an ultra-low power range.

   (b) **Manually-tuned scaling units.** Allows the operator to control both the frequency and the amplitude of the vibrating tip; this ability to adjust either the frequency or energy being used is a direct advantage of using a manually tuned unit[6] (Figure 3–3).

   (c) Some magnetostrictive scalers allow the operator to choose between manually-tuned operations and auto-tuned settings.

b. Piezoelectric ultrasonic scalers (Figure 3–4).

  (1) Characteristics.

   (a) Use crystals or ceramic discs housed in the handpiece to produce rapid mechanical vibrations in the scaling tip.

   (b) Operate between 28,000 and 45,000 cps to remove deposits on tooth structure.

  (2) Operational mechanism.

   (a) An electrical current is applied to the ceramic discs or crystals, causing dimensional changes in the crystals or discs.

   (b) These rapid dimensional changes result in vibrations that are transferred to the tip via a handpiece transducer placed between the discs or crystals and the tip.

   (c) Stroke is primarily linear in nature; however, all tip surfaces are active; lateral surfaces are most efficient.

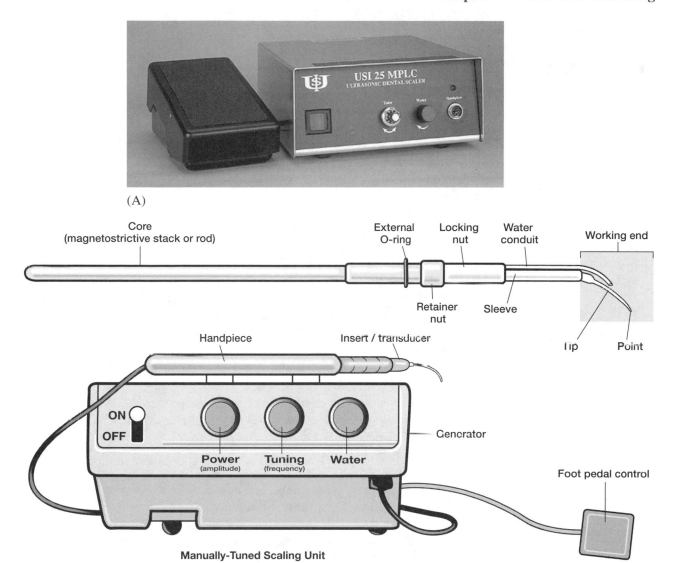

(A)

Core
(magnetostrictive stack or rod)

External
O-ring

Locking
nut

Water
conduit

Working end

Retainer
nut

Sleeve

Tip   Point

Handpiece   Insert / transducer

ON

OFF

Power
(amplitude)

Tuning
(frequency)

Water

Generator

Foot pedal control

Manually-Tuned Scaling Unit

(B)

Figure 3–3   (A) Manually-tuned scaling unit. (B) Parts of a manually-tuned unit. *Photo courtesy of Ultrasonic Services, Inc.*

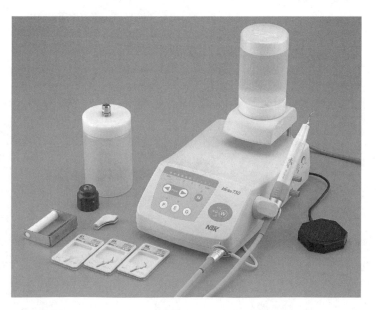

Figure 3–4   Piezoelectric ultrasonic scaler. *Photo courtesy of Brasseler USA.*

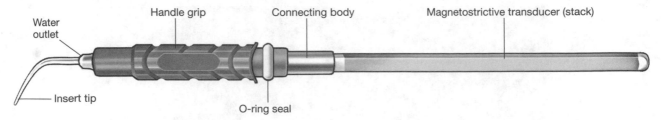

Water outlet

Handle grip

Connecting body

Magnetostrictive transducer (stack)

Insert tip

O-ring seal

Figure 3–5   Components of a magnetostrictive unit.

(d) Length and shape of tip affects stroke and tip movement, as well as amplitude and frequency settings.

III. Ultrasonic Scaling Inserts

There are numerous dental manufacturers of **ultrasonic scaling inserts** and tips. Tips can be designed with a variety of features, but basically all are designed to remove calculus, **plaque** biofilm, and stain. Some tips are limited to supragingival **scaling,** while others are designed to aid in **root planing** allowing access to both the crown and root of the tooth.

A. Anatomy of a magnetostrictive transducer, commonly known as an insert (Figures 3–5 and 3–6).

   1. Designed with a core made from a stack of nickel alloy strips.
   2. Some strips are coated to enhance magnetic properties.
   3. One magnetostrictive scaler uses inserts that contain a ferromagnetic rod that is designed only for use in that scaler.
   4. Inserts available in:
      a. All-metal designs.
      b. Metal/resin combinations.
      c. Metal/silicone grip configurations.
   5. Contains a variety of parts, which can include the following features:
      a. Core. Transforms electrical energy to mechanical energy; composed of a stack of nickel alloy strips or a ferrite ceramic rod.
      b. Working end. Portion of the insert that includes the point, tip, and water conduit.
         (1) Point. Also known as the tip end, the terminal end of the tip—most powerful part of the insert.
         (2) Tip. Portion of the insert that comes in contact with tooth structure; composed of the point, convex, concave, and lateral surfaces (Figure 3–7).

Figure 3–6   Magnetostrictive handpiece and straight insert.

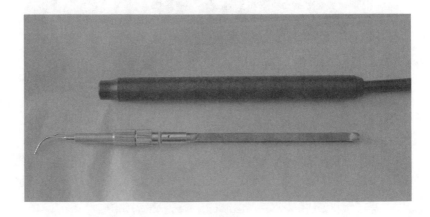

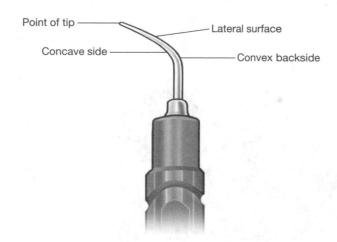

Point of tip — Lateral surface
Concave side — Convex backside

Figure 3–7   Power dispersion of a magnetostrictive insert tip.

(3) Water flow (Figure 3–8).
    (a) External conduit. Provides fluid to the insert tip via a metal conduit also known as a trombone.
    (b) Internal water flow. Fluid flows to the insert tip through a small opening in the insert tip, often referred to as a focused spray or direct flow.
    (c) Sleeve. Covers the portion of the insert that includes the interface of the terminal end of the tip and the insert transducer.
    (d) Locking nut and retainer nut. Locks the water conduit and the working end together in metal magnetostrictive inserts.
    (e) External O-ring. Establishes an interlock between the insert and the handpiece, preventing water leakage.
B. Anatomy of a **piezoelectric scaling tip.** Piezoelectric ultrasonic units use crystals or ceramic discs housed in the handpiece to transform electrical energy to mechanical energy (Figure 3–9).
  1. Tips differ from magnetostrictive inserts because they lack a core.
  2. Tips are small and threaded directly into the handpiece; they should be stored in the holders or cassettes provided by the manufacturer.
  3. Fluid flows through a small hole at the base of the tip to the tip end.
  4. Must use the unit's torque wrench to tighten the tip onto the handpiece to ensure effective tip vibration.

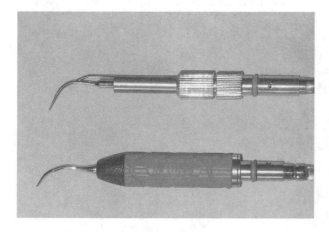

Figure 3–8   Internal vs. external water flow.

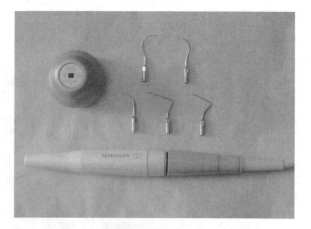

Figure 3–9   Piezo wrench handpiece and tips.

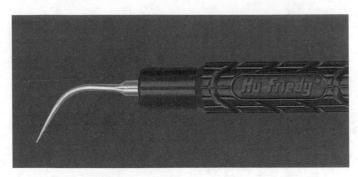

Figure 3–10   Universal straight tip. *Photo courtesy of Hu-Friedy Manufacturing Co., Inc.*

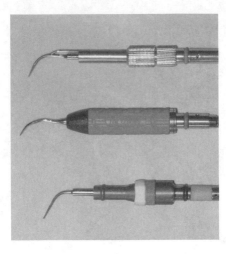

Figure 3–11   Thick debridement instrument tips.

C. Ultrasonic insert tip designs. Many tip designs are available for both magnetostrictive and piezoelectric ultrasonic units. The following basic designs are manufactured for both units.

  1. Basic ultrasonic tip designs.

   a. Universal straight. Designed to adapt to any tooth surface; available in diameters that range from 0.2 to 0.8 millimeters at the tip end (Figure 3–10).

    (1) Supragingival straight debridement. Large-diameter tip specifically designed for scaling gross tenacious deposits and heavy stain; generally more effective in medium-to-high power ranges (Figure 3–11).

    (2) Slim precision straight tips. Designed for scaling light to moderate supragingival deposits, **deplaquing,** or to access deeper periodontal defects; inserts are 0.4 millimeters in diameter at the tip end and most effective when used in low-to-medium **power** (amplitude) ranges. Activating inserts in high power settings can lead to premature tip breakage.[7]

    (3) Slim precision extended straight tips are 0.4 millimeters in diameter; however, the terminal shank of this insert is longer. This dimensional change facilitates root planing with access into

Figure 3–12   Right and left tips. *Photo courtesy of Hu-Friedy Manufacturing Co., Inc.*

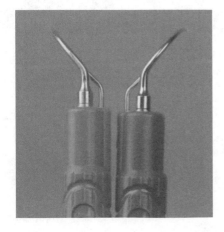

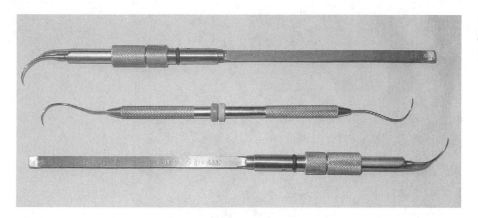

Figure 3–13 Right and left tips compared with Naber's furcation instrument.

deeper periodontal defects without extending the actual length of the tip.

    (4) Beavertail tip. An early design that features a wide tip to be primarily used for scaling large, heavy calculus deposits.

    (5) Triple bend configuration. Designed to be effective in scaling supragingival stain and calculus.

  b. Right and left configurations (Figures 3–12 and 3–13).

    (1) Designed to adapt to buccal and lingual surfaces and areas with limited access, furcations, tight contacts, and malpositioned teeth.

    (2) Slim precision right and left tips are 0.4 millimeters in diameter.

2. Specialty ultrasonic tips.

  a. Diamond-coated tips.

    (1) Designed to remove burnished calculus, not for routine scaling procedures.

    (2) Should be used in specific sites only by highly skilled operators.

    (3) Size of the diamond grit can vary per manufacturer.

      (a) Larger grit coatings are designed for surgical use only.

      (b) Finer grit piezo ultrasonic scaler inserts are used at the end of the procedure to remove the last vestiges of burnished calculus.

  b. Ultra-slim precision tips. Available in either 0.2 millimeter or 0.3 millimeter tip end configurations (Figure 3–14).

    (1) Designed to be used in a manually-tuned magnetostrictive ultrasonic scaler in complex periodontal scaling procedures.

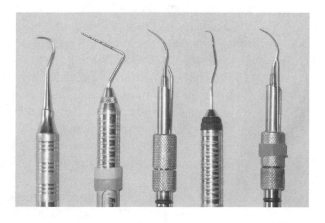

Figure 3–14 Scaler, probe, ultrathin insert, 11-12 explorer, super thin insert.

Figure 3–15   Carbon composite piezo implant tips.

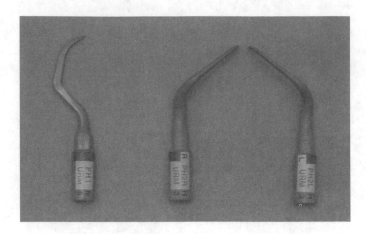

(2) Automatically-tuned ultrasonic scalers create frequency and amplitude ranges that are too high to accommodate this type of tip design.

(3) Operated in low power ranges.

c. Furcation tips. Designed with a 0.8 millimeter ball at the tip end. As the name indicates, these tips are specific to debriding furcas; however, the larger diameter of the tip end may limit access to these areas.

d. Implant tips. Types include:

(1) Magnetostrictive ultrasonic scaler. Special plastic sleeve covers the insert tip to prevent scratching the titanium surfaces of the implant.

(2) Piezoelectric ultrasonic scaler. Special nonmetal composite carbon tip designed for use around implants or fine cosmetic restorations (Figure 3–15).

e. Swivel tips. Magnetostrictive ultrasonic scaler designed with a fingertip swivel that facilitates adaptation of the insert tip on the tooth and reduces awkward hand and finger positioning; also provides unnecessary stopping and manual repositioning of the tip in the handpiece.

f. Titanium-coated tips. Specially designed to resist wear.

IV. Advantages and Disadvantages of Ultrasonic Scalers

A. Advantages.

1. Patient benefits. The development of slimmer tips allows the operator to use an ultrasonic scaler in a wider range of clinical applications than ever before. In addition, both manually-tuned ultrasonic scaler units and the more refined automatically-tuned ultrasonic scaler models provide more opportunities to control patient comfort during ultrasonic scaling procedures. Ultrasonic scalers offer several advantages for the patient.

a. Enhances **periodontal debridement.** A slim ultrasonic scaler insert tip allows instrument access into deep, narrow pockets that may not accommodate the diameter of the blade of a hand instrument.[8,9]

b. Enhances disruption of plaque biofilm.[5]

c. Decreases potential damage to root structure. When properly used, ultrasonic scalers are much less damaging than hand instruments or sonic scalers.

d. Provides continuous periodontal pocket irrigation during scaling.

e. Minimizes anesthesia needs. Little to no anesthesia is required when scaling deeper periodontal pockets when using slimmer insert tips to remove light-to-moderate deposits that are not tenacious.

f. Reduces temporomandibular joint (TMJ) fatigue. Limited lateral pressure on the insert tip and extraoral soft tissue rests reduce stress on the patient's TMJ.

g. Decreases tooth sensitivity. Slimmer tips, operated at low power ranges, create less sensitivity on hypersensitive tooth surfaces such as exposed dentin.

h. Decreases soft tissue discomfort. Slimmer tips, positioned parallel to the tooth and operated at low power ranges, reduce soft tissue distention, resulting in improved patient comfort.

i. Increases acceptance of periodontal debridement procedures because of increased patient comfort and improved efficiency, resulting in more effective use of appointment time.

j. Decreases anxiety in patients who prefer ultrasonic scaling.[10]

k. Reduces tissue trauma. Smooth surfaces of the insert do not create tissue lacerations.

l. Promotes wound healing. Observed by many operators due to bactericidal effect.

m. Provides advanced technology, which some patients prefer.

2. Operator benefits. Instrumentation with an ultrasonic scaling device is dramatically different than scaling with a hand instrument. Operators are more likely to be able to perform complex periodontal procedures, as well as routine scalings, in a shorter period of time with less overall stress to the body. Any time saved can then be reallocated to provide more in-depth patient services that might be otherwise shortened or eliminated. Additional services could include discussion of current treatment needs, evaluation with an intraoral camera, tobacco cessation program information, or customized oral hygiene instruction.[10] Several advantages offered to the operator using ultrasonic scaling include:

a. Facilitates instrumentation in deep or narrow defects.

b. Improves access in areas with complex root anatomy or malpositioned teeth.[3,11,12]

c. Improves visual field through washed visibility.

d. Maintains fragile periodontal patients who elect to be treated with nonsurgical periodontal scaling procedures.

e. Reduces hand and forearm fatigue.

f. Provides less care of inserts since tips do not require sharpening.

g. Provides continuous removal of bloody debris and other types of bioburden due to the lavage effect.

h. Facilitates removal of tenacious calculus.

3. Dental practice benefits.

a. Increases hygiene practice productivity. More complex periodontal debridement procedures can often be performed without anesthesia.

b. Provides efficient use of clinical time by requiring less time for complete debridement.

c. Enhances efficiency through:

(1) Requiring fewer insert tips per procedure.

(2) Not sharpening insert tips.

(3) Limiting tip maintenance.

d. Limits insert retipping or rebuilding, which provides long-term cost savings.

e. Decreases need for anesthesia. Many periodontal debridement procedures and most maintenance procedures can be performed without anesthesia or a limited use of topical anesthetic, if the operator uses newer, slimmer inserts and low-to-medium power ranges.

f. Improves patient acceptance; many patients prefer ultrasonic scaling over hand instrumentation.

g. Provides fewer scheduling challenges. Decreased patient anxiety can result in fewer appointment failures, cancellations, or rescheduling issues.

B. Disadvantages.

1. Patient contraindications include those with:

a. Decalcification. Decalcified areas should be avoided to prevent further enamel destruction.

b. Dental implants. Most ultrasonic inserts or tips are not specifically designed for scaling implants and can cause damage to the titanium surface.

c. Dysphagia. Patients who have difficulty swallowing require close supervision because water will pool in the back of mouth from the water released through the inserts. To help reduce this:[4]

(1) Slightly elevate the patient's head.

(2) Position the saliva ejector in the retromolar pad area to improve water evacuation.

d. Patient reluctance. Some patients are reluctant to try new technology. When dealing with these patients, try to:

(1) Determine the source of concern.

(2) Discuss the advantages of ultrasonic scaling therapy.

(3) Demonstrate how equipment works.

(4) Use anesthesia, if needed.

(5) Apply desensitizing medicaments to hypersensitive tooth structures.

(6) Offer noise reduction devices, such as earphones or earplugs.

2. Operator disadvantages.

a. Lack of availability of ultrasonic scaler.

b. Lack of experience using an ultrasonic scaler; initial learning curve for a manually-tuned scaler may be longer than for an automatically-tuned unit.

c. Time required by an inexperienced operator to tune an insert in a manually tuned unit.

d. Use of insufficient, inappropriate, damaged, or worn ultrasonic scaler inserts or tips.

3. Dental practice disadvantages.

a. Expense.

(1) Initial expense of ultrasonic unit.

(2) Cost of inserts, which are higher than traditional hand instruments.

(3) Cost of disinfecting unit water lines.

b. Patient reluctance.

V. Preparing the Clinical Workstation for Ultrasonic Procedures

A. Ultrasonic unit preparation.

1. Position the ultrasonic unit on the opposite side of the operator's chair.[4]

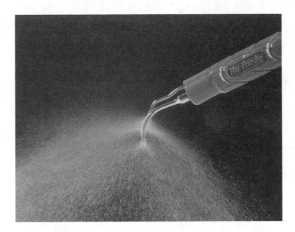

Figure 3–16   Halo-effect spray (in phase). *Photo courtesy of Hu-Friedy Manufacturing Co., Inc.*

2. Plug ultrasonic unit into electrical outlet.
3. Turn the power on.
4. Flush water lines for 2 to 3 minutes to reduce the amount of biofilm buildup in handpiece water lines.[13]
5. Disinfect the surface of the handpiece and wipe dry.
6. Wrap handpiece with a plastic sleeve or barrier.
7. Cover the ultrasonic scaling unit with an appropriate infection control barrier. Keep the unit's ventilation ports open to prevent overheating of the unit during use.
8. Follow the manufacturer's directions for placing the ultrasonic tip into the handpiece; some manually-tuned units require the tip to be placed in a dry handpiece.
9. Hold the handpiece over a sink and adjust water and power levels to the appropriate debridement levels; use appropriate power and water levels for each tip.
    a. Automatically-tuned magnetostrictive ultrasonic unit. Halo-effect indicates sufficient water is cooling the tip, a direct result of the insert operating **in phase** (Figure 3–16).
    b. Manually-tuned magnetostrictive ultrasonic unit. When properly adjusted, water flow appears as a heavy drip flowing from the end of the tip with a small amount of spray, a condition known as tuning **out of phase** (Figure 3–17).
    c. Piezoelectric ultrasonic tip. Proper water flow should be adjusted to a heavy drip.
B. Patient preparation. Since ultrasonic scaling may be a new procedure for some patients, it is advisable to spend a few minutes prior to beginning to

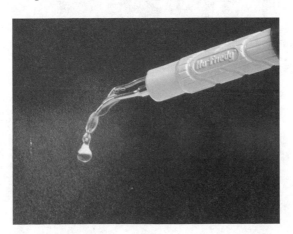

Figure 3–17   Heavy drip flowing (out of phase). *Photo courtesy of Hu-Friedy Manufacturing Co., Inc.*

Table 3–1   Patient/Operator Considerations and Contraindications for Using Ultrasonic Scaler

Patient	Operator
• **Premedication.** Premedicate patient if he/she falls under the current American Heart Association guidelines. • **Cardiac pacemakers.** Patient with a cardiac pacemaker should have a medical consultation directed to the cardiologist prior to using a magnetostrictive ultrasonic scaler.[14,15] • **Ocular or retinal implants.** Patients having ocular or retinal implants should have a medical consult directed to their ophthalmologist. Patients should wear protective eyewear to protect their eyes from bioburden. • **Hearing aids.** Patients who use hearing aids should turn the devices down or off to prevent hearing discomfort. • **Communicable or respiratory diseases.** Patients with either communicable or respiratory diseases are not candidates for ultrasonic instrumentation. Contaminated aerosols can increase the transmission of pathogenic organisms. Aerosolized particles can create an unnecessary respiratory challenge. • **Pregnancy.** There are no studies confirming that ultrasonic scalers affect the health of a pregnant patient or the development of a fetus.	• **Electromagnetic effects (EM).** There is no current significant research indicating health risks to the operator who is exposed to electromagnetic energy. • **Vibrational effects (VE).** There are no current studies that demonstrate that vibration in the ultrasonic handpiece causes neuralgia in the hands, wrists, or arms. • **Pregnancy.** There are no current significant research studies that the clinical use of an ultrasonic scaler poses a hazard to either the operator or developing fetus.

give instructions about the instrumentation concepts. Many may need reassurance that recent advancements in ultrasonic scaling techniques and equipment can result in a more comfortable clinical procedure than what was possible years ago.

1. Review medical history and take vital signs; determine any contraindications for use (Table 3–1).
2. Instruct patient to rinse for 30 seconds with an antimicrobial preprocedural mouth rinse and then expectorate.[16,17]
3. Explain the biological advantages of using ultrasonic scalers, how they differ from hand instrumentation, and what to expect during the scaling procedure.
4. Seat the patient with head slightly elevated (Figure 3–18).
5. Provide patient with protective eyewear.
6. Place the patient napkin.

Figure 3–18   Patient turned with head slightly elevated.

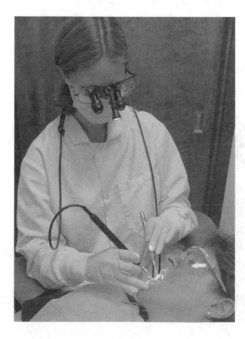

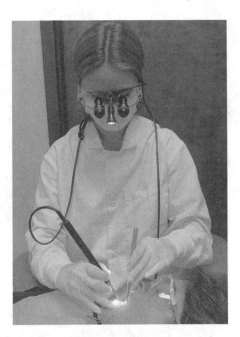

Figure 3–19   Loupes with light.

7. Arrange a signaling mechanism with the patient to indicate current or future needs, such as the raising of a hand.

C. Operator preparation.

1. Complete personal protective equipment.
2. Prepare operator-seating positions, which are the same as for hand instrumentation.
3. Position ultrasonic footswitch for easy access throughout procedure.
4. Place records, such as current radiographs and periodontal charts, in a location that is easy to review during the procedure, but away from the aerosol produced by the ultrasonic scaler.
5. Adjust overhead light to provide adequate illumination.
6. Use magnification and auxiliary illumination during procedure as with all other clinical procedures requiring precise clinical evaluation (Figure 3–19).

VI. Instrumentation

A. Patient positioning.

1. Have patient turn head toward operator.
2. Insert a continuous suction device as close to the work site as possible; instruct the patient NOT to close lips around suction device to prevent "suck-back" in lines.

B. General instrumentation principles.

1. Establish a fulcrum (extraoral or intraoral) to decrease lateral pressure on the ultrasonic scaling tip (Figure 3–20).
2. Activate the ultrasonic tip with the foot control.
3. Place the activated tip lightly on the tooth surface; gently enter sulcus/pocket (Figure 3–21).
4. Keep the tip moving and in contact with the tooth at all times; this can be accomplished by simply gliding the tip across the tooth rather than constantly removing the tip to reposition on another surface of the same tooth (Figure 3–22).

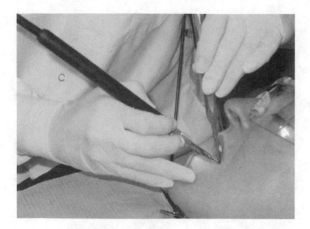

Figure 3–20   Using an extraoral fulcrum.

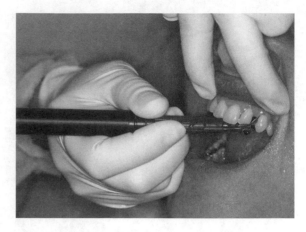

Figure 3–21   Slip insert tip gently into sulcus. *Photo courtesy of Hu-Friedy Manufacturing Co., Inc.*

5. Keep the length of the insert tip as parallel to the tooth surface as possible during scaling, except for instrumentation around cosmetic dental restorations where it is advisable for the angle of the insert to be opened approximately 10 degrees to 15 degrees (Figure 3–23).
6. Use a continuous smooth or light erasure motion, making sure to cover all tooth surfaces with overlapping strokes—horizontal, vertical, or oblique. Avoid using excessive lateral pressure, which dampens tip vibrations and reduces the tip's ability to effectively remove deposits, resulting in burnished calculus and/or damage to the tooth structure.[4]
7. Removing deposits. The operator may observe the following during ultrasonic scaling:
   a. Hard deposits break off in small or large pieces; ultrasonic scaling can pulverize hard deposits, creating a milky appearance in the water.
   b. Deposits are removed in continuous layers rather than in pieces.
   c. Subgingival biofilm is flushed out of the sulcus.
   d. No apparent deposit removal observed, but operator feels reduction in the size of the deposit.
   e. Tenacious, burnished deposits are the most difficult to remove and often require a more robust insert tip, used in medium-to-high power ranges, with additional time spent for deposit removal. Since

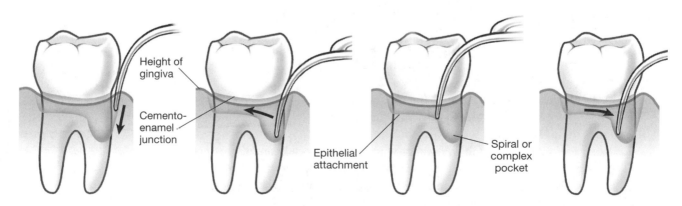

Figure 3–22   Using ultrasonic tip to debride in deep pocket.

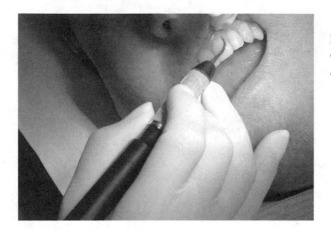

Figure 3–23   Adapt insert tip parallel to tooth surface. *Photo courtesy of Hu-Friedy Manufacturing Co., Inc.*

deposit removal can vary with each patient, the operator may or may not observe clinical manifestations of deposit removal.

8. Subgingival access. Can be easily performed by gently slipping the activated tip under the soft tissue. Care should be taken to avoid tissue distension.

C. Scaling (Figures 3–24 through 3–31).
1. Begin scaling with a universal straight ultrasonic insert.
2. Remove large supra- and subgingival deposits first.
3. Use multiple overlapping strokes starting coronally and progressing to the base of the pocket.
4. Debride interproximal areas. Adapt the tip perpendicular to the long axis of the tooth surface to provide complete coverage (Figures 3–32 and 3–33). Right and left tips are designed to improve access to these surfaces[4] (Figures 3–34 to 3–38).
5. Use the back surface of the tip to maneuver along the epithelial attachment.[4]
6. Instrumentation is complete when:
   a. All areas of the tooth have been instrumented with the activated tip.
   b. No more debris is being flushed from the pocket (Figure 3–39).
   c. No deposits are visible on the tooth surface.
   d. All enamel and root surfaces feel smooth to exploration.

CLINICAL TIP:

Tuning Your Knowledge: It is not necessary to follow with hand instrumentation when all of these requirements have been satisfied.

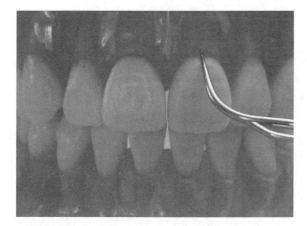

Figure 3–24   Scaling maxillary anterior facial with universal tip.

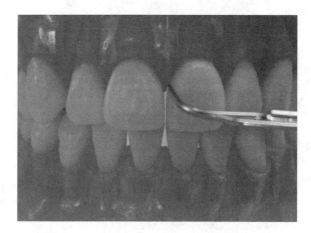

Figure 3–25   Scaling maxillary anterior interproximal with universal tip.

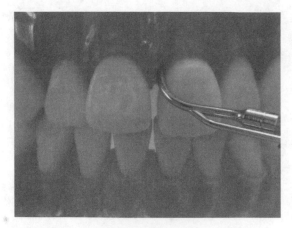

Figure 3–26   Scaling maxillary anterior inter-proximal to the extent of the pocket.

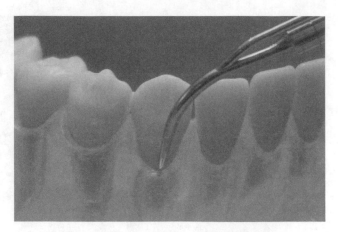

Figure 3–27   Scaling mandibular canine facial surface with universal tip.

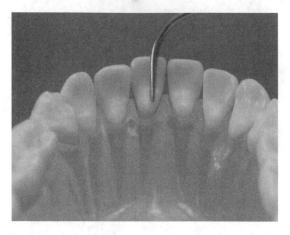

Figure 3–28   Scaling mandibular anterior lingual surface with universal tip.

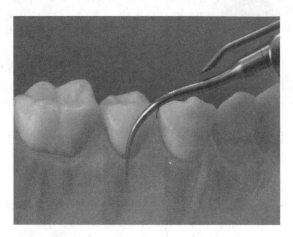

Figure 3–29   Scaling mandibular premolar facial surface with universal tip.

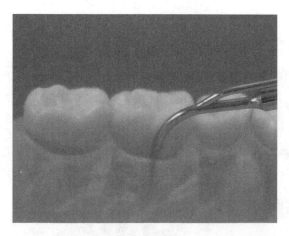

Figure 3–30   Scaling mandibular molar lingual surface with universal tip.

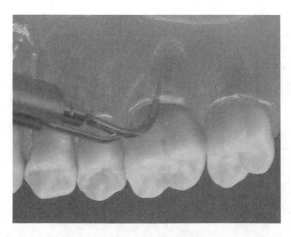

Figure 3–31   Scaling maxillary molar lingual root surface with convex portion of universal tip.

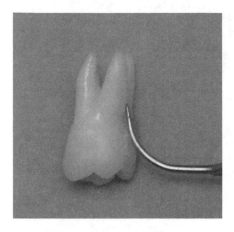

Figure 3–32   Insert tip adapted to tooth anatomy.

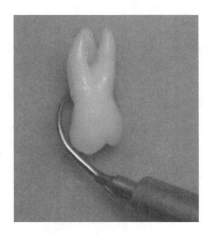

Figure 3–33   Insert tip not adapted to tooth surface.

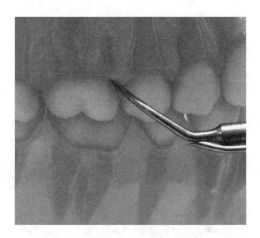

Figure 3–34   Application of right-curved tip.

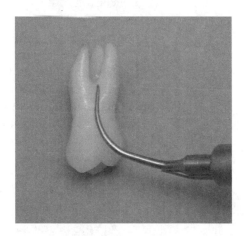

Figure 3–35   Adapting into furcation with a curved insert.

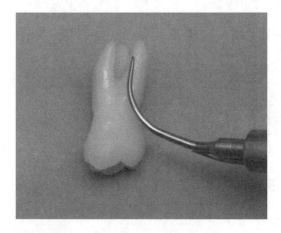

Figure 3–36   Adapting into furcation following root anatomy.

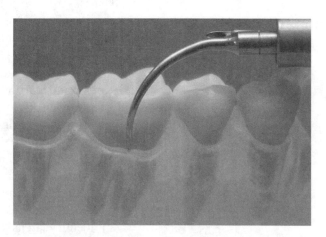

Figure 3–37   Using curved insert into furcation of mandibular molar.

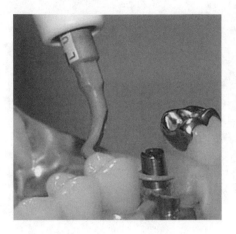

Figure 3–38 Carbon composite implant tip.

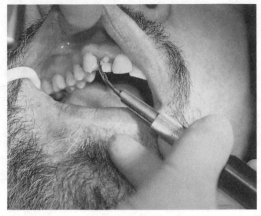

Figure 3–39 Using continuous wash for field visibility.

7. Conclusion of the appointment.
   a. Provide the patient with a post-procedure antimicrobial rinse.
   b. If anesthesia is used, recommend a soft-food diet until the local anesthesia subsides.
   c. Recommend over-the-counter (OTC) analgesic medication for the patient concerned with post-scaling discomfort.
D. Resolving challenging situations.
   1. Removal of tenacious deposits can be accomplished by using the following recommendations.
      a. Exercise patience. Some deposits require repeated instrumentation before being dislodged.
      b. Determine that the ultrasonic tip is properly seated in the handpiece.
      c. Use the more powerful surface of the tip; for example, when scaling with the lateral surface, try the concave or convex surfaces—the insert tip point can be initially used to break a smooth bridge of calculus; it should not be used directly on the tooth structure.
      d. Check scaler power adjustments and increase, if necessary.
      e. Evaluate if the tip or transducer is worn or damaged.
      f. If necessary, use a larger or more robust tip designed for heavy or tenacious deposit removal.
      g. Change the frequency setting of the tip on a manually-tuned unit so it is tuned more in phase.
   2. Sensitivity to ultrasonic scaling procedures.
      It is important that the operator distinguish between tooth discomfort and gingival sensitivity, because the clinical management of these conditions can be quite different. Some patients experience both hard and soft tissue discomfort, so it is important to try to resolve these issues prior to any instrumentation.
      a. Sensitive tooth structure.
         (1) Determine from the patient if there are any areas that have a history of thermal, touch, or air sensitivity.
         (2) Identify areas of exposed root surfaces, cervical abrasion, or erosion.
         (3) Apply an appropriate desensitizing medicament prior to scaling. Products containing various fluoride formulations, light-cured

CLINICAL TIP:

Tuning Your Knowledge: On rare occasions, tenacious deposit removal may not be possible with even with the finest ultrasonic scaler or hand scaling in the hands of a highly skilled operator. Under these circumstances, patients should be referred to a periodontist for further treatment.

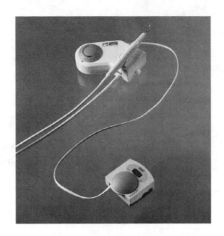

Figure 3–40   Electronic anesthesia P5 and TeamUp. *Photo courtesy of Acteon Group.*

desensitizers, and prophylaxis pastes containing a special calcium carbonate/bicarbonate complex have proven successful in the chairside management of tooth hypersensitivity. Use warm water in a microwave if medicament dispensers are used.

(4) Instruct patient to swish with the warm water prior to scaling.

(5) Consider a professionally applied fluoride treatment at the conclusion of the appointment.

(6) If indicated, prescribe professional home fluorides or FDA-approved desensitizing toothpastes for further sensitivity reduction.

b. Gingival sensitivity.

(1) Apply topical anesthetic in the form of locally applied gels, liquids, sprays, or rinses.

(2) Administer local anesthesia, if necessary.

(3) Use an electronic analgesia device. One piezoelectric ultrasonic scaling unit includes a handheld patient-controlled electronic analgesia device. Follow manufacturer's directions (Figure 3–40).

3. Auditory concerns.

a. Use earplugs, a stereo headset, or noise reduction headphones to modify loud or irritating noises.

b. Turn off or readjust the volume control of hearing aids.

4. Cosmetic dental restoration.[18,19]

a. Avoid contact with tooth-colored restorations with ultrasonic tip.

b. Slightly open the angle to avoid contact with margins of restorations.

c. Operate the power scaler at a low-amplitude setting.

d. Use specifically designed carbon composite tips in the piezoelectric ultrasonic scaler handpiece.

VII. Ergonomics

An operator who chooses to use an ultrasonic scaler should understand there are several factors that can contribute to the development of cumulative trauma disorders when using this type of instrumentation. Although proper use of an ultrasonic scaler can create less stress on an operator's body, it is important to consider such factors as the positioning of the operator, patient, and equipment. In addition, various types of scalers and inserts may contain features that either detract from or improve the overall comfort of the workspace. To date, no one piece of equipment has been developed that provides all of the optimal ergonomic features available.[20,21]

A. Ergonomic features of ultrasonic scalers. Ultrasonic scalers are designed to contain a variety of features that include one or more of the following, and can improve overall operator comfort during scaling.
  1. Scaler handpieces. Features include:
     a. Light weight.
     b. Balanced.
     c. Hose-end swivel device.
     d. Textured and larger diameter grip.
     e. Self-contained light source.
  2. Handpiece cords. Features include:
     a. Light weight.
     b. Flexible.
     c. Sufficient length.
  3. Inserts. Features include:
     a. Grip: Cushioned, large diameter, and textured (Figure 3–41).
     b. Balanced.
     c. Light weight.
     d. Fingertip swivel.
     e. Self-contained light source.
  4. Unit-mounted control switches or dials. Features include:
     a. Easy accessibility.
     b. Simple manipulation.
  5. Footswitches. Features include:
     a. Easy activation.
     b. Resists slipping across the floor.
     c. Easy repositioning.
     d. Cruise control. Amplitude setting remains active without constant foot pressure.
     e. Allows for changes in insert power settings.
  6. Hand-activated power control. The ferrite magnetostrictive ultrasonic scaler features a fingertip-activated power control switch integrated in the handpiece.
B. Operator positioning.
  1. Place the ultrasonic unit on the opposite side of the patient. This allows the operator unrestricted movement and avoids unnecessary twisting, which can contribute to fatigue and the development of cumulative trauma disorders.[20]
  2. Use the same operator-to-patient positioning as with hand instrumentation.

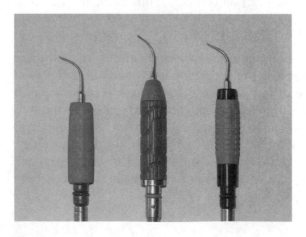

Figure 3–41   Silicone-padded ultrasonic instrument grips.

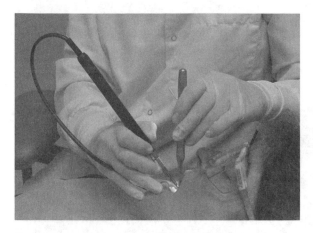

Figure 3–42   Holding cord with "pinky" finger.

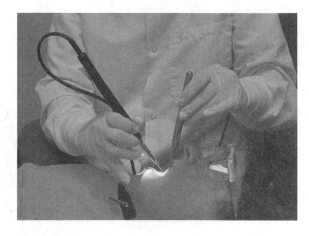

Figure 3–43   Using a palm/thumb cord control.

3. Manage handpiece cord. Effective handpiece cord management minimizes hand and wrist stress created by the weight and drag of the handpiece cord. The following techniques can be used by the operator to minimize such stress.
   a. Hold a loop of handpiece cord between the ring and little finger or between the thumb and palm (Figures 3–42 and 3–43).
   b. Drape the handpiece cord around the neck (Figure 3–44).
   c. Place a loop of excess cord over forearm (Figure 3–45).
   d. Wrap excess handpiece cord around the forearm (Figure 3–46).
   e. Loop excess cord over the overhead light handle; avoid contact with the light reflector (Figure 3–47).
   f. Loop excess cord through metal support attached to bracket table (Figure 3–48).

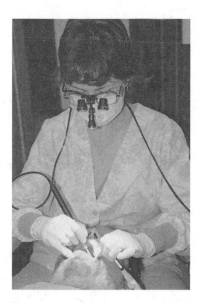

Figure 3–44   Draping cord around the neck.

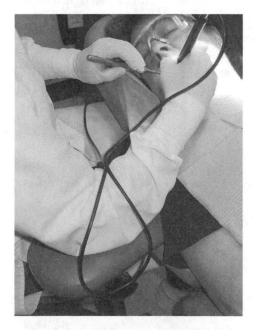

Figure 3–45   Supporting cord with forearm.

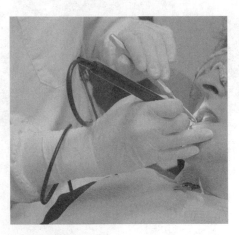

Figure 3–46   Wrapping cord around forearm. *Photo courtesy of R. Moye.*

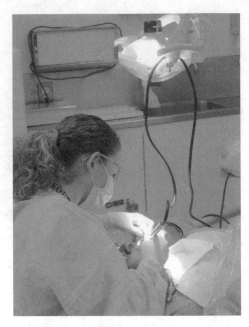

Figure 3–47   Draping cord over overhead light handle.

g. Ask the patient for permission to drape the handpiece cord across his or her chest only if the length of the cord or the room design impedes good operator ergonomics.

C. Patient positioning.
 1. Recline patient chair with back raised slightly.
 2. Practice slight modifications in the patient's head position during the procedure, such as:
   a. Turning head toward the suction.
   b. Tilting chin slightly downward.[4]

D. Applying ergonomic principles to ultrasonic scaling techniques.
 1. Handpiece.
   a. Hold the handpiece using a pen or modified pen grasp (Figure 3–49).
   b. Use a light touch similar to using an explorer or periodontal probe (Figure 3–50).
   c. Lightly rotate the barrel of the handpiece to reposition the ultrasonic tip on the tooth surface during scaling. If limited handpiece rotation

Figure 3–48   Draping cord through metal support cord holder.

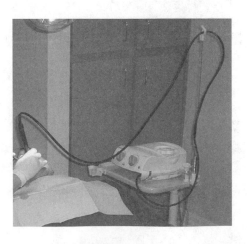

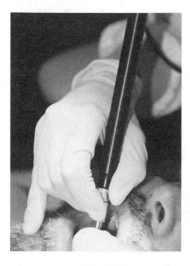

Figure 3–49   Holding the handpiece with a pen grasp.

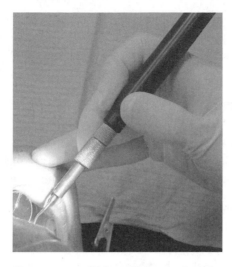

Figure 3–50   Using a light touch with handpiece.

does not provide adequate access to the tooth surface, manually reposition the insert.

2. Instrumentation.
   a. Select an insert that is designed to accommodate the tooth anatomy.
   b. Establish an extra-/intraoral fulcrum or soft tissue rest (Figures 3–51 and 3–52).
   c. Use a light, erasure-type motion.
   d. Limit lateral pressure on tooth surface.
   e. Work with the lowest power levels possible to limit tip vibration.
   f. Defog mouth mirrors by applying commercially prepared solutions or mouth rinses.
   g. Use padded saliva ejectors as cheek retraction devices.
   h. Attach an aerosol suction device when using a magnetostrictive ultrasonic scaler handpiece; however, this device adds weight and reduces maneuverability.

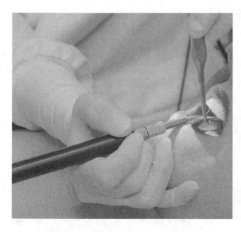

Figure 3–51   Using a multifinger extraoral fulcrum.

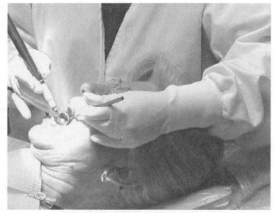

Figure 3–52   Using a cheek fulcrum.

E. Supplemental ergonomic equipment. Many operators find ultrasonic scaling procedures are enhanced by the use of magnification loupes, supplemental illumination, and effective handpiece cord management.
   1. Magnification loupes enhance the operator's visual acuity.[20]
   2. Supplemental illumination enhances the operator's vision, especially when accessing difficult areas such as the distal aspect of maxillary molars.[20]

VIII. Maintenance

A. Care of the ultrasonic scaling unit.
   1. Disinfecting the ultrasonic water lines. Biofilm deposits can form in the small lumen of the ultrasonic unit water lines; disinfection should be completed on a regular basis.
      a. Run a commercially available water line disinfectant through the water lines; follow the manufacturer's directions for correct application.
      b. Use a diluted solution of sodium hypochlorite. Caution should be used because eventually corrosion can develop on any metal fittings in the unit.
      c. Monitor effectiveness of the disinfection procedures by using commercial bacterial testing kits.
   2. In-line water filters. Used to decrease the amount of bacteria running through the lines. They are connected through the water lines and must be changed frequently following the manufacturer's directions.

B. Ultrasonic scaling tips and inserts.
   1. Insert care.
      a. Carefully wash tips with mild soap and warm water.
      b. Place dry tips in autoclave bags or cassettes.
      c. Avoid loading heavy instruments on top of the inserts during sterilization because tips and their components can be damaged.
      d. Use steam autoclaves to sterilize all ultrasonic inserts. Sterilization of inserts in a chemical vapor sterilizer can result in premature o-ring failure. Dry heat, which damages insert o-rings, is contraindicated for sterilizing magnetostrictive ultrasonic scaler inserts.
   2. Tip wear. As with hand instruments, ultrasonic tips have a finite life; replace or retip inserts as needed.
      a. Worn tips lose their efficiency and effectiveness.
         (1) Evaluate tip wear by using manufacturer's guides; these indicate if the ultrasonic insert or tip is still functional in an automatically-tuned unit.
         (2) In contrast, tips that might be considered non-functional in an automatically-tuned ultrasonic unit may still be effective when used in a manually-tuned ultrasonic unit because of the ability to specifically tune the frequency of each tip.
      b. Evaluate damaged, worn, or bent stacks of magnetostrictive ultrasonic scaler inserts for efficiency; replace as needed (Figures 3–53 and 3–54).
   3. External o-ring replacement. The external o-rings on magnetostrictive ultrasonic scaler inserts will deteriorate over time because of the repetitive process of sterilization.
      a. Failed external o-rings cause water to leak from the interface where the insert meets the handpiece and can therefore saturate the patient.
      b. Inadequate water flow causes the handpiece to overheat.
      c. Follow the manufacturer's directions for replacing the external o-ring.

CLINICAL TIP:

Tuning Your Knowledge: It is important to read the manufacturer's instructions for cleaning, sterilizing, and maintaining ultrasonic inserts or tips.

CLINICAL TIP:

Tuning Your Knowledge: Avoid using glutaraldehyde disinfectants. They can damage the nickel alloy strips in magnetostrictive ultrasonic scaler inserts. Resin-hubbed inserts exposed to phenolic disinfectants can cause the resin housing to crack.

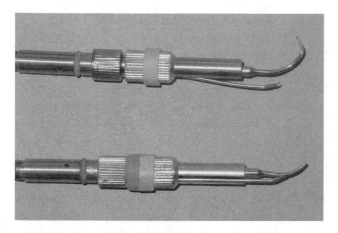

Figure 3–53   Bent tip with poorly positioned water conduit; broken tip.

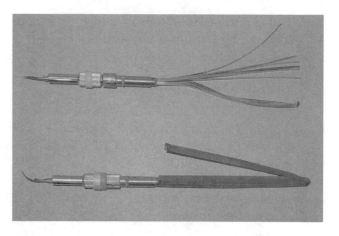

Figure 3–54   Broken and damaged stacks.

Technology impacts our lives in profound ways every day. It is available to assist us, not limit us. It is critical to keep an open mind when considering how to practice dental hygiene. While initially it may be more comfortable for the operator to perform clinical treatment using techniques and procedures that have been used by dental hygienists for years, it is important to evaluate new ways of practicing that will improve the health of our patients and help extend our careers.

Ultrasonic scalers were once considered an adjunct to hand instrumentation. However, with emerging research substantiating the benefits of ultrasonic scaling, changes are becoming evident in this standard of care. Therefore, it is essential operators become well versed and proficient in their clinical skills with the various types of ultrasonic devices available today.

Ultrasonic scaling techniques are dramatically different from hand instrumentation skills; therefore, it is important to take time to learn how to use this technology appropriately. It takes persistence, patience, and practice to become a skilled operator who is capable of utilizing ultrasonic scalers to their fullest extent.

QUESTIONS

1. Which of the following terms describes the action of liquid when it comes in contact with the intensely vibrating tip?
   a. Amplitude
   b. Frequency
   c. Acoustics
   d. Cavitation

2. Ultrasonic scaling devices were primarily used in the 1950s to
   a. deplaque.
   b. cut tooth structure.
   c. remove stain.
   d. debride pockets.

3. Which type of ultrasonic scaling unit allows the operator to control both frequency and amplitude?
   a. Automatically-tuned magnetostrictive
   b. Manually-tuned magnetostrictive
   c. Sonic
   d. Piezoelectric

4. Slim precision tips should be used on all the following settings EXCEPT one. Which one is the EXCEPTION?
   a. High
   b. Medium
   c. Low

5. When inserting an ultrasonic scaling tip into the sulcus, the tip should be activated
   a. prior to sulcus insertion.
   b. within the sulcus.
   c. outside of the patient's mouth.
   d. at a 90 degree angle to the tooth.

6. All of the following are patient considerations for using an ultrasonic scaler EXCEPT one. Which one is the EXCEPTION?
   a. Premedication
   b. Ocular or retinal implants
   c. Cardiac pacemakers
   d. Alopecia
   e. Communicable or respiratory diseases

7. All of the following are general ultrasonic scaler instrumentation principles EXCEPT one. Which one is the EXCEPTION?
   a. Keeping the insert parallel to the tooth.
   b. Using heavy lateral pressure.
   c. Using overlapping strokes.
   d. Keeping the tip moving.

8. On rare occasions, tenacious deposit removal may not be possible with even the finest ultrasonic scaler or hand scaling in the hands of a highly skilled operator. Under these circumstances, patients should be referred to a periodontist for further treatment.
   a. Both statement and reason are correct and related.
   b. Both statements are correct, but *NOT* related.
   c. The statement is correct, but the reason is *NOT*.
   d. The statement is *NOT* correct, but the reason is accurate.
   e. *NEITHER* the statement *NOR* the reason is correct.

9. Glutaraldehyde disinfectants can damage the nickel alloy strips in magnetostrictive ultrasonic scaler inserts. Exposure to phenolic disinfecting compounds affects the integrity of the resin in plastic-hubbed inserts, resulting in cracks and subsequent water leakage.
   a. Both statements are TRUE.
   b. Both statements are FALSE.
   c. The first statement is TRUE and the second statement is FALSE.
   d. The first statement is FALSE and the second statement is TRUE.

10. Supragingival straight debridement inserts have larger diameter tips that are specifically designed to remove gross tenacious deposits and heavy stain. These inserts are generally more effective in medium-to-high power ranges.
    a. Both statement and reason are correct and related.
    b. Both statements are correct, but *NOT* related.
    c. The statement is correct, but the reason is *NOT*.
    d. The statement is *NOT* correct, but the reason is accurate.
    e. *NEITHER* the statement *NOR* the reason is correct.

11. Since ultrasonic scaling may be a new procedure for some patients, it is advisable to spend a few minutes prior to instrumentation to provide information about the procedure. Patients may need reassurance that recent advancements in ultrasonic scaling techniques and equipment can result in a more comfortable clinical appointment.
    a. Both statement and reason are correct and related.
    b. Both statements are correct, but *NOT* related.
    c. The statement is correct, but the reason is *NOT*.
    d. The statement is *NOT* correct, but the reason is accurate.
    e. *NEITHER* the statement *NOR* the reason is correct.

12. Instrumentation with an ultrasonic scaling device is dramatically different than scaling with a hand instrument. When using an ultrasonic scaler, the operator must use a light grasp and keep the tip stationary.
    a. Both statement and reason are correct and related.
    b. Both statements are correct, but *NOT* related.
    c. The statement is correct, but the reason is *NOT*.
    d. The statement is *NOT* correct, but the reason is accurate.
    e. *NEITHER* the statement *NOR* the reason is correct.

13. Recent research indicates that plaque biofilm plays a significant role in the disease process. Debridement with an ultrasonic scaler may be the most efficient way to disrupt this complex community of bacterial pathogens.
    a. Both statement and reason are correct and related.
    b. Both statements are correct, but *NOT* related.
    c. The statement is correct, but the reason is *NOT*.
    d. The statement is *NOT* correct, but the reason is accurate.
    e. *NEITHER* the statement *NOR* the reason is correct.

14. Which of the following terms describes the removal of bacterial plaque and its toxins following the completion of supragingival and subgingival debridement?
   a. Deplaquing
   b. Biofilm
   c. Acoustic turbulence
   d. Acoustic streaming

REFERENCES

1. Zinner, DD. Recent ultrasonic dental studies, including periodontia, without the use of an abrasive. *Journal of Dental Research,* Vol. 34, 1955, 748–749.

2. American Academy of Periodontology. Position Paper: Sonic and Ultrasonic Scalers in Periodontics. *Journal of Periodontology,* Vol. 71, Number 11, 2000, 1792–1801.

3. Checci L, Pelliccioni GA. Hand vs. ultrasonic instrumentation in the removal of endotoxin from root surfaces. *Journal of Periodontology,* Vol. 59, 1998, 398–402.

4. Herremans K. Ultrasonic periodontal debridement. In *Concepts in Nonsurgical Periodontal Therapy.* New York: Delmar Publishers, 1998, pp. 320–343.

5. Scientific American. *Emerging trends in oral care.* New York: Scientific American, 2002, pp. 1–30.

6. Hodges KO. Nonsurgical, supportive, and mechanized periodontal therapies. In *Dental Hygiene Theory and Practice.* St. Louis, MO: Saunders, 2003, pp. 457–492.

7. Trenter SC, Landini G, Walmsley AD. Effect of loading on the vibration characteristics of thin magnetostrictive ultrasonic inserts. *Journal of Periodontology,* Vol. 74, 2003, 1308–1315.

8. Dragoo M. A clinical evaluation of hand and ultrasonic instruments on subgingival debridement. Part I with unmodified and modified ultrasonic inserts. *The International Journal of Periodontics and Restorative Dentistry,* Vol. 12, Number 4, 1992, 311–323.

9. Wylam JM, Mealey BL, Mills MP, et al. The clinical effectiveness of open versus closed scaling and root planing on multi-rooted teeth. *Journal of Periodontology,* Vol. 64, 1993, 1023–1028.

10. Croft LK, Nunn ME, Crawford L, et al. Patient preference for ultrasonic or hand instruments in periodontal maintenance. *The International Journal of Periodontics and Restorative Dentistry,* Vol. 23, Number 6, 2003, 567–573.

11. Walmsley AD, Walsh TF, Laird WRE, Williams AR. The effects of cavitation activity on the root surfaces of teeth during ultrasonic scaling. *Journal of Clinical Periodontology,* Vol. 17, 1990, 306–312.

12. Moore J, Wilson M, Kieser JB. The distribution of bacterial lipopolysaccharide (endotoxin) in relation to periodontally involved root surfaces. *Journal of Clinical Periodontology,* Vol. 13, 1986, 748–751.

13. American Dental Association, Council on Scientific Affairs and the Council on Dental Practice. *Infection Control Recommendations for the Dental Office and the Dental Laboratory,* 1996, pp. 127, 672.

14. Adams D, Fulford N, Beechy J, MacCarthy J, Stephens, M. The cardiac pacemaker and ultrasonics scalers. *Dental Health London,* Vol. 22, 1983, 6–8.

15. Bohay RN, Bencak J, Kavaliers M, Maclean D. A survey of magnetic fields in the dental operatory. *Journal of Canadian Dental Association,* Vol. 60, 1994, 835–840.

16. Harrel S, Barnes J, Rivera-Hildago F. Reduction of aerosols produced by ultrasonics scalers. *Journal of Periodontology,* Vol. 67, 1996, 28–32.

17. Fine D, Yip J, Furgang D, Barnett M, Olshan A, Vincent J. Reducing bacteria in dental aerosols: Pre-procedural use of an antiseptic mouthrinse. *Journal of the American Dental Association,* Vol. 124, 1993, 56–58.

18. Arcoria CJ, Gonzalez JP, Vitasek BA, Wagner MJ. Effects of ultrasonic instrumentation on microleakage in composite restorations with glass ionomer liners. *Journal of Oral Rehabilitation,* Vol. 19, 1992, 21–29.

19. Lee SY, Lai YL, Morgano SM. Effects of ultrasonic scaling and periodontal curettage on surface roughness of porcelain. *Journal of Prosthetic Dentistry,* Vol. 73, 1995, 227–232.

20. Guignon A. Ergonomics. In *Essentials of Dental Hygiene: Preclinical Skills.* New Jersey: Prentice Hall, 2004, pp. 173–197.

21. Morris GA, Kokott MI. A clear view no longer means a stiff neck. *Dental Economics,* Vol. 89, Number 7, 1999, 82–84, 86.

MAGNETOSTRICTIVE ULTRASONIC SCALING PERFORMANCE EVALUATION

Student _____ Date _____

Patient _____ Instructor _____

Re-evaluation
Instr: _____
Date _____

Do not use for patient with unshielded cardiac pacemakers, respiratory problems, communicable diseases, porcelain crowns, titanium implants, decalcification, or dentinal sensitivity.

	S	U	Comments	S	U	Comments
1. Patient approved by dental hygiene clinical instructor.						
2. Provides one preprocedural rinse for 30 seconds.						
3. Positions back of chair slightly more upright.						
4. Drapes ultrasonic unit keeping the back of the unit open.						
5. Attaches handpiece and holds it vertically to bleed for 3 minutes.						
6. Sets power dial according to the insert.						
7. Correctly sets water volume.						
8. Prepares patient by using drape with extra napkins around the neck.						
9. Requires patient to wear protective eyewear.						
10. Operates foot pedal.						
11. Uses correct inserts according to the area of the mouth and deposit.						
12. Uses inserts with a light, continuous erasure motion using fingers.						
13. Demonstrates horizontal, oblique, and vertical strokes using 2–3 mm of tip insert.						
14. Fulcrums at least 1 to 2 teeth away from tooth being scaled.						
15. Pivots to follow contour of tooth.						
16. Re-explores with insert and explorer.						
17. Uses saliva ejector or high volume evacuation throughout entire procedure.						
18. Retracts patient's lips to prevent contact with insert tip.						
19. Moves patient's head from right to left, as needed.						
20. Accomplishes gross removal/pocket debridement/deplaque without trauma.						
21. Correctly disassembles the unit. Disinfects tubing. Places inserts and handpieces in separate paper/plastic bags in autoclave only. Does <u>not</u> place inserts in ultrasonic cleaner.						

Courtesy of Indiana University Purdue University Fort Wayne Dental Hygiene Program.

PIEZOELECTRIC ULTRASONIC SCALING PERFORMANCE EVALUATION

Student _____ Date _____

Patient _____ Instructor _____

Re-evaluation
Instr. _____
Date _____

Do not use for patient with respiratory problems, communicable diseases, porcelain crowns, titanium implants, decalcification, or dentinal sensitivity.

	S	U	Comments	S	U	Comments
1. Patient approved by dental hygiene clinical instructor.						
2. Positions back of chair slightly more upright.						
3. Prepares patient by using drape with extra napkins around the neck.						
4. Requires patient to wear protective eyewear.						
5. Provides one pre-procedural rinse for 30 seconds.						
6. Drapes ultrasonic unit keeping the back of the unit open.						
7. Attaches handpiece to hose (pushing straight in-NOT TWISTING)						
8. Adjusts the power setting: Standard calculus removal = medium setting (10 o'clock on dial)						
9. Selects the correct tip according for the deposit.						
TIP A-supra-and subgingival calculus.						
TIP B-thin deposits on lingual surfaces.						
TIP P-subgingival calculus.						
TIP PS-debridement of root surfaces (pockets up to 10 mm).						
Tightens the tip with the torque, in a clockwise direction.						
10. Positions the length of the tip parallel to the long axis of the tooth at slightly lower setting.						
11. Uses tip with a light stroke and pressure.						
12. Demonstrates overlapping, multidirectional strokes.						
13. Pivots to follow contour of tooth.						
14. Uses only 2 to 3 mm on the sides of the tip.						
15. Uses saliva ejector or HVE throughout entire procedure.						
16. Retracts patient's lips to prevent contact with insert tip.						
17. Moves patient's head from right to left, as needed.						
18. Accomplishes gross removal and/or pocket debridement/plaque without trauma.						
19. Correctly disassembles the unit. Disinfects tubing. Places tips and handpieces in metal container to autoclave (can use nyclave tubing to autoclave container). <u>Does not place tips</u> in ultrasonic cleaner.						

Courtesy of Indiana University Purdue University Fort Wayne Dental Hygiene Program.

Chapter 4

Air Polishing

Mary D. Cooper, RDH, MSEd

MediaLink

A companion CD-ROM, included free with each new copy of this book, supplements the procedures presented in each chapter. Insert the CD-ROM to watch video clips and view a large collection of color images that is also included. This multimedia library is designed to help you add a new dimension to your learning.

KEY TERMS

air embolism
air polisher
Jct Shield™
root detoxification
tag

LEARNING OBJECTIVES

After reading this chapter, the student will be able to:

- discuss the armamentarium for air polishing;
- list medical and clinical indications and contraindications for air polishing;
- list the steps in preparing the patient and operator for air polishing;
- demonstrate how to assemble an air-polishing device;
- demonstrate how to disinfect an air-polishing device;
- list and discuss each procedural step for air polishing.

I. Introduction

The **air polisher,** a powder abrasive device, was first introduced in the late 1970s.[1] Its purpose is to remove extrinsic stain, plaque, and soft deposits with greater ease.[1-3] Literature has supported its efficient and effective means, as well as its safety.[1-6] It requires less time than traditional rubber cup polishing and removes stain three times faster than scaling with curettes with less fatigue to the operator.[1] Air polishers are available as handpiece units that attach directly to the air/water connector on the dental unit, in combination with an ultrasonic, or as separate units.

II. Mechanism of Action

A. Uses fine particles of specially treated powder (sodium bicarbonate or sodium-free [aluminum trihydroxide] formulation), pressurized air, and water, creating a fine slurry as its polishing agent.

   1. Air pressure varies from 65 to 100 lbs/sq inch (psi);[4] controlled by the operator.

CLINICAL TIP:

Polishing Your Knowledge: The amount of tooth structure removed using an air polisher is less than 10.68 microns—a hand curette removes 27.09 microns.[6]

115

Figure 4–1   Cavijet unit.

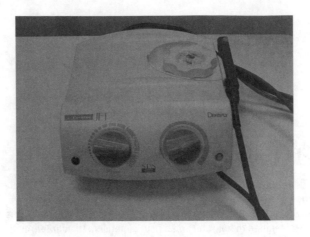

2. Water pressure is 25 to 60 psi;[4] controlled by operator.

B. Slurry removes surface deposits by continuous mechanical abrasion.

III. Unit

The air polishing unit houses the controls for turning the machine on and off and adjusting the water control, as well as the reservoir for the air powder abrasive. Follow manufacturer's directions for proper assembly (Figure 4–1).

A. Parts.

    1. Handpiece—lightweight; includes air hose, water hose, and nozzles (tips) (Figure 4–2).

        a. Nozzles. Connect to air hose and water hose where air, water, and powder mix are released. Types include:

           (1) Straight rod nozzle (i.e., Cavijet). Eliminates the need for connecting tubes; has male/female attachment (Figure 4–3).

           (2) Air/water nozzle (i.e., Prophy-jet). Connects to matching color air/water hoses.

        b. Hoses. Connect to main unit.

           (1) Air. Forces compressed air through air polishing unit.

           (2) Water. Forces water through air polishing unit.

    2. Reservoir (chamber). Holds air abrasive powder.

        a. Reservoir cap. Maintains powder in reservoir.

           (1) Control valve. Situated on top center of the reservoir cap; allows for adjustments of powder flow, depending on patient's needs (Figure 4–4).

               (a) Turn control knob to H ([heavy powder flow or high stream], 12:00 o'clock position) for heavy stain removal.

               (b) Turn control knob to L ([light powder flow or low stream], 6:00 o'clock position) for light stain removal.

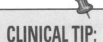

CLINICAL TIP:

Polishing Your Knowledge: Store the powder in a dry, cool location to prevent moisture contamination.

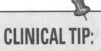

CLINICAL TIP:

Polishing Your Knowledge: The sodium bicarbonate formulation is water-soluble.

Figure 4–2   Lightweight handpiece.

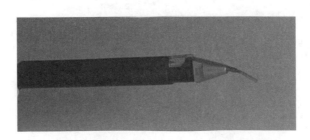

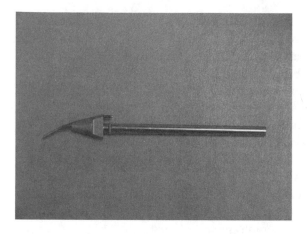

Figure 4–3   Straight rod nozzle (tip).

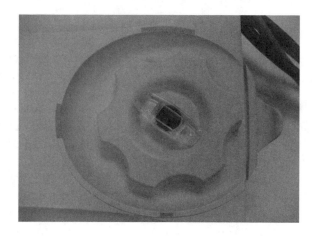

Figure 4–4   Reservoir cap with control valve.

3. Foot pedal. Depress into compression levels:
   a. As soon as unit is turned on, there is a steady stream of air; can be used to dry the tooth.
   b. Halfway compression produces a stream of water and air; useful for rinsing.
   c. Full compression releases aerosolized powder, water, and air.
B. Assembling unit. Follow manufacturer's directions (Figure 4–5).

CLINICAL TIP:

Polishing Your Knowledge: When using a handpiece with tubing, make sure to match tubing lines. Mixing water and air lines can cause serious damage to the unit.

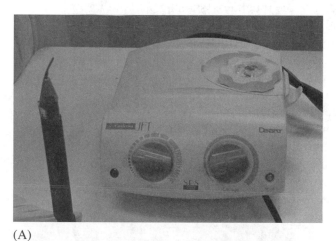

(A)

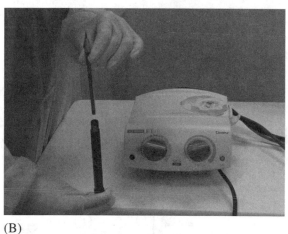

(B)

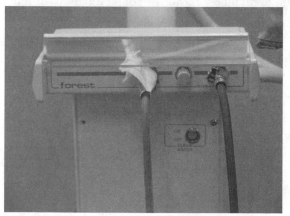

(C)

Figure 4–5   (A) Assembled unit. (B) Insert nozzle into handpiece. (C) Attach hoses to unit.

IV. Contraindications/Indications for Use

Contraindications and indications for use are concerned with patient selection and preparation, operator preparation, and clinical technique.

A. Patient selection. Since there are several contraindications and indications for use, proper patient selection is critical.

1. Review patient's medical history to determine any conditions, diseases, or illnesses that may contraindicate the use of air polishing, as well as any other medical considerations. Avoid use for patients with:

   a. Known infectious diseases. Danger of airborne contaminants, such as HIV and Hepatitis B.

   b. Respiratory complications. Microorganisms may be aspirated into the lungs and, therefore, can complicate breathing for persons with asthma, tuberculosis, or emphysema.

   c. Renal disease or metabolic disorders, such as Cushing's disease or Addison's disease. Air polishing can disrupt acid/base balance.

   d. Use of diuretics or long-term steroid therapy. Air polishing can disrupt acid/base balance.

   e. Hypertension (sodium-restricted diets). Operator can use a sodium-free (aluminum trihydroxide) formulation for patients with hypertension.

2. Examine hard and soft tissues and dental history to determine possible dental contraindications. Avoid use on:

   a. Composite resins. Susceptible to surface roughness or pitting.[1]

   b. Porcelain restorations. Margins may be altered by extensive exposure, along with surface roughness, staining, and pitting.[1]

   c. Cementum and dentin. Structures are not as mineralized as enamel and therefore more susceptible to abrasion. Use caution when polishing root surfaces.

   d. Margins of all restorations. May result in loss of marginal integrity; margins should be hand instrumented.[1]

   e. Sealants. Susceptible to abrasion.

   f. Active periodontal conditions where soft, spongy tissue is present. Can cause **air embolism,** or small blood clots.

   g. Deciduous teeth or newly erupted permanent teeth. Due to the immature enamel, spray could erode teeth.

3. Indications for use.

   a. Removes extrinsic stain (i.e., smoking, coffee/tea, and chlorhexidine) and plaque.

   b. Maintains orthodontic appliances. Easier to adapt versus traditional rubber cup polishing, which requires physical contact with tooth surface being cleaned. Avoid use on gold wires and brackets—can leave material with a dull, matte finish. Application to orthodontic appliances: Direct tip 90 degrees to tooth to avoid disruption of the bond interface.[7]

   c. Assists in **root detoxification** during periodontal surgery by removing endotoxins, plaque, and stain and leaving a uniformly smooth surface, clean and free of diseased tissue.[1,8,9]

   d. Aids with care of dental implants.[10] Removes plaque and stain with minimal alteration of implant.[1] This is still controversial and additional information is indicated.

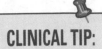

CLINICAL TIP:

Polishing Your Knowledge: A majority of patients, 94%, prefer air polishing to traditional rubber cup polishing.[6]

CLINICAL TIP:

Polishing Your Knowledge: When polishing restorative dental materials, follow manufacturer's recommendations to avoid prolonged or excessive use.

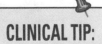

CLINICAL TIP:

Polishing Your Knowledge Aluminum trihydroxide is too new to conclude if it is indicated for use prior to sealant placement.[11]

    e. Aids with sealant placement and acid-etch procedures.
      (1) Increases resin **tag** formation.
      (2) Decreases bond failure between tooth and sealant.
      (3) Cleanses enamel more evenly and completely than traditional polishing and scaling.

B. Patient preparation. Use the following steps to prepare the patient for air-powder polishing.
  1. Explain procedure, review medical history, and take blood pressure.
  2. Place disposable/plastic drape over patient's clothing.
  3. Position patient more upright.
  4. Provide safety glasses to the patient and wrap face with a clean towel.
  5. Instruct patient to use an antimicrobial preprocedural rinse, such as 0.12 percent chlorhexidine, which reduces bacterial contamination of aerosols.
  6. Apply a nonpetroleum lubricant to the lips to protect from abrasive spray that can dry the lips.

CLINICAL TIP:

Polishing Your Knowledge: Tags are finger-like depressions created by the etchant. They are essential for the retention of the sealant.

C. Operator preparation. The operator should be properly protected when performing air-powder polishing. Use standard precautions, which include wearing:
  1. Fluid-resistant protective apparel.
  2. Face shield or protective safety glasses with side shields.
  3. Gloves.
  4. Well-fitting mask with high filtration capabilities.

D. Clinical technique.
  1. Preparation.
    a. Connect air/water hoses.
    b. Turn unit on for 15 seconds to eliminate residual powder or moisture in the lines.
    c. Hold handpiece over sink or cup; drain and flush water line as recommended by the Centers for Disease Control and Prevention guidelines by activating foot control.
    d. Turn unit off and remove reservoir cap.
    e. Shake powder in jar to mix and create an even consistency.
    f. Fill chamber with powder to the top of the center tube; place finger over tube in the middle of chamber to prevent powder from blocking air line (manufacturer's flavoring can be added to mask saline taste).
    g. Replace reservoir cap.
    h. Turn unit on.
    i. Depending on type of air polisher:
      (1) Attach nozzle (insert) into handpiece (i.e., Cavijet), or
      (2) Slide a sterilized handpiece sheath onto air/water tubing (i.e., Prophyjet).
        (a) Attach a sterilized nozzle onto tubing matching color coding.
        (b) Thread handpiece sheath on to sterilized nozzle.
    j. Use control on top of reservoir cap to adjust powder flow according to patient's needs. For patients with:
      (1) Heavy stain: Turn control knob to H (heavy powder flow), 12:00 o'clock position.
      (2) Light stain: Turn control knob to L (reduced powder flow), 6:00 o'clock position.

CLINICAL TIP:

Polishing Your Knowledge: Some operators instruct patients to remove contact lenses (if applicable) due to the amount of spray generated, regardless of wearing safety glasses.

2. Technique recommendations without **Jet Shield**™
   a. Position patient slightly upright at 45 degrees with patient's head toward operator to access areas with direct vision; recline patient to treat maxillary lingual surfaces.
   b. Place a moistened 2″ × 2″ gauze square over tongue or on patient's lip near working area. This helps reduce burning and stinging experienced by some patients from the force of the air/water/powder mixture.
   c. Use high-volume evacuation (HVE), with assistant, if possible, or saliva ejector to provide adequate evacuation.
   d. Establish and maintain a systematic pattern.
   e. Adapt appropriate distance of nozzle to tooth—3 millimeters to 4 millimeters—slightly apical to the incisal/occlusal to the middle third of tooth to prevent subcutaneous air emphysema or localized epithelial abrasion. Holding the nozzle further away from the tooth surface minimizes the abrasive action and increases the aerosols. Use the following angulations while polishing (Figure 4–6):
      (1) Posterior teeth. Direct nozzle at 80-degree angle to the tooth.
      (2) Anterior teeth. Direct nozzle at 60-degree angle to tooth.
      (3) Occlusal surfaces. Direct nozzle at 90-degree angle to occlusal surface.
   f. Cup lip with index finger and thumb to pool water in vestibule to minimize aerosol and ease evacuation.
   g. Use intermittent slurry with a rapid, constant sweeping (circular) motion from interproximal to interproximal.
   h. Polish one to two teeth at a time (1 to 2 seconds or less per tooth) at full compression to increase efficiency and patient comfort. Avoid loss of tooth structure by subjecting tooth to no more than 10 seconds of air polish agent slurry. Use less time on root surfaces because they abrade more rapidly than enamel.
   i. Rinse teeth and tongue often by pressing foot pedal halfway after every one to three teeth (increases efficiency and minimizes saline taste).

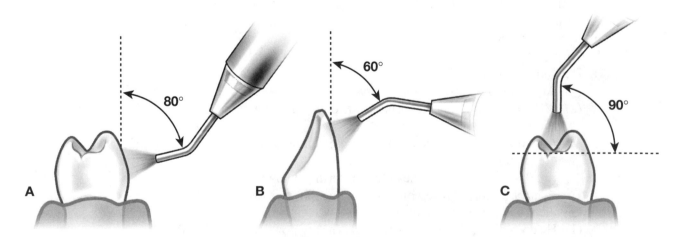

Figure 4–6   Proper placement of nozzle from teeth is 3 mm to 4 mm. (A) Posterior teeth. Direct nozzle at 80-degree angle to tooth. (B) Anterior teeth. Direct nozzle at 60-degree angle to tooth. (C) Occlusal surface. Direct nozzle at 90 degrees.

j. At completion of procedure, rinse thoroughly, floss, and inspect teeth for stain. If stain is present, reinstrumentation and/or use of air polisher may be indicated again.

k. Wipe debris from patient's face with moist towel; offer patient lip balm.

3. Technique recommendation with Jet Shield™. After proper assembly:

a. Follow manufacturer's instructions on assembling and disassembling.

b. Apply cup to the middle third of tooth with light pressure to flare cup.

c. Pivot nozzle inside cup to adapt to all areas—incisal, gingival, mesial, and distal surfaces.

d. Apply 2 seconds of spray for each segment of tooth.

4. Aerosol considerations. Minimize contamination risks by using proper armamentarium and technique, which include:

a. Preprocedural antimicrobial rinse (i.e., 0.12 percent chlorhexidine) helps reduce airborne oral microbes.

b. HVE/saliva ejector helps contain aerosol.

c. Recommended angulations and appropriate distance from nozzle tip to tooth reduce amount of aerosol spray.

d. Safety glasses for patient and operator protect from aerosol spray.

e. Aerosol-reduction device, such as a high bacterial filtration efficiency (BFE) mask, can filter out at least 98 percent of all particles 3μ or larger. Jet Shield™ (Figure 4–7) reduces or eliminates the visible aerosol normally produced during air polishing.

(1) System.

(a) Contains two parts—a disposable cup and clear tube extension (Figure 4–8) that is attached to the air polisher nozzle.

(b) Additional tubing attaches to the saliva ejector or HVE (Figure 4–9).

(2) Advantages.

(a) Eliminates the use of exact angulations with cup/nozzle.

(b) Eliminates use of gauze, hand cupping, and patient positioning.

CLINICAL TIP:

Polishing Your Knowledge: Remember, there is always a steady stream of air from the nozzle when the unit is activated.

CLINICAL TIP:

Polishing You Knowledge: If spray escapes during air polishing with the Jet Shield™, readjust the cup to maintain flat contact with tooth surface.

CLINICAL TIP:

Polishing Your Knowledge: *In vitro,* spatter was reduced by 97% when using a Jet Shield™.[5]

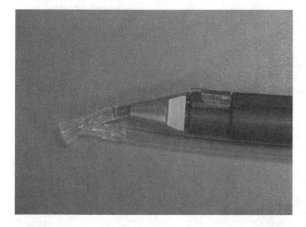

Figure 4–7   Jet Shield™.

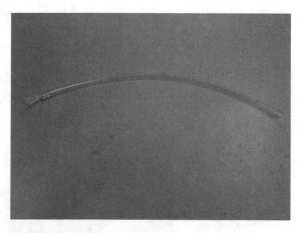

Figure 4–8   Clear tube extension (Jet Shield™).

Figure 4–9   Tubing attached to saliva ejector.

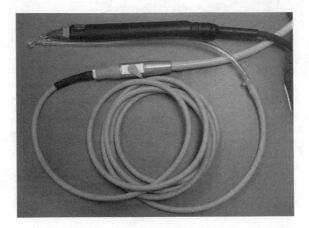

(c) Minimizes the possibility of tooth abrasion since the cup is placed on the tooth as with traditional polishing techniques.
(3) Application.
    (a) Use light pressure to flare cup slightly.
    (b) Pivot nozzle inside of cup to ensure removal of deposits.

V. Suggested Maintenance of Air Polishing Unit

A. Follow manufacturer's instructions.
B. Perform on a daily basis.
  1. Beginning of day.
    a. Unscrew powder reservoir (chamber should be empty).
    b. Turn unit on for 15 seconds to remove any residual powder or moisture in lines.
  2. Completion of procedure.
    a. Clean nozzle after each use with a wire-cleaning tool to prevent clogging (Figure 4–10). Place nozzle (tip) in ultrasonic cleaner, then:
      (1) Replace cleaning tool in nozzle (Figure 4–11).
      (2) Package and autoclave.
      (3) Package and autoclave handpiece, i.e., Prophyjet.
    b. Disinfect unit with an Environmental Protection Agency (EPA)–approved disinfectant. Using a disposable barrier will help minimize disinfecting time; e.g., wiping cords and unit.
    c. Disinfect foot pedal and air/water hoses.
  3. End of day.
    a. Turn unit off.
    b. Follow procedures listed previously under 2.
    c. Remove reservoir cap.
    d. Remove powder from chamber and pour into powder storage jar to prevent clogging of lines. Keep powder chamber and air line free of moisture, which can cause system to fail.

Figure 4–10   Wire cleaning tool.

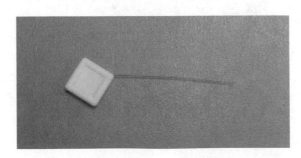

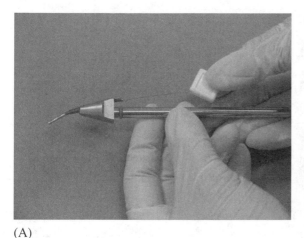
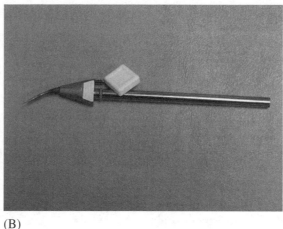

(A)   (B)

Figure 4–11   (A) Inserting cleaning tool into nozzle. (B) Wire tool fully inserted prior to packaging and sterilizing.

    e. Remove any residual powder with HVE.
    f. Activate the system for 15 seconds to clear powder chamber.
    g. Replace and secure lid.
    h. Disinfect and clean unit and sterilize air-polishing nozzle and cleaning wire according to manufacturer's instructions.

Before polishing, thorough instrumentation should be performed to remove calculus and as much extrinsic stain as possible. Polishing tooth surfaces, whether with traditional rubber cup or air polishing to remove stain, is a cosmetic (selective) procedure. Air polishing does efficiently and effectively remove extrinsic stain and plaque. However, before polishing, every patient should be evaluated and assessed to determine the need before performing the procedure.

QUESTIONS

1. All of the following methods minimize aerosol during air polishing EXCEPT one. Which one is the EXCEPTION?
   a. Rinse with a preprocedural antimicrobial rinse prior to air polishing.
   b. Use HVE during air polishing.
   c. Hold the nozzle tip 4 mm to 5 mm from the tooth surface.
   d. Use an aerosol-reduction device.

2. Which of the following is the proper angulation, in degrees, to place the nozzle (tip) when air polishing the anterior teeth?
   a. 90
   b. 80
   c. 60
   d. 45

3. All of the following are dental contraindications for using the air polisher EXCEPT one. Which one is the EXCEPTION?
   a. Composite restorations
   b. Cementum
   c. Porcelain restorations
   d. Orthodontics

4. The nozzle tip should be placed 3 mm to 4 mm from the tooth surface during air polishing. The tip should also be angled slightly toward the cervical third of the tooth.
   a. Both statements are TRUE.
   b. Both statements are FALSE.
   c. The first statement is TRUE. The second statement is FALSE.
   d. The first statement is FALSE. The second statement is TRUE.

5. All of the following are medical contraindications for using an air polisher EXCEPT one. Which one is the EXCEPTION?
   a. Addison's disease
   b. HIV
   c. Cushing's disease
   d. Arthritis

6. Which of the following patients would be a good candidate for air polishing?
   a. Asthmatic
   b. Emphysemic
   c. 5-year-old with brown stain
   d. 13-year-old in full orthodontics

7. All of the following are advantages of using a Jet Shield™ EXCEPT one. Which one is the EXCEPTION?
   a. Minimizes tooth abrasion.
   b. Eliminates use of exact angulations of cup.
   c. Eliminates use of hand cupping.
   d. Decreases use of powder mixture.

8. Proper maintenance of an air polisher is important. It is essential to clean the nozzle after each use to prevent clogging.
   a. Both statements are TRUE.
   b. Both statements are FALSE.
   c. The first statement is TRUE. The second statement is FALSE.
   d. The first statement is FALSE. The second statement is TRUE.

9. All of the following are steps in preparing the patient for air polishing EXCEPT one. Which one is the EXCEPTION?
   a. Place a nonpetroleum lubricant on the lips.
   b. Place protective eyewear on operator.
   c. Instruct patient to use a preprocedural rinse.
   d. Review patient's medical and dental histories.

10. All of the following are part of the techniques used in air polishing EXCEPT one. Which one is the EXCEPTION?
    a. Position patient slightly upright to polish mandibular arch.
    b. Direct the nozzle at 60 degrees for the posterior teeth.
    c. Polish one to two teeth at a time.
    d. Establish a systemic pattern.

REFERENCES

1. Gutmann ME. Air polishing: A comprehensive review of the literature. *Journal of Dental Hygiene,* Vol. 72, Number 3, 1998, 47–56.
2. Gerbo LR, Lacefield WR, Barnes CM, Russell CM. Enamel roughness after air-powder polishing. *American Journal of Dentistry,* Vol. 6, Number 2, 1993, 96–98.
3. Brown DM, Barnhart RC. A scientific foundation for clinical use of air polishing systems: Part I. A review of the literature. *Journal of Practical Hygiene,* Vol. 4, Number 3, 1995, 36–40.
4. Toller-Watts SL, Thomson-Lakey EM. Clinical application of the air polisher. *Journal of Practical Hygiene,* Vol. 1, Number 4, 1992, 27–32.
5. Harrel SK. Advances in air polishing techniques. *Dental Connection,* Vol. 1, Number 1, 1998, 1–8.
6. Fong C. Dispelling air polishing myths. *Journal of Practical Hygiene,* Vol. 9, Number 1, 2000, 25–27.
7. Ramaglia L, Sbordone L, Ciaglia RM, Barone A, Martina P. A clinical comparison of the efficacy and efficiency of two professional prophylaxis procedures in orthodontic patients. *European Journal of Orthodontics,* Vol. 21, 1999, 423–428.
8. Satah E, Wu CH, Suzuki T, Hara K, Amizuka N, Ozawa H. The effectiveness of the air-powder abrasive device for root planing during periodontal surgery. *Periodontal Clinical Investigation,* Vol. 14, Number 1, 1992. 7–13.
9. Agger MS, Horsted-Bindslev P, Hovgaard O. Abrasiveness of an air-powder polishing system on root surfaces in vitro. *Quintessence International,* Vol. 32, Number 5, 2001, 407–411.
10. Mongel R, Buns C-E, Mengel C, Flores-de-Jacoby L. An in vitro study of the treatment of implant surfaces with different instruments. *The International Journal of Oral and Maxillofacial Implants,* Vol. 13, Number 1, 1998, 91–96.
11. Clinical Research Associates Dental Hygiene Newsletter, Vol. 3, Number 3, 2003, May-June.

AIR POLISHING PERFORMANCE EVALUATION

Student _____

Date _____

Patient _____

Instructor _____

Do not use for patient with hypertension, chronic respiratory problems, on a sodium-free diet.
Avoid spray on soft tissues, highly polished restorations, dentin or cementum, and sulci.

Re-evaluation

Instr. _____

Date _____

	S	U	Comments	S	U	Comments
1. Patient approved by dental hygiene clinical instructor.						
2. Provides patient with protective eyewear.						
3. Drapes towel around the patient's face and neckline.						
4. Coats patient's lips with nonpetroleum jelly.						
5. Correctly assembles unit.						
6. Adjusts powder flow rate (high-low) to accommodate needs of the patient.						
7. Uses cup or sink to bleed powder through hose.						
8. Contains spray by cupping patient's lip.						
9. Centers spray on the middle third of the tooth.						
10. Places nozzle (tip) 3 to 4 mm from tooth surface.						
11. On buccal/lingual surfaces of posterior teeth—directs spray, 80° angle toward gingiva.						
12. On facial/lingual surfaces of anterior teeth—directs spray 60° angle toward gingiva.						
13. On occlusal surfaces—directs spray at 90°.						
14. Uses constant circular motion.						
15. Cleans two to three teeth at a time, then rinses.						
16. Uses saliva ejector/HVE throughout procedure.						
17. Uses direct vision throughout procedure.						
18. Correctly disassembles unit. Disinfects unit. Properly prepares materials for autoclaving.						

Chapter 5

Tobacco Cessation

Nancy K. Mann, RDH, MSEd

MediaLink

A companion CD-ROM, included free with each new copy of this book, supplements the procedures presented in each chapter. Insert the CD-ROM to watch video clips and view a large collection of color images that is also included. This multimedia library is designed to help you add a new dimension to your learning.

KEY TERMS

abrasion

addiction

bidi

carbon monoxide (CO)

carcinogenic

carcinoma

chewing tobacco

chronic obstructive pulmonary disease (COPD)

craving

dependence (physiological)

dipping

drug

halitosis

hookah

kretek

leukoplakia

nicotine ($C_{10}H_{14}N_2$)

N-nitrosamines

oral cancer

Preterm Low Birth Weight (PLBW)

secondhand smoke

smokeless (spit) tobacco

snuff

surgeon general

tobacco

tolerance

withdrawal syndrome

LEARNING OBJECTIVES

After reading this chapter, the student will be able to:

- identify the role of the dental hygienist in tobacco education and cessation;
- define nicotine and its effect on the body;
- discuss the forms of tobacco and two characteristics of each form:
  a. cigarettes
  b. bidis
  c. kreteks
  d. cigars
  e. pipes
  f. smokeless tobacco
- using statistical information, name two facts about the harmful effects of tobacco that might be motivating in helping a patient quit tobacco use;
- list and recognize the precancerous oral side effects of tobacco;
- name five hazardous chemicals released in tobacco smoke;
- name and discuss the most common oral cancer;
- discuss the side effects of the treatment of oral cancer;

- differentiate between normal and abnormal oral conditions;
- define brush biopsy;
- describe the clinical signs of smoking-related chronic periodontitis;
- state the ingredients of smokeless tobacco products and their effects on the oral cavity;
- list and describe the effects of the major ingredients in secondhand smoke;
- name a possible side effect of smoking during pregnancy;
- explain the five As in tobacco cessation;
- list and describe the first-line pharmacotherapies that can be prescribed for patients who want to quit using tobacco;
- differentiate between the pharmacotherapies that are available over the counter and those requiring a prescription;
- list strategies to help in coping with withdrawal symptoms;
- discuss motivational strategies for helping patients quit tobacco.

I. Introduction

Quote: "**Tobacco** use is an oral health problem and the dental office is a logical place for a tobacco cessation program . . . and the entire office team should be involved."[1] . . . Because dental hygienists treat patients and update medical histories frequently, many health problems can be detected. The dental hygienist is the ideal dental professional to take on the role of tobacco prevention and education in the dental office because he or she teaches disease prevention and promotes health.[2]

Studies have shown that oral healthcare professionals can be effective in helping their patients stop using tobacco and are an untapped resource for providing cessation services.[3] When dental professionals assist their patients with tobacco cessation, they eliminate an important causative/contributing factor for a number of oral conditions, including cancer and periodontal diseases.[1]

When the American Dental Hygienists' Association National Dental Hygiene Research Agenda was revised in October 2001, tobacco prevention and cessation were specifically named as research topics that should be given priority. The third section is entitled "Health Promotion/Disease Prevention," and III.A.1. states that dental hygienists "Assess their effectiveness in counseling patients regarding prevention and cessation of tobacco use."[4]

A. By assisting patients with tobacco use cessation, dental professionals can improve the outcome of dental treatment and, at the same time, add years and quality to their patients' lives.[1]

B. Tobacco dependence is now increasingly recognized as a chronic disease, one that typically requires ongoing assessment and repeated intervention. Dependence can be physiological and/or psychological.

C. Data strongly indicates that effective tobacco interventions require coordinated interventions.[5]

D. The dental team plays an important role in screening, assessing, treating, and referring for tobacco-related conditions. Code 1320 is the CDT-5 code that can be utilized for tobacco counseling in the dental office every six months.[3]

II. Nicotine

Nicotine's chemical symbol is $C_{10}H_{14}N_2$.

A. Definition: "A colorless, oily, water-soluble, highly toxic, liquid alkaloid, found naturally in tobacco and valued as an *insecticide*."[7] (See the photo of the flowering tobacco plant below.)

B. Characteristics of nicotine.
    1. A **drug** that turns brown when burned and acquires the odor of tobacco when exposed to air.

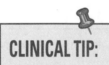

CLINICAL TIP:

Igniting Your Knowledge: Tobacco use is the #1 public health problem in the United States.[6]

Flowering tobacco plant

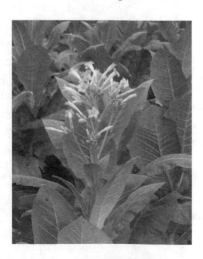

2. Five to ten times more addictive than crack cocaine.[1]
3. Absorbed through the skin and mucosal lining of the mouth and nose or by inhalation in the lungs, reaching the brain in 10 seconds.

C. Effects of nicotine.
1. Pathophysiology of nicotine.
   a. Acts as both a stimulant and a sedative to the central nervous system (CNS).
   b. Ingestion of nicotine results in an almost immediate "kick," because it causes a discharge of epinephrine from the adrenal cortex, stimulating the CNS and other endocrine glands, causing a sudden release of glucose.
   c. Depression and fatigue follow, leading the abuser to seek more nicotine.
   d. Absorbs readily from tobacco chew or smoke in the lungs. The tobacco smoke can be from cigarettes, cigars, or pipes.
   e. With regular use of tobacco, levels of nicotine accumulate in the body during the day and persist overnight. Therefore, daily smokers or chewers are exposed to the effects of nicotine for 24 hours each day.
   f. Takes only seconds for nicotine to reach the brain and has a direct effect on the body for up to 30 minutes.[9]
   g. Stress and anxiety affect nicotine tolerance and dependence.
      (1) The stress hormone corticosterone reduces the effects of nicotine, therefore
      (2) More nicotine must be consumed to achieve the same effect.
      (3) As a result, **tolerance** to nicotine is increased, which leads to increased physiological **dependence.**[9]
2. Immediate effects of nicotine include:
   a. Increase in heart rate, blood pressure, and respiration.
   b. Decrease in skin temperature.
   c. Narrowing of arteries.
   d. Thickening of blood.
   e. Stimulation of the CNS.
3. Long-term effects of nicotine include:
   a. **Addiction.**
   b. Damaged immune system.
   c. Blocked blood vessels.
   d. High blood pressure (HBP).
   e. Bronchitis and/or emphysema.
   f. Stomach ulcers.
   g. Production of abnormal sperm in males.
   h. Dryness and wrinkling of the skin.[6]
   i. Impotence.

III. Types of Tobacco Use
A. Cigarettes.
1. Facts.
   a. Most prevalent form of nicotine addiction in the United States.
   b. Contain 10 milligrams of nicotine per cigarette.
   c. Through inhalation, the average smoker takes in 1 to 2 milligrams of nicotine per cigarette.
   d. Ten puffs per cigarette equals 200 hits of nicotine to the brain per pack.

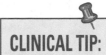

CLINICAL TIP:

Igniting Your Knowledge: "No one has ever become a cigarette smoker by smoking cigarettes without nicotine."[8]

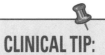

CLINICAL TIP:

Igniting Your Knowledge: Nicotine does not cause cancer. It is the additives in tobacco products that cause cancer.[10]

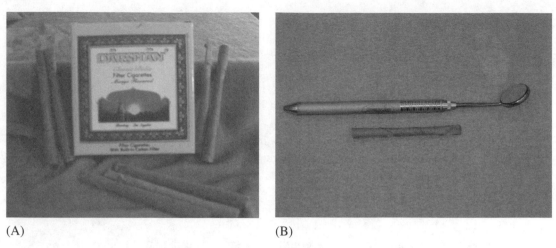

(A)   (B)

Figure 5–1   (A) Bidi (beedies or beadies). (B) Size of a bidi compared to a dental mirror.

e. Results in rapid distribution of nicotine throughout the body, reaching the brain within 8 to 10 seconds of inhalation.[9]

2. Types.

a. **Bidis** (sometimes spelled *beedies* or *beadies*). Hand-rolled, often unfiltered cigarettes filled with finely flaked tobacco bundled in a fuzzy leaf and tightly bound with a colored thread (Figure 5–1).

(1) Imported from India.

(2) Size. About half the diameter of major-brand cigarettes.

(3) Contain up to 8 percent nicotine—three times the nicotine—and five times the tar of name-brand cigarettes; considered more dangerous than regular cigarettes.

(4) Bidi smokers have twice the lung cancer risk of smokers of filtered cigarettes, partly because of the nonporous nature of the tendu, or ebony, leaves that serve as bidi wrappers.

(5) Resemble marijuana joints and come in flavors like mango, wild cherry, chocolate, strawberry, cardamom, cinnamon, clove, grape, lemon lime, mint, regular, vanilla, black licorice, and mandarin orange.[12]

b. **Kretek** (Figure 5–2). Cigarette made of a blend of 60 percent tobacco and 40 percent cloves; may have multiple varieties of tobacco with flavorings. Often, the tip of the rolling paper is dipped in saccharine, which adds to the sweetness of the kretek and increases the subtle blend of flavors.[13]

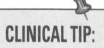

CLINICAL TIP:

Igniting Your Knowledge: To keep the bidi sticks lit, smokers must take deep drags more frequently.[11]

Figure 5–2   Kreteks.

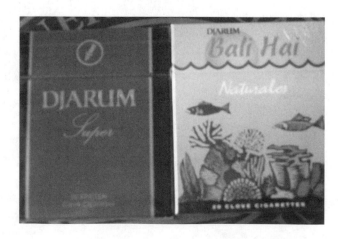

B. Cigars.
  1. Average cigar emits three times as much **carcinogenic** cancer-causing matter and 30 times as much **carbon monoxide** as one cigarette.
  2. **Secondhand smoke** adversely effects the health of nonsmokers including children, adults, and pets.
  3. Cigar smokers have an increased risk of periodontal disease and often suffer from badly stained teeth, dental restorations, chronic bad breath, and impaired wound healing.

C. Pipes.
  1. Pipe tobacco is shredded tobacco leaf in loose form that has been aged and possibly sprayed with chemical flavorings.
  2. The largest risk for pipe smokers may be in developing lip cancer.
  3. Since pipe tobacco burns at a lower temperature than that contained in cigarettes, pipe smoke may have higher concentrations of carbon monoxide and cancer-causing substances.
  4. **Hookah.**
      a. Flavored tobacco placed in the ceramic top of the pipe. As many as three people can smoke from one pipe, and the tobacco lasts about two hours. The tobacco is put in a bowl on top of fruit so the smoke goes from the bowl through the fruit and picks up the fruit's flavor.
      b. A charcoal disk heats the imported tobacco, which has been soaked in molasses or honey and mixed with fruit pulp. Each smoker gets a disposable plastic mouthpiece, and inhales through a long hose that is passed around. The smoke is chilled and filtered as it bubbles through the glass water chamber.
      c. First introduced as a popular social practice in India nearly 400 years ago, and quickly spread to Iran and the rest of the Middle East. Later, hookahs became part of the Turkish coffee shop culture.
      d. An estimated 200 to 300 hookah houses have opened nationwide in the past three to five years, and are usually popular around college campuses.

D. Smokeless or spit tobacco (ST) products. Types include:
  1. **Snuff** (moist **dipping**) (Figure 5–3)
      a. Finely ground or shredded form of tobacco.
      b. Sold in a small, round tin can; also available in sachets.
      c. Placed between lower lip or cheek and gingiva as a "dip" (pinch).

CLINICAL TIP:

Igniting Your Knowledge: One lighted cigar smoked in an unventilated room produces air pollution smoke equivalent to 43 cigarettes.[14]

CLINICAL TIP:

Igniting Your Knowledge: Pipe smokers have increased rates of chronic cough and phlegm.[15]

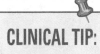

CLINICAL TIP:

Igniting Your Knowledge: There is no safe form of tobacco.

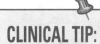

CLINICAL TIP:

Igniting Your Knowledge: Nicotine is NOT filtered out in the water.

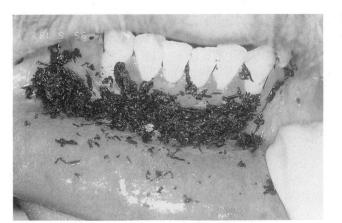

Figure 5–3   Snuff.

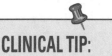

CLINICAL TIP:

Igniting Your Knowledge: The nicotine in **smokeless tobacco** is absorbed directly into the bloodstream and is addicting.

CLINICAL TIP:

Igniting Your Knowledge: Risk of death comparisons include:

1. From terrorism: 1 in a million.
2. As a pedestrian: 1 in 40,000.
3. From auto accident: 1 in 5,000.
4. From tobacco use: 1 in 3.[1]

2. Chew (wad).
   a. Coarsely cut or shredded leaves.
   b. Packaged in loose or plug form.
   c. Contains at least 28 known cancer-causing chemicals and nicotine.
   d. Can cause cancers of the lip, tongue, cheek, throat, gingiva, palate, floor of mouth, or larynx.
      (1) Surgery to treat **oral cancer** is often extensive and disfiguring and may involve removing parts of the face, tongue, cheek, or lip. Oral cancer can spread quickly to other parts of the body.
      (2) On average, half of oral cancer victims are dead within five years of diagnosis.[16]
3. Plug. Shredded tobacco leaves, which are pressed into a hard block and placed between the cheek and gingiva.
   a. An average size dip in the mouth for 30 minutes contains as much nicotine as two to three cigarettes.
   b. Can cause gingival recession, verrucous, and **leukoplakia.**
   c. Increases loss of taste and smell, which causes loss of appetite and, in turn, results in poor nutrition and health.

IV. Epidemiology

A. Statistics.
   1. Tobacco kills more than 440,000 Americans every year.[17]
   2. Tobacco use causes more premature deaths than the combined total resulting from cocaine, heroin, alcohol use, fires, auto accidents, homicides, suicides, and AIDS.
   3. Smoking costs the United States approximately $157.7 billion each year in healthcare costs and lost productivity.[17]
   4. Directly responsible for:
      a. Eighty-seven percent of lung cancer cases.
      b. Thirty-eight percent of all United States cancer deaths.
      c. Thirty percent of coronary heart disease.
      d. Eighty percent to 90 percent of **chronic obstructive pulmonary diseases (COPD)** (i.e., emphysema and bronchitis).[1]
      e. Cataracts, pneumonia, acute myeloid leukemia, abdominal aortic aneurysm, stomach cancer, pancreatic cancer, cervical cancer, kidney cancer, and periodontitis.[17]
   5. More females have started smoking, making lung cancer surpass breast cancer as the leading cause of female cancer death.
      a. Pregnant women who smoke have an increased risk of:
         (1) Spontaneous abortions.
         (2) Fetal and infant deaths.
         (3) Premature births or **Preterm Low Birth Weight (PLBW).**
         (4) Underweight children.
         (5) Children with decreased lung function.
         (6) Triggering development of cleft lip/palate.
      b. Secondhand (passive) smoke is almost as detrimental to fetal development as active smoking pregnant women.

B. Environmental tobacco smoke (secondhand, passive) and caries implications.
   1. Secondhand smoke is:
      a. The third leading cause of preventable early death, following smoking and alcohol.[1]

Table 5–1 Chemicals Released from Cigarette Smoke[1]

Compound Released	Additional Information about Compound
Acetone	Main ingredient in fingernail polish remover.
Ammonia	Used for stripping wax from floors and removing varnish; often a toilet bowl cleaner.
Arsenic	Poison.
Butane	Cigarette lighter fluid.
Cadmium	Found in batteries.
Carbon Monoxide	Bonds with oxygen in blood cells to cause suffocation; found in car exhaust fumes and faulty furnaces.
Cresol	Main ingredient for industrial plastics and adhesives.
DDT	A pesticide that has been banned from use.
Formaldehyde	Embalming fluid.
Hydrogen cyanide	A fumigation poison banned from international use.
Isoprene	Natural base for tire rubber.
Methanol	Used as rocket fuel.
Naphalene	Moth balls.
Nicotine	Insecticide; also an addictive drug.
Nitrobenzene	Gasoline additive.
Pyrene	A main constituent of coal tar.
Toluene	Industrial solvent.

    b. Linked to tooth decay in children by not only hampering the immune system, but also causing mouth breathing and reduction of saliva flow.[18]

  2. Children whose parents smoke have more colds, bronchitis, pneumonia, worsened asthma, impaired development of lung function, and risk of ear infections.

  3. Nonsmokers living with smokers have an increased risk of developing lung cancer and dying early of heart disease; for every eight smokers who die from smoking, one innocent bystander dies from exposure to passive smoke.[1]

C. Hazardous chemicals in smoke. With each puff of smoke, the body is exposed to over 4,000 chemicals, over fifty of which are known to cause cancer (Table 5–1).

V. Tobacco-Induced and Associated Oral Conditions

Tobacco causes many health hazards and its use has serious side effects. Of particular note to the dental professional are the tobacco-induced oral conditions, since tobacco use begins in the mouth. When tobacco and alcohol use are combined, the risk of oral cancer increases fifteen times more than for non-users of tobacco and alcohol products.[19] Remember this when recommending alcohol-based mouthrinses for patients who smoke or use other forms of tobacco.

A. Cancer.
  1. Types.
    a. Pre cancer.
      (1) Verrucous. Rough, wart-like in appearance (Figure 5–4).
      (2) Leukoplakia. White plaque that cannot be scraped off. Appears either as a smooth, white patch or as leathery-looking wrinkled skin; results in cancer in 3 percent to 5 percent of all cases (Figure 5–5).
      (3) Erythroplakia. Red patch, persistent, and velvety that cannot be identified as any other specific red lesion such as inflammatory erythemas or those produced by blood vessel anomalies or infection.[20]

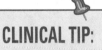

CLINICAL TIP:

Igniting Your Knowledge: Breathing in secondhand smoke can cause asthma.[2]

CLINICAL TIP:

Igniting Your Knowledge: The toxins from cigarette smoke go everywhere the blood flows.[17]

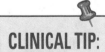

CLINICAL TIP:

Igniting Your Knowledge: Tobacco also alters taste and smell.

Figure 5-4   Verrucous.

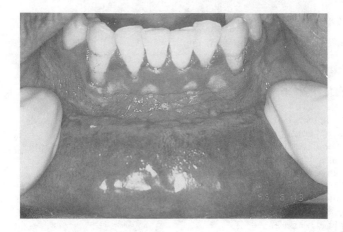

(4) Erythroleukoplakia. Mixture of leukoplakia interspersed with erythroplakia or vice versa that are likely to be premalignant or malignant.[21]

b. Oral cancer (**carcinoma**) (i.e., squamous cell). Cancer that originates from epithelial tissue and comprises about 90 percent of all oral cancers (Figure 5–6). These lesions can occur anywhere in the mouth and can be white, red, or red and white.

c. Complications during radiation and chemotherapy.
(1) Ulcerations.
(2) Tissue inflammation.
(3) Bleeding.
(4) Infections.
(5) Salivary flow dysfunction.

d. Results of these complications include xerostomia (dry mouth) and caries, as a result of the radiation, gingival breakdown, delayed healing, and bone infections.

2. Identification.
a. Perform thorough and complete intra- and extraoral examinations to determine any lesions from the norm including the lips, labial mucosa, buccal mucosa, gingiva, tongue, floor of mouth, and palate.

b. Recognition. Denote normal versus abnormal tissues.[22]

c. Referral for medical examination and possible biopsy.
(1) Medical doctor.
(2) Oral surgeon.

Figure 5-5   Leukoplakia.

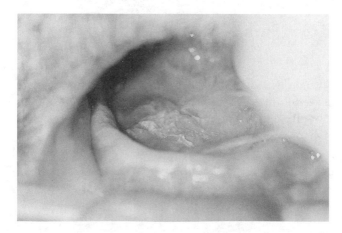

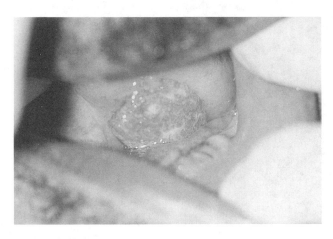

Figure 5–6   Carcinoma.

(3) In-office cytology smear or brush biopsy (Figure 5–7). To perform a brush biopsy:
(a) Slightly moisten the biopsy brush with the patient's saliva,
if the lesion is dry.
(b) Press the biopsy brush firmly against the lesion (Figure
5–8).
(c) Rotate 5 to 10 times (depending on the thickness of the lesion) until pink tissue or pinpoint microbleeding is observed.
(d) Rotate and drag the brush lengthwise, transferring as much
material from the brush to the slide as possible.
(e) Spread the cellular sample from the brush onto the glass
slide (Figure 5–9).
(f) Apply fixative agent to the slide and send to the laboratory
(Figure 5–10).
(g) Kits are available with all supplies necessary; check with a
dental supplier.[23]

B. Nicotine stomatitis. Red pin dots that often appear on the palate of smokers. Palate appears white and leathery with the red pin dots sprinkled
throughout (Figure 5–11).
C. Periodontal diseases. Discussed in greater detail in section VI.
D. Recession. Injured gingiva pull away from the teeth, exposing root surfaces
and leaving teeth sensitive to heat and cold.
   1. Results from constant irritation to the area in the mouth where a small
      wad of **chewing tobacco** is placed, causing permanent damage to peri-
      odontal tissue.
   2. Can damage the supporting bone structure.

CLINICAL TIP:

Igniting Your Knowledge:
Warning signs of cancer, if
symptoms persist more than
two weeks, include:

A sore that does not heal.
A lump or thickening of the
  cheek.
White patch, red patch, or combination red/white patch.
A prolonged sore throat or
  feeling that something is
  caught in the throat.
Difficulty in chewing, swallowing, or moving the
  tongue.
Restricted movement of the
  tongue or jaws.

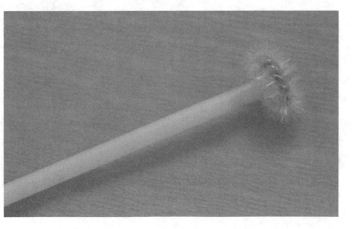

Figure 5–7   Brush biopsy.
*Photo courtesy of CDx
Laboratories.*

Figure 5–8   Rotate brush against lesion.   *Photo courtesy of CDx Laboratories.*

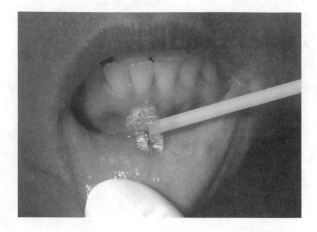

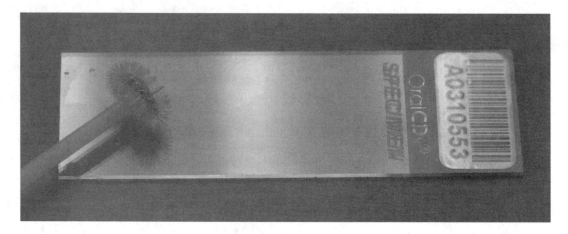

Figure 5–9   Apply brush to slide.   *Photo courtesy of CDx Laboratories.*

Figure 5–10   Apply fixative agent to slide.   *Photo courtesy of CDx Laboratories.*

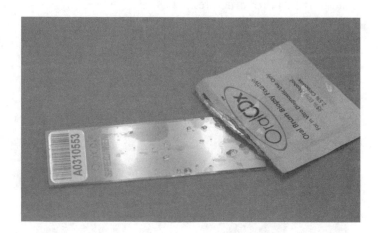

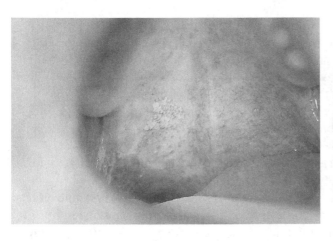
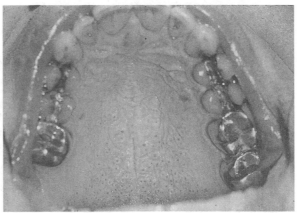

Figure 5–11   Nicotine stomatitis. *Photos courtesy of Dr. Arden G. Christen, Indiana University School of Dentistry, Department of Oral Biology.*

E. **Black hairy tongue.** Results when cells of the top layer of the tongue get enlarged but do not slough off, forming a thick mat.
 1. Cause. Unknown; benign condition.
 2. Characteristics. Extra tissue can get stained by food materials, bacteria, or tobacco and become yellowish, brown, or black.
F. **Halitosis** (oral malodor or bad breath).
G. **Staining of teeth and restorative materials.**
 1. Cause. Results from tar from the tobacco products, which adheres to plaque biofilm and calculus, leaving a light brownish-black extrinsic stain.
 2. Location. Usually found on gingival one-third and extends toward incisal/occlusal area, depending on severity.
H. **Abrasion.** Caused by grit and sand in smokeless tobacco products that scratch teeth and wear away enamel, i.e. spit tobacco. Premature loss of tooth enamel can cause added sensitivity. Gritty materials also scratch the soft tissue in the mouth, allowing the nicotine and other chemicals to get directly into the blood stream.
I. Caries. Caused from the sugar added to smokeless tobacco during the curing and processing to improve its taste. Sugar reacts with bacteria found naturally in the mouth, causing an acidic reaction, which leads to decay.[1]
J. Cleft lip/palate. Congenital condition associated with tobacco use during pregnancy, probably due to hypoxia.[24]

VI.   Tobacco and Periodontal Diseases
A. Smoking is a major risk factor for periodontal diseases.[17]
 1. Both current and former smokers show an increased prevalence and severity of periodontal diseases.
 2. There is a significant positive association between the amount of tobacco smoked and the severity of periodontitis.
 3. There is a linear and direct correlation between smoking and attachment loss with effects even at a low level of smoking.
 4. The periodontal status of former smokers ranks between current smokers and those who have never smoked.
 5. Eighty-six percent to 90 percent of refractory periodontitis cases are smokers.[1]

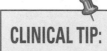

CLINICAL TIP:

Igniting Your Knowledge: **N-nitrosamines** are cancer-causing chemicals found in cured tobacco products.

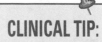

CLINICAL TIP:

Igniting Your Knowledge: Smoking also causes osteoporosis.[2]

B. Clinical appearance of smoking-associated periodontitis.

1. Gingiva. Tends to be fibrotic with thickened rolled margins. Minimal gingival redness or edema relative to disease severity as well as relatively severe and widespread disease (attachment and tooth loss) compared to a person the same age who never smoked.

2. Pocketing. Proportionately greater in anterior and maxillary lingual sites and gingival recession in anterior segments with no association between periodontal status and plaque or calculus scores.[25]

3. Recession. Using smokeless (spit) tobacco increases the risk of localized recession, but its effect on periodontitis is unclear.

4. Nicotine and other tobacco products produce local and systemic effects.
   a. Local effects include cytotoxic and vasoactive substances from tobacco smoke and can inhibit tissue perfusion and cell proliferation and metabolism.
   b. Systemic effects. Smoking causes immuno-suppression and impairment of soft tissue and bone cell function.

C. Microbiology. Some studies show there may be increased levels of periodontal pathogens in smokers versus nonsmokers; the possibility that smoking might favor a specific periopathogenic microflora is still unclear.[26]

D. Wound healing. Impaired healing and poorer clinical results to both non-surgical (i.e., scaling/root planing and locally delivered antibiotics) and surgical periodontal therapy for smokers versus nonsmokers.

1. Results for smokers versus nonsmokers.
   a. Decreased bleeding on probing (smoking constricts blood vessels) and increased probing depths, even with good oral hygiene.
   b. Decreased gain of attachment.
   c. Smokers have decreased success with open flap debridement, osseous resection, soft tissue and bone graft procedures, and guided tissue regeneration procedures.
   d. Implants. Failure rate in smokers is significantly higher than in non-smokers.
   e. Cigar and pipe smoking has similar adverse effects on periodontal health as cigarette smoking.

2. Factors that may contribute to impaired wound healing.
   a. Smoking impairs revascularization of bone and soft tissue.
   b. Polymorphonuclear (PMN) leukocytes alter chemotaxis, phagocytosis, and adherence.
   c. Altered antibody production.
   d. Negative effect on bone metabolism may influence osteoporosis and periodontitis by similar mechanisms.

E. Periodontal diagnosis, prognosis, and treatment planning.

1. Smoking status should be considered in dental hygiene assessment, diagnosis, prognosis, treatment planning, and evaluation because it is a clinically useful predictor of future disease activity.

2. In addition, smoking cessation should be considered a part of periodontal treatment.

F. Benefits of smoking cessation.

1. Stabilizes periodontal status for a majority of patients and ceases or slows attachment loss.

2. Decreases the risk of:
   a. Lung and many other cancers.

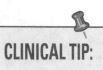

CLINICAL TIP:

Igniting Your Knowledge: American Cancer Society phone number: (800)-ACS-2345

   b. Coronary diseases.
   c. Stroke.
   d. Chronic obstructive lung diseases.
   e. Periodontal disease.
3. Reduces the risk of:
   a. Tooth loss. It may take a number of years after cessation before the rate of tooth loss is similar to that of nonsmokers.
   b. Damage to children's health.
   c. Ulcers.
   d. Premature wrinkling of skin.
   e. Infertility in women.
   f. Impotence in men.
   g. Cataracts.
   h. Macular degeneration.
4. Reduces the enormous cost of tobacco use. Healthcare costs of treating tobacco-related diseases and cost of lost earnings due to disability and early death approach $100 billion a year in the United States.[1]

G. Role of the dental hygienist.
   1. Identify the tobacco user. Accomplished by asking on medical history form.
   2. Personalize the risk. Accomplished during the intraoral, extraoral, and periodontal examinations, preferably with the patient holding a mirror and observing conditions pointed out by the dental hygienist.
   3. Encourage patient to set a stop date.
   4. Provide and monitor pharmacologic therapy.
   5. Follow up, encourage, and continue to support patient.
   6. Refer patient to a cessation class, support group, or nicotine dependence center.

H. Identification and assessment of tobacco use status. Take vital signs, including blood pressure, respiration and heart rates, temperature, and perform tobacco assessment. When taking the vital signs for patients, the tobacco question is part of the initial assessment and information gathering.[27] Tobacco questions to ask include the following:
   1. "Do you use tobacco?" "If so, what kind, how often, and how much?"
   2. "Do you want to quit?" If yes, the dental hygienist may begin intervention.
      a. Patients who use tobacco and are willing to quit should be treated using the five As of intervention—Ask, Advise, Assess, Assist, and Arrange (see section VII).
      b. Patients who use tobacco, but are unwilling to quit at this time, should be treated with the 5 Rs—Relevance, Risks, Rewards, Roadblocks, and Repetition[5] (see section VII).
      c. Patients who have recently quit should be provided with relapse prevention information[5] (see section VII).

VII. Intervention

A. Five As of intervention.[5] The five As give a logical, systematized sequence of steps for the dental hygienist to follow in broaching the topic of tobacco with patients (Table 5–2).
B. ADHA Smoking Cessation Intervention. In January 2004, the ADHA launched a nation-wide program for dental hygienists to get more involved with tobacco prevention and control. The purpose of the ADHA SCI Network is to enhance communication between ADHA, constituent

CLINICAL TIP:

Igniting Your Knowledge: Most patients try several times before they quit for good.[2]

CLINICAL TIP:

Igniting Your Knowledge: Mark Twain once said giving up smoking was easy; he'd done it thousands of times!

CLINICAL TIP:

Igniting Your Knowledge: Teach patient oral self-examination techniques.

Table 5–2   Five As of Intervention

Ask about tobacco use.	Identify and document tobacco use status for every patient at every visit.
Advise to quit.	In a clear, strong, and personalized manner, urge every tobacco user to quit.
Assess willingness to make a quit attempt.	Determine if the tobacco user is willing to make an attempt to quit at this time.
Assist in quit attempt.	For the patient willing to make a quit attempt, use counseling and pharmacotherapy to help him or her quit.
Arrange followup.	Schedule follow-up contact, preferably within the first week after the quit date.

organizations, and the dental hygiene community on issues related to smoking cessation.

Because of time constraints for the dental hygienist at chairside, the five As protocol was shortened to:

1. *Ask* tobacco status.
2. *Advise* tobacco users to quit.
3. *Refer* patient to telephone quitlines.

C. Pharmacotherapy. First-line pharmacotherapies have been found to be safe and effective for tobacco dependence treatment and have been approved by the United States Food and Drug Administration (FDA) for this use. First-line medications have established empirical record of efficacy and should be considered first as part of tobacco dependence treatment, except in cases of contraindications.

1. Bupropion SR (Zyban).
   a. First non-nicotine medication shown to be effective for smoking cessation and approved by the FDA for that use.
   b. Initial dose is 150 milligrams per day for three days, then a dose of 150 milligrams twice a day, initiated one week before the patient's stop date.[10]
   c. Best to refer to family physician to prescribe due to side effects consisting of seizures in 1 out of every 1,000 people.[28]

2. Nicotine gum (Figure 5–12).
   a. Currently available exclusively as an over-the-counter (OTC) medication.
   b. Packaged with instructions on correct usage, including chewing instructions. Operators should offer 4 milligrams rather than 2 milligrams nicotine gum to highly dependent smokers.

3. Nicotine inhaler.
   a. Available exclusively as a prescription medication.

CLINICAL TIP:

Igniting Your Knowledge: A complete list of telephone quitlines in each state can be found at www.smokefree.gov

CLINICAL TIP:

Igniting Your Knowledge: Consult the *Physicians' Desk Reference* for side effects and risks of Zyban.

CLINICAL TIP:

Igniting Your Knowledge: Nicotine gum can cause upset stomach and a sore mouth.[5]

Figure 5–12   Nicotine gum.

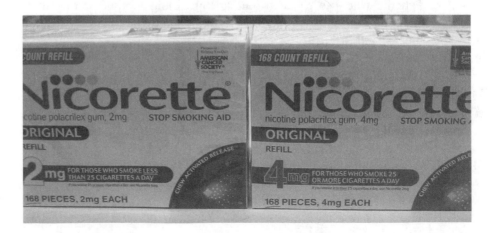

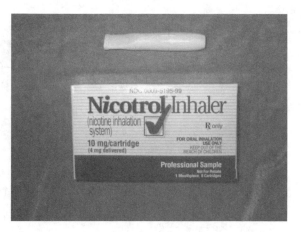

Figure 5–13   Nicotine inhaler.

b. Device resembles a cigarette and holds a cotton plug impregnated with 10 milligrams of nicotine; however, 80 puffs are needed to obtain 2 milligrams of nicotine (Figure 5–13).

c. Patient can use the inhaler for approximately three months.

4. Nicotine nasal spray.

a. Available exclusively as a prescription medication.

b. Dose:

(1) Since each spray contains 0.5 milligrams of nicotine, a one-dose spray in each nostril provides a 1 milligram dose.

(2) Patients can use 1 to 2 doses each hour for a total of 12 to 16 doses per day.

(3) Dose should be tapered after three months of use.

5. Nicotine patch.

a. Available both as an OTC and as a prescription medication.

b. Following strengths are available: 22 milligrams, 21 milligrams, 15 milligrams, 14 milligrams, 11 milligrams, and 7 milligrams per dose.

(1) Initially, the patient must be given the appropriate dose to effectively halt the **cravings** and to quit successfully.

(2) There are approximately 10 milligrams of nicotine in every cigarette, and 1 to 3 milligrams are absorbed by the smoker in each cigarette.

(3) A one-pack-a-day smoker would therefore need to receive about 20 to 23 milligrams of nicotine daily via a patch; dispensing a 14 milligram patch, for example, would be underdosing the patient and thereby risking relapse because the patient will still crave nicotine (Figure 5–14).

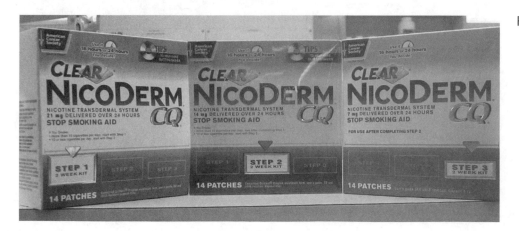

Figure 5–14   Nicotine patch.

Figure 5–15 Nicotine patch step-down program.

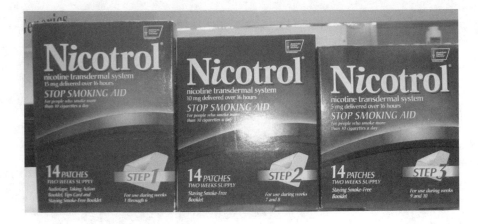

6. Nicotine step-down patch program.
   a. Available in three strengths: 15 milligrams, 10 milligrams, and 5 milligrams.
   b. Designed to gradually reduce the amount of nicotine absorbed until it is no longer needed. Have the patient:
      (1) Start with the 15 milligram patch and use for six weeks.
      (2) Then switch to the 10 milligram patch for two weeks.
      (3) Lower the dose to the 5 milligram patch for two more weeks (Figure 5–15).
7. Nicotine lozenge.
   a. Available OTC in 2 or 4 milligrams.
      (1) Use 4 milligrams if first cigarette of day is smoked within first half hour of rising.
      (2) Use 2 milligrams if first cigarette of day is after first half hour of rising.
   b. Delivers 25 percent more nicotine than gum.[29]
   c. Use 8 to 9 lozenges daily for the first six weeks, then taper over the next six weeks (Figure 5–16).
8. Combination nicotine replacement therapy. Combining the nicotine patch with a self-administered form of nicotine replacement therapy—either the nicotine gum or nicotine nasal spray—is more efficacious than a single form of nicotine replacement. Patients should be encouraged to use such combined treatments if they are unable to quit using a single type of first-line pharmacotherapy (Figure 5–17).

Figure 5–16 Lozenges used as a stop-smoking aid.

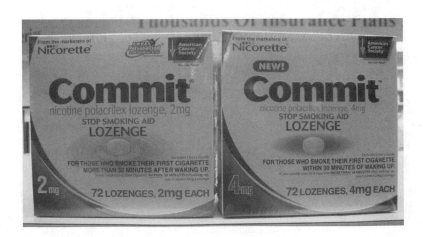

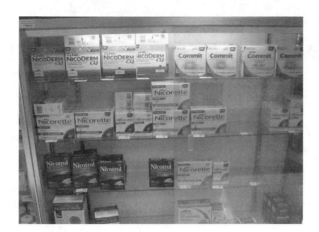

Figure 5–17   Combination therapies are readily available over the counter.

9. Other.
   a. Prescription medications, such as Nortriptyline and Clonidine, are also efficacious but are not considered first-line pharmacotherapies.
   b. Reduced nicotine cigarettes are available in 0.6 milligram, 0.3 milligram, and .05 milligram nicotine content, but they still have 10 milligrams of tar per cigarette and are not recommended for use in quitting smoking.[30]

D. Four Ds. Used to help patients cope with **withdrawal syndrome,** which is common with this addiction.
   1. Deep breaths. Help the patient relax and make the craving dissipate.
      a. Instruct patient to breathe in and exhale slowly, as if smoking a cigarette.
      b. When breathing, the patient should inhale deeply, hold it for several seconds, and then slowly exhale.
   2. Drink water. Instruct patient to drink plenty of water all day long, especially during a craving.
      a. Drinking water helps flush the toxins out of the system and keep hands and mouth busy if that is what is missing from smoking.
      b. Some ex-smokers prefer to drink through a straw, which also helps with the oral fixation.
   3. Do something else. Instruct patient to become more active.
      a. Suggestions include going for a brisk walk or meeting with a friend.
      b. Changing the environment can lessen the urge to smoke and provide a distraction.
   4. Delay. Most smokers falsely assume that each craving lasts a long time—perhaps up to 45 minutes. Actually, cravings come and go quickly.
      a. Average craving only lasts about 5 to 10 minutes.
      b. Suggest the patient wait 10 minutes; to help those 10 minutes go by, practice the other Ds.[31,32]

E. Withdrawal symptoms (see Table 5–3).
F. Helping in the stages of change. The following steps may help the patient in various stages of change:
   1. Precontemplation.
      a. Increase awareness of need to change.
      b. Give personalized information of the benefits of quitting.
      c. Encourage patient to think about change.

Table 5–3   Common Withdrawal Symptoms[31,32,33]

Common Withdrawal Symptoms	How to Help Relieve Symptoms
Dry mouth, sore throat	Chew gum or drink water or orange juice. Use throat sprays and cough drops only if necessary.
Headache	Do deep breathing and other relaxation techniques, nap, take a bath or hot shower. Take headache medicine only if needed, and take it with food.
Difficulty sleeping	Avoid caffeine in the evening, do relaxation techniques, stay more active during waking hours by getting *physical activity,* do deep breathing or read a relaxing book to help fall asleep.
Irregularity	Drink water and eat high-fiber foods.
Feeling tired during the day	Do deep breathing, take a nap, try to get more sleep at night.
Hunger	Drink water, eat low calorie snacks, eat smaller but more frequent meals during the day.
Cravings	Practice *the Four Ds.*
Tension, anxiety, irritability	Do relaxation exercises, drink water and fruit juices, do something enjoyable, ask those around to be patient.
Numbness/tingling in arms and legs	Get up and move around.
Difficulty concentrating	Take a quick walk, do deep breathing, and avoid alcohol.
Feeling lightheaded or dizzy	Recommend deep breathing and regular physical activity.
Coughing	Recommend hot herbal teas, cough drops, or sugarless hard candy. The lungs are working overtime to cleanse themselves. The cough may get worse before it gets better. If the coughing persists, consult physician.

      d. Counsel patient about risks of smoking.
      e. Offer to help if the decision is made.
  2. Contemplation.
      a. Motivate and increase confidence.
      b. Emphasize benefits of change with the assurance that the advantage of quitting will be more significant than inconvenient.
      c. Explore concerns and fears, as well as obstacles.
      d. Help resolve ambivalence and offer confidence that the smoker can achieve success.
  3. Preparation.
      a. Help individualize a plan for change—ask smoker to set quit date.
      b. Set realistic goals, such as tapering amount, then set quit date.
      c. Provide options, such as pharmacotherapy and motivation.
      d. Provide and have patient seek social support, such as through a support group.
  4. Action.
      a. Reaffirm commitment and follow-up.
      b. Teach behavioral skills.
      c. Provide educational materials.
      d. Note benefits: Suggest smoker use strategies for at least three months.
      e. Celebrate success and use rewards.
      f. Continue follow-up.
  5. Maintenance.
      a. Encourage plan for potential difficulties, such as holidays or family reunions.
      b. Recommend a support group.

   c. Reinforce reasons for quitting.
   d. Reinforce self-confidence in quitting and encourage rewards.
  6. Relapse.
   a. Assist in coping and facilitate another attempt.
   b. Check adequacy of nicotine replacement therapy dosage.
   c. Overcome shame and guilt.
   d. Use relapse as a learning experience.
   e. Analyze what went wrong.
   f. Emphasize persistence.[5]

G. Motivational intervention for patients who are unwilling to quit. The five Rs are designed to motivate smokers who are unwilling to quit at this time. They include relevance, risks, rewards, roadblocks, and repetition.
  1. Relevance. Motivational information has the greatest impact if it is relevant to a patient's disease status, risk, family, or social situation, health concerns, age, or gender.
  2. Risks. Include:
   a. Acute. Shortness of breath, asthma, harm to pregnancy, impotence, infertility, and increased carbon monoxide.
   b. Chronic. Heart attack, stroke, lung as well as other cancers, COPD, long-term disability, and need for extended care.
   c. Environmental. Secondhand smoke and all the side effects.
  3. Rewards. The dental team member may highlight those rewards that seem most important to the patient such as improved health, saving money, feeling better, and improving complexion, taste, smell, and breath.
  4. Roadblocks. May include barriers such as withdrawal symptoms, depression, fear of failure, enjoyment of tobacco, lack of support, and weight gain.
  5. Repetition. The motivational intervention should be repeated every time the patient comes in and involves reassuring patients that most make repeated quit attempts before they are successful.[5]

CLINICAL TIP

Igniting Your Knowledge: Cigarette smoke is capable of destroying the antioxidants found in saliva, leaving behind a mixture of compounds that can hasten oropharyngeal cancer development.[35]

VIII. Resources[5]
A. Action on Smoking and Health: www.ash.org
B. Addressing Tobacco in Managed Care: www.aahp.org/atmc.htm
C. Agency for Healthcare Research and Quality: www.ahrq.gov
D. American Academy of Family Physicians: www.aafp.org
E. American Cancer Society: www.cancer.org
F. American Dental Association: www.ada.org
G. American Legacy Foundation: www.americanlegacy.org
H. American Lung Association: www.lungusa.org
I. American Medical Association: www.ama-assn.org
J. American Psychological Association: www.apa.org
K. Americans for Nonsmokers' Rights: www.no-smoke.org
L. Centers for Disease Control and Prevention: www.cdc.gov/tobacco
M. National Cancer Institute: www.nci.nih.gov
N. National Center for Tobacco-Free Kids: www.tobaccofreekids.org
O. National Guideline Clearinghouse: www.guideline.gov
P. National Heart, Lung, and Blood Institute: www.nhlbi.nih.gov/index.htm
Q. National Institute on Drug Abuse: www.drugabuse.gov
R. Office on Smoking and Health at the Centers for Disease Control and Prevention: www.cdc.gov/tobacco

CLINICAL TIP

Igniting Your Knowledge: When saliva and cigarette smoke get together, a potentially lethal synergistic effect occurs.[35]

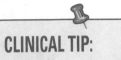

CLINICAL TIP:

Igniting Your Knowledge: In May 2004 the Surgeon General, Dr. Richard Carmona, released a new document entitled *The Health Consequences of Smoking: A Report of the Surgeon General.* It is available by calling 1-800-CDC-1311, or going to www.surgeongeneral.gov OR www.cdc.gov/tobacco

S. Office on Smoking and Health at the Centers for Disease Control and Prevention: State highlights including lists of State tobacco control contacts: www.cdc.gov/tobacco/statehi/statehi.htm
T. Robert Wood Johnson Foundation: www.rwjf.org
U. Society for Research on Nicotine and Tobacco: www.srnt.org
V. Southern Illinois University: www.siu.edu/tobacco
W. **Surgeon General:** http://www.surgeongeneral.gov/library/smokingconsequences/
X. World Health Organization: www.who.int

Tobacco dependence is a chronic disease that deserves treatment. The oral effects of tobacco have been discussed. Effective treatments have been identified and should be applied to every tobacco user.[34] The ADA and ADHA mandates that members take more of a leading role in tobacco education and cessation. Many materials are available for dental office–based tobacco interventions. "Dental offices provide a unique opportunity to expand the reach of health care and self-help cessation programs."[3] Dental hygienists can take a leading role.

QUESTIONS

1. Which of the following is NOT one of the five As of intervention in tobacco cessation counseling?
   a. Arrange
   b. Assess
   c. Aware
   d. Assist
   e. Ask

2. Which of the following medications for nicotine replacement therapy requires a prescription?
   a. Patch
   b. Inhaler
   c. Gum
   d. Lozenge

3. Nicotine causes oral cancer. The most common oral cancer is squamous cell carcinoma.
   a. Both statements are TRUE.
   b. Both statements are FALSE.
   c. The first statement is TRUE. The second statement is FALSE.
   d. The first statement is FALSE. The second statement is TRUE.

4. Which of the following is the BEST advice the dental hygienist can give to the patient seeking assistance in quitting cigarettes?
   a. Switch from cigarettes to a pipe.
   b. Switch from cigarettes to cigars.
   c. Stop tobacco cold turkey.
   d. Taper off cigarettes, set a quit date, and be ready to wear a nicotine patch for nicotine replacement therapy.

5. The dental hygienist examines a patient who uses smokeless tobacco—approximately one pouch per week for five years. Which of the following is the LEAST likely to be noted during the oral exam?
   a. Absence of stained teeth.
   b. Stained tongue.
   c. White wrinkled patches in the vestibule.
   d. Leukoplakia on the buccal mucosa.
   e. Gingival recession.

6. The best advice to give someone trying to quit tobacco includes all of the following EXCEPT one. Which one is the EXCEPTION?
   a. Practice deep breathing exercises.
   b. Drink water.
   c. Exercise.
   d. Eat healthy food.
   e. Test resolve in a smoking atmosphere.

7. A 26-year-old patient just informed the dental hygienist she is three months pregnant. Which of the following is a possible side effect of smoking for this patient's pregnancy?
   a. Development of a pyogenic granuloma.
   b. Preterm low birth weight delivery.

c. Overdue delivery.

d. Herpes simplex, type I.

8. Which of the following is considered the greatest risk factor for periodontal disease?

    a. Tobacco use

    b. Gender

    c. Age

    d. Socioeconomic status

9. Why is secondhand smoke considered to be so dangerous?

a. Eye irritation.

b. Bone resorption.

c. Contains around 4,000 hazardous chemicals.

d. Premature skin wrinkling.

10. Which of the following is NOT a clinical appearance of smoking-associated chronic periodontitis?

    a. Bleeding

    b. Fibrotic gingival with thickened margins

    c. Recession

    d. Minimal gingival redness

REFERENCES

1. Stafne EE, Bakdash B. University of Minnesota, Division of Periodontology: <http://www.umn.edu/perio/tobacco/hazardouschemicals.html>. Accessed August 1, 2003.

2. Slomski A. Waiting to inhale. *Access,* Vol. 5, Number 17, May-June 2003, 40–49.

3. Gordon, JS, Severson, HH. Tobacco cessation through dental office settings. *Journal of Dental Education,* Vol. 65, Number 4, 2001, 354–363.

4. Gadbury-Amyot CC, Doherty F, Stach DJ, et al. Prioritization of the national dental hygiene research agenda. *The Journal of Dental Hygiene,* Vol. 76, Number II, 2002.

5. Fiore MC, Bailey WC, Cohen SJ, et al. *Treating tobacco use and dependence.* Clinical Practice Guideline. Rockville, MD: U.S. Department of Health and Human Services. Public Health Service. June 2000.

6. Centers for Disease Control. <http://www.cdc.gov/tobacco/quit/guideline.htm> Accessed May 15, 2003.

7. *The Random House Dictionary of the English Language,* 2nd ed. New York: Random House, 1987, p. 1298.

8. Dunn WL. 1972. Quoted in *Federal Register,* August 11, 1995, p. 41596.

9. Hanson, GR. NIDA's continued commitment to nicotine research. *NIDA Notes,* Vol. 17, Number 6, 2003, pp 1–3 <http://www.drugabuse.gov?NIDA_Notes> Accessed August 1, 2003.

10. Dale, LC, Fisher, P. *Tobacco use and dependence intervention in the office setting.* Seminar given at Lutheran Hospital, Fort Wayne, IN, April 2003.

11. Asma S. Tobacco Information and Prevention Source, http://www.cdc.gov/tobacco/quit/guideline.htm. Accessed August 1, 2003.

12. Centers for Disease Control and Prevention's Morbidity and Mortality Weekly Report, Vol. 49, Number 33, 2000, 755–758.

13. <http://www.indonesianclovecigarettes.com/kretek.htm> Accessed August 1, 2003.

14. Fehrenbach, M. Cigar smoking. *RDH,* Vol. 23, Number 2, 2003, 42–50.

15. <http://www.drugs.indiana.edu/publications/iprc/factline/cigar.html> Accessed August 15, 2003.

16. National Institute of Dental and Craniofacial Research and National Cancer Institute, National Institutes of Health, "Spit Tobacco: Know the Score," November 1999.

17. U.S. Department of Health and Human Services. *The health consequences of smoking: A report of the Surgeon General.* U.S. Department of Health and Human Services, Centers for Disease Control and Prevention, National Center for Chronic Disease Prevention and Health Promotion, Office on Smoking and Health, 2004.

18. Danner V. Secondhand smoke linked to tooth decay. *The Journal of Dental Hygiene,* Vol. 77, Number II, 2003, p.78.

19. The Oral Cancer Foundation. Accessed at <www.oralcancer.org> on July 2, 2003.

20. Wood NK, Goaz PW. *Differential diagnosis of oral and maxillofacial lesions* (5th ed.). St. Louis, MO: C.V. Mosby, 1997, p. 57.

21. Melrose, RJ. Premalignant oral diseases. *Journal of the California Dental Association* 2001.

22. Cooper MD, Wiechmann, L. In*: Essentials of Dental Hygiene: Preclinical Skills.* Upper Saddle River, NJ: Prentice Hall, 2004.

23. Svirsky JA, Burns JC, Page DG, Abbey LM. Computer-assisted analysis of the oral brush biopsy. *The Compendium of Continuing Dental Education,* Vol. 22, 2001, 99–106.

24. Fried, JL. Women and tobacco: Oral health issues. *Journal of Dental Hygiene,* Vol. 74, Number 1, 2000, 49–55.

25. Haber J. Cigarette smoking: A major risk factor for periodontitis. *Compendium of Continuing Education* Vol. XV, Number 8, 1994, 1002–14.

26. American Academy of Periodontology position paper: Tobacco use and the periodontal patient. *Journal of Periodontology,* Vol. 70, Number 11, 1999, 1419–1427.

27. Fiore, MC. The new vital sign. Addressing and documenting smoking status. *The Journal of the American Medical Association,* Vol. 266, December 11, 1991, p. 3183.

28. Jones, K., RRT, Coordinator of Nicotine Dependence Center, Lutheran Hospital, Fort Wayne, IN. Personal interview, August 18, 2003.

29. Shiffman S, Dresler CM, Hajek P, Simon J, Gilburt A, Targett DA, Strahs KA. Efficacy of a nicotine lozenge for smoking cessation. *Archives of Internal Medicine,* Vol. 162, 2002, 1267–1276.

30. Vector Tobacco, Inc. Accessed at <www.questcigs.com> on June 13, 2003.

31. American Cancer Society. Freshstart Smoking Cessation Program Participant's Guide. 1998.

32. Strecher, VJ, Rimer, B. *Freedom from smoking.* American Lung Association, 1999.

33. National Cancer Institute, <http://rex.nci.nih.gov/NCI_Pub_Interface/Clearing_the_Air/symptoms.html.>. Accessed on June 20, 2003.

34. Christen, AG. Tobacco cessation, the dental profession, and the role of dental education. *Journal of Dental Education,* Vol. 65, Number 4, 2001, 368–374.

35. Nunn P. Saliva: You might be surprised what it can do. *Access,* Vol. 19, Number 2, February 2005, 16–21.

Chapter 6

Dental Sealants

Shirley Gutkowski, RDH, BSDH

MediaLink

A companion CD-ROM, included free with each new copy of this book, supplements the procedures presented in each chapter. Insert the CD-ROM to watch video clips and view a large collection of color images that is also included. This multimedia library is designed to help you add a new dimension to your learning.

KEY TERMS

biofilm	glass ionomer	operculum
bonding agent	hydrophilic	polymerization
caries risk	hydrophobic	sealant
curing	mechanical retention	transitional sealants
enameloplasty		
etchant		

LEARNING OBJECTIVES

After reading this chapter, the student will be able to:

- compare and contrast the different sealant materials used;
- know how to place dental sealants;
- understand caries risk;
- gain an understanding of how to assess caries risk;
- list the benefits of sealing the occlusal surface of the tooth;
- understand the benefits of protecting the surfaces of the tooth other than the occlusal surface.

I. Introduction

A **sealant** is referred to as a composite resin, or plastic material that is most commonly placed on the occlusal surfaces of posterior teeth. While composite resin is still the first choice by all recommendations,[1,2] **glass ionomer** sealants have evolved to become a worthy consideration for nontraditional patients—those with circumstances that make traditional sealants inadequate. Sealants have helped decrease the decay rate in western civilizations; however, the literature is replete with admonitions to use sealants more. The U.S. government *Healthy People 2010* document has set a goal for sealants to be placed on 50 percent of the children by 2010.

II. Purpose of Placing Sealants

As a surface protectant, a sealant acts as a barrier between the enamel and the oral environment. Traditionally sealants are placed on the occlusal surface. Future discussions will center around sealants' therapeutic benefits as well as its

Figure 6–1   Microscopic view of an occlusal surface—showing pits and fissures.

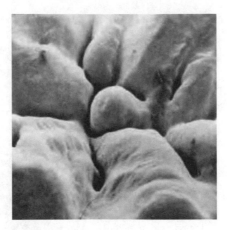

ability to block pathogens from the vulnerable enamel. Sealants act as a barrier against:

A. Bacterial invasion. Sealant acts as a physical barrier that blocks the bacteria from coming into contact with the enamel, particularly in pits and fissures. Although the occlusal surface accounts for only 13 percent of the total surfaces, occlusal decay accounts for nearly 50 percent of decay (Figure 6–1).

B. Bacterial by-products, such as lactic acid.

C. Environmentally low pH as occurs in high caries individuals. Lactic and other acids (as by-products of bacterial metabolism) create an environment that is hospitable to cariogenic bacteria as well as disruptive to the enamel.

III. Tooth Surfaces Protected by Sealants

A. Occlusal. With traditional application, the bioacceptable sealant material fills the pits and fissures. A bioacceptable material is one that is harmless to the surrounding tissue and functions in a way that does not harm the host. Material flows into the occlusal anatomy, pits, and fissures, which blocks bacteria from invading areas that are inaccessible to the toothbrush or other mechanical means for disrupting **biofilms.**

1. Creates mechanical block. Protects pits and fissures from biofilm formation and bacterial by-products that initiate and perpetuate the enamel decay process.

2. Eliminates nutrients from the bacteria, if any are still present, in the pits or fissures.

3. Cuts off air supply to the bacteria that remain in the pits and fissures after thorough cleaning, effectively creating a hostile, oxygen-free environment that kills bacteria.

4. Provides fluoride continuously for the life of the material when using glass ionomer sealant materials.

    a. Occurs by a perpetual chemical reaction between the powder and liquid components of the material.

    b. Chemical reaction cures (hardens) the material and provides fluoride to the surrounding enamel.[3]

B. Broad or vertical surfaces. Newer sealant materials bond directly to the tooth by a chemical bond rather than a mechanical bond and are more viscous, allowing the operator to apply sealant material on the sides of the tooth where plaque may accumulate; these surfaces include buccal, lingual, mesial, and distal.

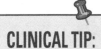

CLINICAL TIP:

Sealing Your Knowledge: Recent estimates state that providing a single surface restoration requires 2.5 times more effort than does placing sealants.

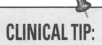

CLINICAL TIP:

Sealing Your Knowledge: Glass ionomer is one material used on the broad surfaces of teeth because it bonds directly without etching the tooth surface and is more viscous than traditional resin sealants.

IV. Armamentarium and Patient Preparation
  A. Armamentarium.
   1. Mouth mirror. Retracts tongue and cheek.
   2. Explorer.
       a. Helps remove organic debris from the pits and fissures.
       b. Checks sealant integrity at the end of the placement sequence.
   3. Slow-speed handpiece. Cleans the surface of the tooth to be sealed.
   4. Pumice. Helps remove stain and organic matter.
   5. Prophy brush. Removes stain and organic matter from pits and fissures.
   6. Sealant material. Fills pits and fissures.
   7. Applicator. Places sealant material; comes in a variety of styles.
   8. **Etchant.** Prepares the tooth for **mechanical retention.**
   9. **Bonding agent.** Increases bond strength.
  10. Microbrush. Small plastic wand with a flocked end that aids in material distribution.
  11. Bib. Worn by patient to protect clothing.
  12. Cotton rolls. Isolate teeth and absorb water and/or saliva.
  13. Dri Angles or Dri Tips. Small paper triangles used to block Stensen's ducts, absorb water and/or saliva, as well as keep the buccal mucosa from coming in contact with the tooth.
  14. Saliva ejector. Helps evacuate water and saliva from the mouth.
  15. High-volume evacuation (HVE). Removes copious amounts of water after rinsing.
  16. Amber safety glasses. Worn by the patient to protect the retina during **polymerization** of certain sealants materials with the ultraviolet (UV) light.
  17. Articulating paper. A marking paper used to check occlusion after sealant placement; indicates the need for adjustment of sealant material as necessary.
  18. UV light. Initiates polymerization of resin sealants.
  B. Prepare patient. It is important to always review the patient's health history before beginning any treatment.
   1. Explain procedure to the patient in common terms; when working with children, it is helpful to have them feel and view the materials that will be used.
   2. Place bib to protect patient's clothing.
   3. Recline patient to a level where operator's arms are parallel to the floor.
   4. Provide protective amber eyewear to the patient.
   5. Turn patient's head toward the operator, allowing for:
       a. Better lighting.
       b. Water/saliva to pool in a small area for easy removal.
       c. Better ergonomics for the operator.

V. Types of Materials
There are two major types of sealant materials used—composite resins and glass ionomers. Each is used in specific cases, depending on the case presentation.
  A. Composite resin. First choice for an occlusal sealant;[1] developed to be used as a sealant material on occlusal surface; excellent flowability; largest selling type of sealant material.
   1. Constituents. The nature of sealant material is chemical.
       a. Bis-GMA acrylic acid monomer and copolymers. Component that some say releases a synthetic estrogen. American Dental Association (ADA) position states that the amount released is negligible.

CLINICAL TIP:

Sealing Your Knowledge: Moisture contamination is the most likely cause of sealant failure. However, inadequate etching can also be a cause of sealant failure. Enamel rod breakage is another potential cause for sealants to be lost prematurely.

CLINICAL TIP:

Sealing Your Knowledge: All sealants have slight differences between them. It is important the operator read the manufacturer's directions before using a new material. It is also recommended to read the package inserts once a year to note any changes in the material or directions for use.

CLINICAL TIP:

Sealing Your Knowledge: If any etchant should come in contact with the skin, rinse well with water. It won't burn immediately, but will eventually cause a chemical burn on the skin.

b. Some composite resin sealant materials are filled with inorganic fillers.
   (1) Microscopic fillers give material some body and reduce occlusal wear, which has become less of a consideration because the most important aspect is for the sealant to be placed in the pits and fissures where wear is not a factor.
   (2) Most manufacturers have eliminated the fillers because they made the product difficult to use—they increased surface tension, which in turn, decreased the material's flowablity.
c. Unfilled resins contain no inorganic fillers.
   (1) Resin material flows freely into the pits and fissures.
   (2) Display superior handling properties.
   (3) Placement into the pits and fissures is easy.
   (4) Minimal occlusal adjustment is needed; if there is an area where the material is excessive, it would wear and come into occlusion.
2. **Curing** of composite resin sealants. Achieved by using ultraviolet light polymerization.
   a. Monomer, or molecule, within the resin readily combines with another monomer when activated with a curing light, creating a polymer.
   b. Solid polymer. Created once the material is fully cured; this is advantageous, because bacteria and/or their by-products cannot penetrate through a solid mass.
   c. Self-polymerization occurs with different kinds of materials.
      (1) Effect can be set in motion by visible light, or by a chemical reaction that is initiated by mixing two components together before applying to the tooth.
      (2) In the United States composite resin sealants, which are activated by ultraviolet light, are most popular to use (Figure 6–2).
3. Bonding or attachment to the tooth. Imperative for a successful composite resin sealant. There are two ways to accomplish this—mechanically and chemically. Mechanical means prepares the tooth to accept the material by removing the matrix between the enamel rods. This is accomplished by applying a phosphoric acid, in a gel or liquid form, on the tooth, which removes the matrix and leaves only the enamel rods intact, creating a surface for the material to engage, or hold onto, once it is polymerized (Figure 6–3).
4. Advantages of composite resin sealants include:

Figure 6–2   Percentages of light-cured versus self-cured dental sealants in the year 2000.

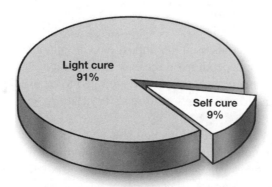

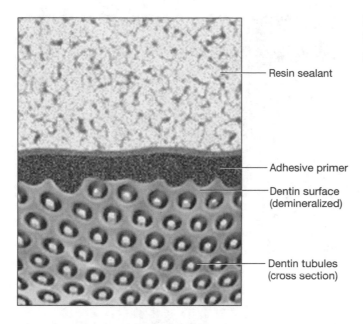

Figure 6–3   Mechanical bonding (or attachment) to tooth.

Resin sealant

Adhesive primer

Dentin surface (demineralized)

Dentin tubules (cross section)

a. Long history of use. This is the most popular type of sealant material being used today; material and the mechanical bond can last up to ten years.

b. Inexpensive. Although the cost of sealants can vary greatly, the cost is competitive.

c. Requires no mixing. Ready to dispense. Some materials come in cartridges with a cannula (a small hollow tube used for delivering materials) on the tip for dispensing directly into the pits and fissures (Figure 6–4); others are available in a single-use dispenser tip (Figure 6–5). This is advantageous because it eliminates a step when trying to place the material on a partially cooperative young child.

d. Not time sensitive. Material is workable until cured with the light source; therefore, there is no limit on the working time.

e. Provides acceptable esthetics. Most of the materials are clear or a color-tinted amber or opaque white. These colors are acceptable to operators and patients.

5. Disadvantages of composite resin sealants include:

a. Must obtain a dry field during preparation. The theory behind this is that the minerals in the saliva will rebuild the etched portion of the tooth, creating ineffective or inferior mechanical bonds.

CLINICAL TIP:

Sealing Your Knowledge: Newer one-step etch and bond materials are coming into the market. The material is rubbed onto the tooth, then dried, making the tooth ready to accept the resin sealant.

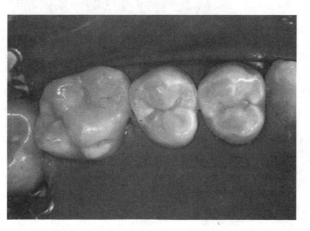

Figure 6–4   The pits and fissures of these teeth are cleaned, then isolated with a rubber dam. Although recommended for superior isolation, most operators use cotton rolls. Also note the fissure of the lingual cusp on the first molar.

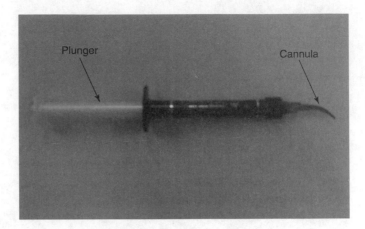

Figure 6–5   Premeasured sealant cartridge.

b. Material is **hydrophobic** (repels water). If the tooth has moisture on it, the water molecules will repel the sealant material, creating an ineffective seal.

c. Requires multiple steps. Placement requires six to eight steps. In some cases, such as with an uncooperative patient, multiple steps can be a hindrance. In certain circumstances, such as a severely mentally challenged child, sealants may be placed while the patient is having other procedures completed under general anesthesia. In these cases, the dentist may likely perform the procedure.

d. Requires a bonding agent. While most operators do not use a bonding agent during sealant placement, it is recommended and has been found to increase bond strength between the tooth and the sealant material. This adds two additional steps to the procedure—applying the bonding agent and drying it. As with all materials, directions must be checked and the substance applied as recommended by the manufacturer.

e. Must be applied on fully erupted occlusal surface. An **operculum** is a contraindication to sealant placement. Due to the material's hydrophobic nature, any tissue tags must be removed surgically (laser, cautery, or scalpel), or the sealant must be placed once the tooth has erupted further, which may be past a critical window of opportunity.

f. Has been tested only on pits and fissures. The material is so fluid that it has not been tested for use on the broad surfaces of the tooth, such as the buccal and lingual surfaces. Until recently, the only surface that has had sealants placed on it is the occlusal, protecting the most common area of tooth decay. There are materials that can be placed on vulnerable vertical surfaces if the patient is unable to keep these areas clean.

g. Shrinkage during polymerization. Can result in undesirable consequences.

h. Provides little fluoride release. When included, there is minimal fluoride release that has not been shown to decrease decay or remineralize the tooth.[2,4]

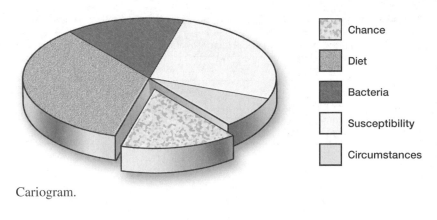

Chance

Diet

Bacteria

Susceptibility

Circumstances

Cariogram.

CLINICAL TIP:

Sealing Your Knowledge: For a full explanation on caries risk assessment access Malmo University in Sweden at http://www.db.od.mah.se/car/cariogram/cariograminfo.html. This website provides a precise exercise in building a cariogram, which will allow for accurate caries risk assessment for patients (see figure to the left).

6. Case selection. Evaluate the following patient criteria prior to applying resin sealants. Consider **caries risk** factors.[2,5] Caries is an infectious disease that has a number of mitigating factors including diet, family history, fluoride use, saliva qualities, oral flora, host response, oral hygiene, and tooth composition. All of these factors must be taken into consideration when treatment planning for sealant placement.

   a. Caries risk must be low to moderate. The patient and/or family history shows no or few caries.

   b. Possess light-to-moderate biofilm. For resin sealants a patient with little disclosable plaque biofilm is a better candidate than one with a heavy layer of biofilm on the teeth. Often patients with heavy biofilm on their teeth will present with gingivitis; the associated bleeding can contaminate the tooth after etching, effectively undermining the mechanical retention. For such a case presentation, a glass ionomer sealant is a better choice.

   c. Practice a diet low in simple sugars. When establishing caries risk factors, a patient with a diet low in simple sugars will decrease risk for decay.

   d. Practice infrequent acid challenges. This category is linked to diet. Frequent acid challenges do not only come with food intake, but also carbonated liquids, which expose teeth to carbolic acid and other acids such as citric and malic.

   e. Use daily fluoride. Patients who live in an area with fluoridated water and use products with fluoride have a lower risk of decay.

   f. Brush effectively, a minimum of once per day. Daily biofilm removal is important.

   g. Good quantity and quality of saliva. Important for establishing caries risk factors (Table 6–1).

      (1) Assists in maintaining mucosal integrity, facilitating speech, breaking down complex carbohydrates, flushing toxins, releasing chemicals that provide taste in the food, and diluting and buffering acids.

      (2) Provides buffering capacity. When choosing a sealant material for a patient, it is important to know and understand the patient's saliva buffering capacity.

CLINICAL TIP:

Sealing Your Knowledge: People with low caries risk, i.e., better oral hygiene and normal diet and saliva, are good candidates for resin sealants. Glass ionomer sealants are recommended for those who have poor oral hygiene, or high caries risk factors.

CLINICAL TIP:

Sealing Your Knowledge: To perform an easy saliva quantity test: Hold the lower lip with a piece of gauze and dry with a second piece of gauze. Take a time reading when the saliva erupts from the ducts. Anything less than sixty seconds is excellent.

CLINICAL TIP:

Sealing Your Knowledge: Saliva quantity can be measured in ml/min. as the patient continually spits into a medicine dose cup with either unstimulated or stimulated (chewing a paraffin pellet) saliva. A good amount of saliva is about 600 milliliters per day or 1 to 3 millimeters per minute stimulated.

Table 6–1   Characteristics of saliva in children with and without caries experience.

Unstimulated and stimulated salivary pH and flow rate in patients with and without caries.

	With Caries	Without Caries
Unstimulated salivary pH	6.55 +/− 0.07	7.12 +/− 0.05
Stimulated salivary pH	7.72 +/− 0.09	7.21 +/− 0.06
Unstimulated salivary flow (ml/min)	0.43 +/− 0.03	0.73 +/− 0.09
Stimulated salivary flow (ml/min)	0.60 +/− 0.05	1.12 +/− 0.10

(a) Composite resin sealant materials. Best for the uncompromised patient with healthy saliva that buffers well.

(b) Glass ionomer material. Better choice for patients with poor quality saliva.

(3) pH range of 6.5 or higher. pH of saliva can be checked easily chairside. Composite resin sealants provide excellent barriers to bacteria and their by-products. Patients who have physiological complications, such as poor saliva, are excellent candidates for sealants.

h. Low bacterial counts. Biofilms with low *Streptococcus mutans* counts are not as cariogenic as those with high counts. Bacterial counts are difficult to establish at this time; companies are experimenting with chairside tests to establish the types of bacteria and detect the presence of lactic acid.

i. Eruption. For the bond to attach to the tooth, the occlusal table must be fully accessible. As mentioned earlier, an operculum covering the distal pit will make it impossible to seal the entire tooth.

Note: Also remember enamel is maturing over time. Immature enamel will not respond to the etching and result in an inferior bond.

j. Patient cooperation must be high.

(1) Sealant placement is technique sensitive; a sudden movement by the patient can cause unpleasant experiences, such as:
 (a) Tasting some of the etchant or sealant material.
 (b) Contaminating the occlusal table with saliva.
 (c) Placing the etchant on the skin or mucosa, causing a mild chemical burn.

(2) Often a dental hygienist is called upon to place sealants alone, without an assistant and the use of four-handed dentistry. With four-handed dentistry, an assistant helps with cheek retraction, tongue management, saliva control, and handing materials to the operator.

k. Patient's oral hygiene. Should be good to excellent. Poor oral hygiene can predispose a patient to caries, and nontherapeutic sealants will not provide the level of protection needed by those with high caries risk.

l. Fluoridated municipal water supply. Patients who live in areas with adequate water fluoridation are excellent candidates for resin sealants. This decreases caries risk and facilitates remineralization of the teeth on an ongoing basis.[7]

m. Insured population.[8] When determining the need for resin sealants, insurance availability can play a part in treatment planning.

(1) Insured population has a lower incidence of decay, and therefore are good candidates for sealant placement.

(2) Insurance plays a dual role in treatment plans.

(a) Often patients will choose to forgo treatment recommendations that are not a covered insurance benefit or third party payment plan.

(b) To practice ethical dental hygiene, the patient must be given the best treatment options for the risk factor and clinical presentation—second and third choices can be explored if the patient cannot afford or is not willing to pay for the first option choice.

n. Individuals with moderate-to-low income benefit from sealant placement; however, they may benefit more from a therapeutic sealant material because low income falls into the moderate-to-high caries risk; studies support that children from low-income homes have a higher incidence of decay.

7. Preparing the tooth for application. Proper preparation is essential for sealant longevity. Cleaning the tooth before etching assures that any biofilm, or organic material, is removed so the etchant can attach to the enamel. The following directions are for single-operator application, or two-handed dentistry, and are of a general nature. For specific directions of a particular manufacturer's material, follow the directions included with the material.

a. Clean the occlusal surface.

(1) Use pumice with prophy brush, or an air polisher. Avoid using materials such as prophy paste because the flavoring oils can interfere with the mechanical bond.

(2) If using a prophy brush, apply intermittent pressure to occlusal surface; this can increase removal of organic matter.

(3) Rinse with water and air/water spray, enough to remove the debris left by the polishing procedure.

(4) Use HVE or saliva ejector to remove water, debris, and saliva.

b. Isolate the tooth with cotton rolls. When working alone, cotton rolls help with moisture control as well as retracting the tongue and cheek. Saliva contamination can cause the etched tooth to become remineralized and interfere with the mechanical bond between the tooth and the material, which can lead to premature sealant loss or a sealant bomb. A sealant bomb, a result of an improperly placed sealant, allows bacteria and nourishment for the bacteria access under the sealant where decay can progress undetected. Extensive decay is discovered once the sealant is no longer retained. To isolate the tooth:

(1) Place one cotton roll on the buccal side of the tooth in the vestibule.

(2) Place another cotton roll under the tongue. This helps the operator retract the tongue, as well as absorb the saliva from Wharton's duct.

(3) Instruct patient not to move his or her tongue; it should be relaxed on the floor of the mouth.

(4) Place Dri Angle or Dri Tip onto the buccal mucosa; this step blocks the Stensen's duct and passively holds the mouth open.

CLINICAL TIP:

Sealing Your Knowledge: The Dri Angle should be placed against the buccal mucosa with the narrow end placed distally.

(5) Dry the tooth with air to remove excess saliva and allow the etchant to touch the tooth; this step takes approximately 1 second.

(6) Place saliva ejector in patient's mouth for continual evacuation. Instruct patient not to close around the tip of the saliva ejector, because negative pressure can result in a backflow situation where the contents of the evacuation hose enter the patient's mouth and the tooth surface may get contaminated.

(7) Apply etchant. Material is usually a phosphoric or other acid that dissolves the interprismatic matrix leaving only the enamel rods, which are extremely delicate and can be broken with little effort. This arrangement, with the microscopic enamel rod towers, is what provides the mechanical means for sealant attachment (Figure 6–6).

    (a) Read and follow manufacturer's directions for the amount of time to etch tooth.

    (b) Phosphoric acid, as an etchant, comes in gel or liquid in most sealant kits.

        i. Gel etchants are used by most operators because they are easier to control. They were initially developed for use with adhesive restorative and esthetic restorations when placement was needed on vertical surfaces for extended periods. It has grown in popularity for sealant placement as well.

        ii. Liquid etchants have the added benefit of penetrating pits and fissures, allowing for the mechanical bond to penetrate deeper.

(8) Rinse with water or air/water combination for 15 seconds; this will dilute and remove the etchant from the tooth surface. Too much rinsing can damage the delicate enamel rods or increase the mineral content, which can negatively affect the mechanical bond. Use HVE to evacuate water from the mouth and cotton rolls—this is the easiest way to evacuate the rinse water from the mouth.

    (a) When using HVE, turn the bevel of the tube flush against the cotton roll to remove the water; this will save time, elim-

CLINICAL TIP:

Sealing Your Knowledge: If a tooth becomes contaminated with saliva after the etching step, re-etch for half the time recommended by the manufacturer.

Figure 6–6   Gel etchant is applied to the teeth, including the lingual cusp on the first molar.

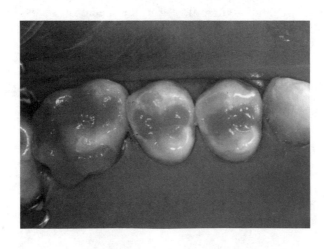

inate a step (replacing the cotton rolls), and keep the tongue from lifting and wetting the newly etched tooth with saliva.

(b) If HVE is not avaiable to dry the cotton roll, it is advisable to place another dry roll on top of the wet one instead of trying to remove the wet one and risking contaminating the tooth with saliva.

(c) Instruct patient not to swallow material or water.

(9) Place another cotton roll on top of the existing roll on the lingual side of the tooth. A second cotton roll will help keep the tongue aside, as well as absorb additional saliva.

(10) Dry the tooth. Using the air/water syringe, press the air button, directing the airflow against the gloved hand to expel any remaining moisture from the hose before attempting to dry the tooth, then:

(a) Direct the air onto the etched tooth until it appears frost-like; this appearance results when the etch is sufficient to allow for a mechanical bond (Figure 6–7).

(b) If the tooth does not appear frost-like, re-etch the tooth.

(11) Apply composite resin sealant material.

(a) Place a small amount of material only into the pits and fissures. Avoid covering the entire occlusal surface because excess material can interfere with occlusion.

(b) Apply material beginning at the mesial and allowing it to flow distally; this helps distribute the material.

(c) If necessary, dab with a microbrush to distribute the material. Avoid using an explorer for this task, because enamel rods are fragile, and the explorer can break the rods and shorten sealant life expectancy.

(12) Light cure. Follow manufacturer's directions for using the ultraviolet curing light to polymerize the material.

(13) Check the cured sealant to assure complete bonding by exploring around the margins; if voids in the material become evident, follow manufacturer's directions for filling them.

(14) Remove cotton rolls.

(15) Rinse tooth and mouth. Use copious amounts of water for this task to assist in removing the taste resulting from the material.

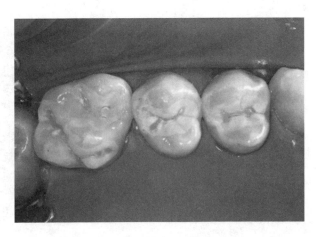

Figure 6–7 Notice the frost-like appearance of the etched teeth.

(16) Use HVE to evacuate water.

(17) Repeat procedure on all teeth receiving sealants.

(18) Instruct patient to close to check occlusion; if the patient feels an area of prematurity upon biting, the occlusion will need to be adjusted by using:

(a) Articulating paper to mark the high spots (articulating paper is a piece of paper with a color coating).

   i. Dry the teeth with the air syringe.

   ii. Place the paper between the upper and lower teeth.

   iii. Ask the patient to close, and tap teeth together—high spots in the material will be marked by the colored paper.

   iv. If the paper leaves a mark on the sealant, adjust that portion.

(b) Use a slow-speed handpiece and a stone or other abrasive to adjust the marked portion of the material, then remark.

   i. Continue this exercise until the patient is comfortable with the bite or the articulating paper no longer leaves a mark.

   ii. Avoid adjusting the tooth itself; adjust only the material.

8. Variations on resin sealants. The popularity of resin sealants has researchers finding ways to improve them.

  a. Some manufacturers have added photo-active color to the material.

    (1) One such material goes on with a pink color and cures opaque white (see Figure 6–8).

    (2) Another material turns green in the presence of UV light, allowing the operator to determine if the material is still present at subsequent examinations.

  b. Another modification is a resin sealant that has **hydrophilic** properties, as well as a low pH. This is called an integrated composite.

    (1) At a molecular level, the material seeks out water and, when it finds it, the pH drops even lower, effectively creating a "self-etching" state.

    (2) The majority of the material's working conditions is identical to traditional resin sealants.

    (3) Benefit of the hydrophilic nature. It penetrates the pits and fissures, seeking out minute amounts of water and creating a bond that is superior to one without this feature. The hydrophobic

Figure 6–8   Resin-based sealant application. *Photo courtesy of Dr. Chris Bryant.*

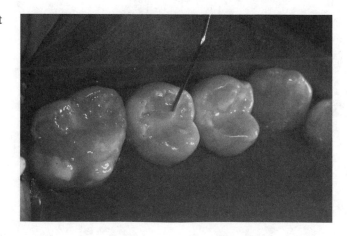

nature of resins without this feature causes the material to repel in the presence of water, creating a bubble-like effect at the margins. More information on this material is available at www.pulpdent .com.

B. Glass ionomer. Second choice of sealant material to use if resin sealant is not adequate.[9] This is true if the patient presents with high caries risk, xerostomia, or other conditions that preclude the use of resin sealants.

1. Constituents of glass ionomers (vary among different companies).
   a. Possess a chemical reaction different from other materials, making them an excellent choice for a certain category of patient; produce a material that provides a barrier against decay and releases fluoride to the surrounding hard tissue.
   b. Constituents include the following:[10]
      (1) Aluminum.
      (2) Calcium.
      (3) Salt.
      (4) Fluoride.
      (5) Phosphorus.
      (6) Silica.
      (7) One, or a combination, of the following acids:
         (a) Polyacrylic.
         (b) Tartaric.
         (c) Maleic.
2. Curing. Achieved by chemical reaction when the powder and liquid portions are mixed.
   a. Reaction is perpetual. The fluoride is not a structural component of the fully cured material, allowing it to move freely in and out of the sealant.
   b. Essentially, glass ionomers act as a rechargeable battery, releasing fluoride continually. When the fluoride gradient is such that there is more fluoride in the environment than in the material, it accepts the fluoride molecules.[4]
   c. Traditional resin sealant materials cure in the presence of light energy; glass ionomers cure as the mixed components react.
3. Bonding occurs chemically with enamel. The acid in the material breaks down the enamel at the site and fuses with the glass ionomer, creating a bond that is much stronger than the traditional mechanical bond. Because it fuses to the enamel, there is less chance of marginal breakdown or a poor bond.

   Note: In comparing Figure 6–3 with Figure 6–9, Figure 6–9 shows how the material's bond to the enamel is superior to the cohesive bond of the material.
4. Advantages.[11,12]
   a. Provides continual fluoride release for more than two years;[11,12] rechargeable with environmental fluoride.[11,12]
   b. Requires no etching or bonding agent. The low pH of the material liberates enamel molecules and allows for a fusion between the enamel and the glass ionomer (Figure 6–10).
   c. Can be used in nontraditional applications.
      (1) On broad surfaces of the tooth, such as the buccal, lingual, mesial, and distal.

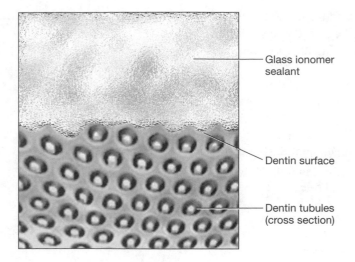

Figure 6–9 Chemical bonding (or attachment) to the tooth.

Glass ionomer sealant

Dentin surface

Dentin tubules (cross section)

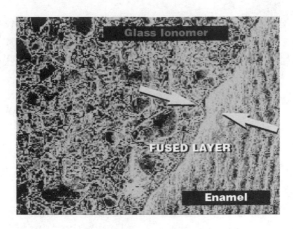

Figure 6–10 Glass ionomer attachment to tooth. *Photo courtesy of Dr. Hien Ngo.*

(a) Traditional sealants are too fluid to be placed on any surface other than the occlusal.

(b) If a patient presents with psychological, physical, or physiological limitations that precludes him or her from accessing all surfaces of all the teeth, a glass ionomer surface protectant is recommended.

(2) In a moist environment. Although glass ionomers cannot be placed in a puddle of saliva, they can be placed in a moist environment; isolation of the tooth is only important to keep the tongue at bay and excessive moisture off the tooth (Figure 6–11).

(3) On a partially erupted tooth. Traditional resin sealants cannot be placed under an operculum due to moisture concerns and immaturity of the enamel. However, glass ionomers can be placed under these conditions and have shown great promise in this application[3] (Figure 6–12).

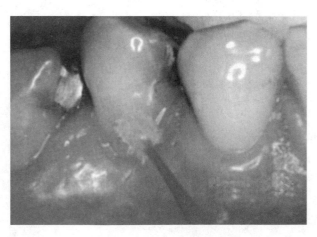

Figure 6–11 Glass ionomer can be placed in a moist environment. *Photo courtesy of Dr. Hien Ngo.*

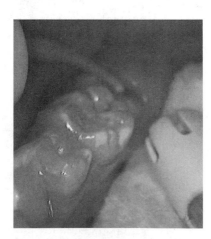

Figure 6–12 Placement of glass ionomer under an operculum. *Photo courtesy of Dr. Hien Ngo.*

d. Can actively remineralize enamel by fluoride passing through the material as well as other components of enamel repair, such as calcium and phosphates. Incipient decay has been shown to be deactivated after placement of glass ionomer with the tooth becoming remineralized.[13,14]

e. Able to view in pits and fissures with scanning electron microscope after visibly worn[15]—glass ionomers have a reputation for being soft. Early studies have given glass ionomers short shrift as a sealant material due to this characteristic. Later studies have found that, although the material is not visible to the naked eye, scanning electron microscopy provides proof that the material is still present, providing a physical barrier to decay while continually releasing fluoride.[4]

f. Thermal expansion. Similar to that of enamel.[4]

g. No shrinkage occurs during polymerization, which provides a more stable bond.[1]

h. Permeable by calcium and phosphorus.

i. Does not allow biofilm growth. Due to the nature of the material, biofilm cannot grow on the material for extended periods of time, increasing its effectiveness as a surface protectant.[16,17]

j. Buffers lactic acid in the vicinity of the material. This benefit is magnified by the fact that in an acidic environment, even more fluoride is released.[4,18]

k. Material is hydrophilic. Without this property, the material can fracture (Figure 6–13).

l. Requires little cooperation from the patient. Since glass ionomers are not sensitive to moisture, they are easier to place in a pre-cooperative patient. While in place as a surface protectant, the patient with the above-mentioned disability can experience a lower caries rate.

m. Biocompatibility. In dentistry all materials strive to be biocompatible—their presence does not cause damage or disease.
   (1) Example: Tissue does not respond favorably to amalgams placed at the gingival surface.
   (2) However, glass ionomers can be used as a surface protectant at the gingival surface without causing complications to the soft tissue.

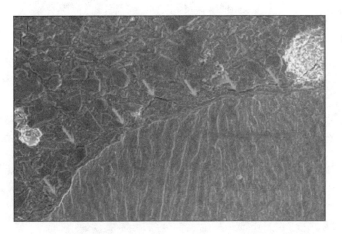

Figure 6–13 Glass ionomer material is hydrophilic.

5. Disadvantages.[9]
   a. Possesses difficult handling properties—material must be mixed. It is dispensed in capsules and mixed in a triterator.
   b. Wears with time. Because the overriding purpose of a sealant is to block the pits and fissures, which are not in occlusion, it is not contraindicated in patients who brux; material will remain where it is needed most.
   c. Working and curing times are dependent on chemical reaction, which may vary; for example, on a hot, humid day the material may take longer to cure because of the material's hydrophilic nature.
6. Case selection. The following patient criteria must be evaluated prior to choosing glass ionomer as the sealant material. Because of its unique properties, patients who present with the following attributes are good candidates for this sealant material. Caries risk factors (for a full discussion on caries risk establishment, refer to the section on composite resin sealants) include:
   a. Must be moderate-to-high risk. This sealant material is recommended for patients whose risk for decay is higher than for patients considered for resin sealants.
   b. Possess moderate-to-heavy biofilm. Because this material reduces attached biofilm, it is a good choice for patients who cannot manage their own biofilm removal.
   c. Poor diet, such as:
      (1) Frequent acid challenges from food, beverages, and/or bacterial by-products.
      (2) Making poor dietary choices, such as a high simple sugar diet.
      (3) Consuming simple carbohydrates and soft foods frequently.
      (4) Limiting the variety of raw foods.
   d. Uninsured. The uninsured population is statistically at higher risk for decay.[8]
   e. Physically challenged. May not be able to maintain adequate oral hygiene.
   f. Ineffective oral hygiene. Not properly or thoroughly removing plaque and food particles.
   g. Insufficient topical fluoride. Those not receiving low doses throughout the day.
   h. Low income. This group is at risk for caries.[8]
   i. Erupting teeth. Teeth with an operculum and immature enamel can still be sealed.
   j. Incipient decay determined by laser or light device. Research has proven that detecting decay with an explorer lacks sensitivity.[19] Newer devices can give objective feedback that allows operators to detect accurate levels of demineralization; one such product is the DIAGNOdent (KaVo USA).
      (1) Sealants placed over incipient decay are proven to be effective; the American Association of Pediatric Dentistry (AAP) also supports the practice.
      (2) Difficulty arises when establishing parameters for incipiency; using an explorer as a tool for detecting decay limits the operator's ability to detect decay.[1] With the advent of more accurate diagnostics, the practice should be more accepted.

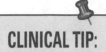

CLINICAL TIP:

Sealing Your Knowledge: Newer glass ionomers have increased retention and the ability to resist wear and fracture.

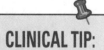

CLINICAL TIP:

Sealing Your Knowledge: A tutorial for DIAGNOdent is available at www.kavo.com.

k. Dependent elderly. Fall in the same classification as children. If they have teeth, someone is taking care of the teeth for them. Studies support that those providing oral care in dependent living situations want to help take care of the teeth, yet fall short of that goal. Glass ionomers are indicated for this cohort.

7. Surfaces for placing glass ionomer sealant/surface protectant. Because of the chemical bond and its viscosity, it is easy to place this material on all surfaces, not just the pits and fissures. Advantages, such as fluoride release and ability for calcium and phosphates to penetrate it, makes it an excellent product to protect surfaces that have never been considered for sealants before.

a. Occlusal. Traditional placement.

b. Broad surfaces: Facial, lingual, mesial, distal.

8. Preparing for placement of the glass ionomer sealant.

a. Clean the surfaces of the teeth receiving the glass ionomer surface protectant.

(1) Use an appropriate means to remove organic matter, such as prophy paste with prophy brush or cup, or an air polisher.

(2) Rinse with water, using the air/water syringe, enough to remove the debris left by the polishing procedure.

(3) Use HVE or saliva ejector to remove water and saliva.

b. Isolate the tooth with cotton rolls. When working alone, cotton rolls help with moisture control, as well as hold the tongue and cheek away. Total saliva management is not as important for glass ionomer sealants as it is for resin sealants. The chance for a sealant bomb is unlikely with this material because of the superior bond, fluoride release, and ability of the material to allow calcium and phosphates to penetrate.

(1) Place one cotton roll in the buccal vestibule of the mandibular teeth.

(2) Place another cotton roll under the tongue. This helps retract the tongue, as well as absorb the saliva from Wharton's duct.

(3) Instruct patient not to move his or her tongue; it should be relaxed on the floor of the mouth.

(4) Place Dri Angle or Dri tip onto the buccal mucosa; this step blocks the Stensen's duct and passively holds the mouth open.

(5) Remove visible water from the tooth with suction and a sweeping motion from the air syringe, enough to allow clear visualization of the tooth.

c. Mix the glass ionomer according to manufacturer's directions. The material comes in premeasured capsules, containing the correct ratio of powder and liquid (Figure 6–14).

(1) Direct application. This is one way to deliver the product to the tooth. The indirect method of placing glass ionomer follows in section 2 on page 166.

(a) Once mixed, place the capsule into the applier (the gun) from the kit (see directions that came with the material for a drawing). If placed correctly, as the handle is squeezed, a plunger will emerge, penetrating the capsule's plunger, which forces the material out of the tip (Figure 6–15).

Figure 6–14   Mixing glass ionomer material in a premeasured capsule.

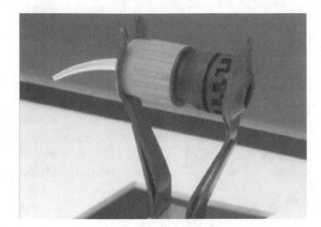

(b) Squeeze a small amount onto the indicated areas one at a time (Figure 6–16).

(c) Set the applier on the bracket table and wet the index finger of the dominant hand from the buccal mucosa or from the air/water syringe.

(d) Press the glass ionomer into each tooth with the wet gloved finger, one at a time, with moderate pressure. This has been shown to increase penetration and retention of the material.

(e) Remove cotton rolls and Dri Angles.

(f) After approximately 60 to 90 seconds from the mixing time, ask the patient to close together; this step adjusts the occlusion, removing excess material from the cuspal slopes.

(2) Indirect method.

(a) Tooth preparation is similar to the preparation necessary for the occlusal surface; tooth must be clean of obvious debris.

(b) Extrude material onto a treated paper pad, also known as a mixing pad.

(c) Dab a microbrush (flocked plastic stick) into the sealant material.

(d) Dab the loaded brush onto the tooth's surface, placing the material into the grooves (Figure 6–17).

CLINICAL TIP:

Sealing Your Knowledge: Using an explorer to maneuver the material into the pits and fissures may only accomplish breaking the enamel rods, increasing chances for complete sealant failure.

Figure 6–15   Using an applier (gun) to dispense glass ionomer material.

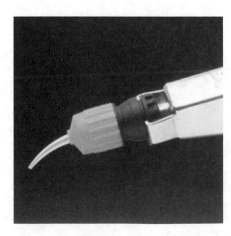

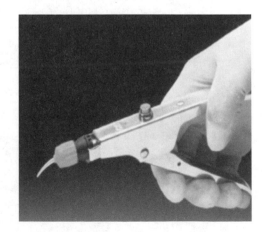

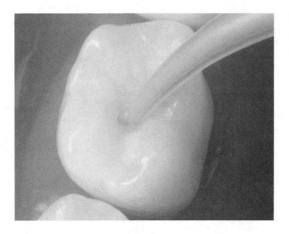

Figure 6–16   Squeeze small amount of material onto occlusal surface.

(e) After 20 to 30 seconds of setting time, wet the gloved index finger of the dominant hand and press the glass ionomer onto the tooth with moderate pressure.

(f) Remove cotton rolls and Dri Angles.

(g) After approximately 60 to 90 seconds from the mixing time, ask the patient to close together; this step adjusts the occlusion, removing excess material from the cuspal slopes.

(h) Indirect method for surfaces other than the occlusal.

   i. Tooth preparation is similar to the preparation necessary for the occlusal surface; tooth must be clean of obvious debris.

   ii. Apply the glass ionomer with a microbrush in a thin coat over the surface needing protection (see Figure 6–10).

- Avoid bulky application at the gingival/cervical area although glass ionomers are biocompatible. Improper placement with excessive material can allow debris to become trapped at the gingival area.

- At about the 90-second mark, use an instrument such as a sickle scaler to remove excess that may have accumulated near the gingival area before the material fully cures.

CLINICAL TIP:

Sealing Your Knowledge: Primary teeth have not been seen as candidates for sealants in the past. The position paper from the AAP encourages sealants on all teeth, even primary teeth.[2]

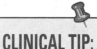

CLINICAL TIP:

Sealing Your Knowledge: It is not necessary to avoid fluoride application before applying resin sealants.

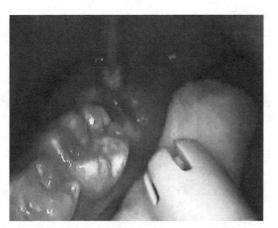

Figure 6–17   Dab loaded brush onto tooth surface.

9. Recommendations from the Academy of Pediatric Dentistry (APD)[2] regarding sealants.
    a. Effectiveness and safety.
        (1) Bonded composite resin sealants, placed by appropriately trained dental personnel, are safe, effective, and underused in preventing pit and fissure caries on at-risk surfaces.
        (2) Effectiveness is increased with good technique and appropriate follow-up and resealing as necessary.
    b. Benefits.
        (1) Increased by placement on surfaces judged to be at high risk or surfaces that exhibit incipient carious lesions.[2]
        (2) Placing sealant over minimal enamel caries has been shown to be effective in inhibiting lesion progression.
        (3) Appropriate follow-up care, as with all dental treatment, is recommended.
    c. Evaluation of risk. Performed by an experienced operator using indicators of tooth morphology, clinical diagnostics, past caries and fluoride history, and present oral hygiene care.
        (1) Caries risk and potential sealant benefit. May exist in any tooth with a pit or fissure, at any age, including primary teeth of children and permanent teeth of children and adults.
        (2) Placement methods. Should include careful cleaning of the pits and fissures without removal of any appreciable enamel; some circumstances may indicate use of a minimal enameloplasty technique.
        (3) Retention. A low-viscosity, hydrophilic material bonding layer as part of, or under, the actual sealant has been shown to enhance long-term retention and effectiveness.
        (4) Glass ionomer materials have been shown to be ineffective as pit and fissure sealants, but could be used as **transitional sealants.**
        (5) The profession must be alert to new preventive methods effective against pit and fissure caries; these may include changes in dental materials or technology.
    d. Additional information presented in the position paper.
        (1) Caries risk can change over time.
        (2) Sealing primary teeth is worthwhile.
        (3) No anticaries advantage. There is no fluoride in the traditional composite resin sealant.
        (4) Sealants can be placed after a fluoride treatment. The notion that fluoride application directly prior to sealant placement interferes with the etching process has been disproved. The position of the APD is that it is acceptable to place sealants directly after an office fluoride treatment.
10. Advancements in glass ionomer materials. Any dental material is in a continual process of evolution; glass ionomers are no exception.
    a. In the future, attempts will be made to increase flowability and compressive strength.
    b. Another advancement is to add substances to the material, such as Recaldent®, which provides the building blocks for possible tooth remineralization.

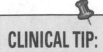

CLINICAL TIP:

Sealing Your Knowledge: There are no long-term studies to show that enameloplasty is effective.[1]

CLINICAL TIP:

Sealing Your Knowledge: Caries risk can change with time. A stroke can cause a patient who was diligent with home care to suddenly become ineffective, increasing the risk. A child gaining manual dexterity can become less of a risk for decay, or a patient who gets dental insurance is in a cohort who, statistically, has less of a caries risk.

(1) Recaldent is an amorphous calcium phosphate encased in casein phosphopeptide-amorphous calcium phosphate (CPP-ACP), making the components for tooth remineralization available from the glass ionomer.

(2) One study published in 2003 suggested that this marriage of products produced a "superior material (to glass ionomer alone) with improved anticariogenic potential."[20]

VI. Controversies Concerning Sealants

There are a number of controversies in dentistry.

A. Amalgam. Some are lobbying to remove the use of mercury in restorative materials.

B. Municipal water fluoridation. Some still do not want fluoride in water systems. Fluoride works best in low, frequent doses; systemic fluoride has lost favor over the last few years.

C. Sealants. The American Dental Association (ADA) has a position paper on this; an overview of the controversy follows:[21]

1. Resin sealants and estrogen.

a. Components of sealants are said to release an estrogen-like substance that, in theory, contributes to breast cancer and testicular cancer.

b. The official declaration made in the January 2000 issue of the *Journal of the American Dental Association* (JADA).

(1) Eleven out of twelve sealants did not emit the problem substance.

(2) Further studies are anticipated.

c. Sealants should be carefully placed in the pits and fissures to decrease any chance for wear.

2. **Enameloplasty**[2,22] (removal of enamel using microdentistry techniques, such as air abrasion or fissurotomy burs).

a. Justification. Removing incipient decay will allow a better seal and less microleakage; the following are justifications dentists use to perform enameloplasty:

(1) Decay under sealants.

(2) Unsure of fissure anatomy.

(3) Incipient decay.

b. Unwarranted. Study after study has proven this practice to be unnecessary due to:[2]

(1) Unknown safety.

(2) Unnecessary to have decay-free fissure.

(3) Weakens tooth.

c. Not a preventive procedure. The entire idea behind placing sealants is not to perform surgery on the tooth and enameloplasty is surgery; sealants preserve tooth structure, whereas enameloplasty removes tooth structure.

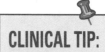

CLINICAL TIP:

Sealing Your Knowledge: For additional information, conduct an Internet search using key phrases *estrogen, sealants,* and *sealant controversy.*

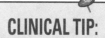

CLINICAL TIP:

Sealing Your Knowledge: With enameloplasty, the pits and fissures are opened using air abrasion, a special bur called a fissurotomy bur or laser.

Sealants have been proven as an adjunct to the total oral care dental hygienists can provide for their patients. Critical thinking skills are important in assessing the patient for the best possible sealant material to use. Caries risk is an important risk assessment tool that can help the operator make the best choice for which material should be used.

ADA Position and Statement

Estrogenic Effects of Bisphenol A Lacking in Dental Sealants

A 1996 study conducted by researchers in Spain and published in *Environmental Health Perspectives* found that a chemical, bisphenol A (BPA), which can potentially mimic human estrogen, leached out of dental sealants.[1] Although the study did not show any causal effect between the presence of BPA and any health condition, the ADA was sufficiently concerned about this research to conduct its own evaluation.

Of the 12 brands of dental sealants that currently carry the ADA Seal of Acceptance, 11 of the 12 materials leached no detectable BPA on first analysis; on second analysis, one sealant leached a trace amount of BPA within the test sensitivity (5 parts per billion). The manufacturer of this sealant was contacted. After additional quality control procedures were implemented in the manufacturing process, detectable BPA was successfully eliminated in the final product. (BPA is not a direct ingredient of dental sealants; it is a starting raw chemical that appears in the final product only when the raw materials fail to fully react.)[2]

Hence, none of the dental sealants that carry the ADA Seal release detectable BPA, although it must be emphasized that there is no evidence to suggest a link between any adverse health condition and BPA leached out of dental sealants.

The ADA also looked beyond product chemistry for the presence of BPA in dental sealants. The Association tested the blood of dentists who had dental sealants on their teeth and those who did not. The ADA examined 40 blood samples: 30 were from dentists with one to 16 sealed surfaces, and ten samples were from dentists who had no sealants. BPA was not found in any of the blood samples from either group, suggesting that if BPA is leached from dental sealants it is not detectable in blood tests; thus, it does not present an estrogenic hazard.[3]

In addition to its laboratory studies, the ADA worked with researchers at University of Nebraska Dental School on a clinical project to measure BPA exposure during and after sealant application. Dental sealants were applied to test subjects, then saliva and blood samples were collected at various time intervals after sealant application. This study showed that BPA released orally from a dental sealant may either not be absorbed or is not detectable at or above 5ppb when measured in systemic circulation.[4]

An article in the Journal of American Dental Association corroborates ADA findings regarding BPA and dental sealants. Researchers at Boston University School of Dental Medicine who tested seven brands of sealants confirmed that none released any BPA.[4,5]

1. Olea N, Pulgar R, Perez P, Olea-Serrano, Rivas A, Novillo-Fertrell, Pedraza V, Soto A, Sonnenschein C. Estrogenicity of resin-based composites and sealants used in dentistry. *Environmental Health Perspectives,* Vol. 104, 1996, 298–305.
2. Bowen RL. Use of epoxy resins in restorative materials. *Journal of Dental Research,* Vol. 35, 1956, 360–369.
3. Siew C, Miaw CL, Chou HN, Gruninger SE, Geary R, Fan PL, Meyer DM. Determination of bisphenol A in dentist serum samples (Abstract 1070). *Journal of Dental Research,* Vol. 77, 1998 (Special Issue A).
4. Fung EYK, Ewoldsen NO, St.Germain HA, Marx DB, Miaw C-L, Siew C, Chou H-N, Gruninger SE, Meyer DM. Pharmacokinetics of bisphenol A released from a dental sealant. *Journal of the American Dental Association,* Vol. 131, 2000, 51–58.
5. Nathanson D, Lertpitayakun P, Lamkin M, Edalatpour M, Chou LL. In vitro elution of leachable components from dental sealants. *Journal of the American Dental Association,* Vol. 128, Number 11, 1997, 1517–1523.

August 04, 1998   Page Updated: June 05, 2002

QUESTIONS

1. Sealants are appropriate for which age group?
   a. Children under 6 years of age.
   b. All age groups.
   c. Children with erupting teeth.
   d. Dependent elderly.

2. Where should a Dri Angle be placed?
   a. On the tongue.
   b. Against the palate.
   c. Against the oral mucosa, with the widest portion positioned mesially.
   d. Against the oral mucosa, with the widest portion positioned distally.

3. Which of the following is the best list of the advantages of resin sealants?
   a. Good esthetics, fluoride release, long history.
   b. Long history, no mixing, occlusal adjustments.
   c. No mixing, long history, not time sensitive.
   d. Chemical bond, no etching, insensitive to moisture.

4. Before placing the composite resin sealant material, which is the correct order the following steps should be completed?
   a. Clean the tooth, rinse, etch, and rinse.
   b. Clean the tooth, apply fluoride, and place cotton rolls.
   c. Apply fluoride, place cotton rolls, etch, and rinse.
   d. Etch, rinse, and dry.

5. Resin sealants release enough fluoride to remineralize teeth. Glass ionomers have the ability to recharge with fluoride.
   a. Both statements are TRUE.
   b. Both statements are FALSE.
   c. The first statement is TRUE. The second statement is FALSE.
   d. The first statement is FALSE. The second statement is TRUE.

6. Which sealant material would be BEST to use for a 30-year-old developmentally challenged patient with no incidence of caries, high biofilm levels, or poor diet?
   a. Resin sealant.
   b. Glass ionomer sealant.
   c. No sealant necessary.
   d. Would address the diet before making a sealant decision.

REFERENCES

1. Berg JH. The continuum of restorative materials in pediatric dentistry—A review for the clinician. *Pediatric Dentistry,* Vol. 20, Number 2, 1998.

2. Feigal RJ. The use of pit and fissure sealants. *Pediatric Dentistry,* Vol. 24, Number 5, 2002.

3. Taifour D, Frencken JE, van't Hof MA, Beiruti N, Truin GJ. Effects of glass ionomer sealants in newly erupted first molars after 5 years: A pilot study. *Community Dental Oral Epidemiology,* Vol. 31, Number 4, 2003, Aug, 314–9.

4. Freedman R, Diefenderfer KE. Effects of daily fluoride exposures on fluoride release by glass ionomer-based restoratives. *Operative Dentistry,* Vol. 28, Number 2, 2003.

5. Tinanoff N, Kanellis MJ, Vargas CM. Current understanding of the epidemiology, mechanisms, and prevention of dental caries in preschool children. *Pediatric Dentistry,* Vol. 24, 2002, p. 6.

6. Sanchez GA, Fernandez De Preliasco MV. Salivary pH changes during soft drink consumption in children. *International Journal of Paediatric Dentistry,* Vol. 13, 2003, 227–251.

7. Featherstone J. Prevention and reversal of dental caries: Role of low level fluoride. *Community Dental Oral Epidemiology,* 1999, p. 27.

8. Dennison JB, Straffon LH, Smith RC. Effectiveness of sealant treatment over five years in an insured population. *Journal of the American Dental Association,* Vol. 131, Number 5, 2000.

9. Berg JH. Glass ionomer cements. *Pediatric Dentistry,* Vol. 24, Number 5, 2002.

10. Katsuyama S, Ishikawa T, Fujii B. *Glass Ionomer Dental Cement—The Materials and Their Clinical Use.* St. Louis, MO: Ishiyaku, 1993.

11. Croll RP, Nicholson JW. Glass ionomer cements in pediatric dentistry: Review of the literature. *Pediatric Dentistry,* Vol. 24, 2002, p. 5.

12. Forsten L. Short- and long-term fluoride release from glass ionomers and other fluoride-containing filling materials in vitro. *Scandinavian Journal of Dental Research,* 1990, p. 98.

13. van Amerongen WE. Dental caries under glass ionomer restorations. *Journal of Dental Public Health,* Vol. 56, Number 3, 1996, special issue.

14. ten Cate JM, van Duinen RN. Hypermineralization of dentinal lesions adjacent to glass ionomer cement restorations. *Journal of Dental Research,* 1995.

15. Weerheijm KL, Kreulen CM, Gruythuysen RJM. Comparison of retentive qualities of two glass-ionomer cements used as fissure sealants. *Journal of Dentistry for Children,* 1996, July-August.

16. Berg JH, Farrell JE, Brown LR. Class II glass ionomer/silver cement restorations and their effect on interproximal growth of mutans streptococci. *Pediatric Dentistry,* Vol. 12, Number 1, 1990.

17. Friendl KH, Schmalz G, Hiller KA. Resin-modified glass ionomer cements: Fluoride release and influence on *Streptococcus mutans* growth. *European Journal of Oral Sciences,* Vol. 105, Number 1, 81–5, 1997.

18. Carey CM, Spencer M, Gove RJ, Eichmiller FC. Fluoride release from a resin-modified glass-ionomer cement in a continuous-flow system. Effect of pH. *Journal of Dental Research,* Vol. 82, Number 10, 2003, October, 829–32.

19. Chong MJ, Seow WK, Cheng E, Wan V. Visual-tactile examination compared with conventional radiography, digital radiography, and DIAGNOdent in the diagnosis of occlusal occult caries in extracted premolars. *Pediatric Dentistry,* Vol. 25, Number 4, 2003, July–August, 341–9.

20. Mazzaoui SA, Burrow MF, Tyas MJ, et. al. Incorporation of casein Phosphopeptide-amorphous calcium phosphate into a glass-ionomer cement. *Journal of Dental Research,* Vol. 82, Number 11, 2003.

21. Estrogenic Effects of Bisphenol a Lacking in Dental Sealants, http://www.ada.org/prof/resources/positions/statements/seal_est.asp. Accessed 8/10/04.

22. Blackwood JA, Dilley DC, Roberts MW. Evaluation of pumice, fissure enameloplasty and air abrasion on sealant microleakage. *Pediatric Dentistry,* Vol. 24, Number 3, 2002.

SEALANT PERFORMANCE COMPETENCY

Student _____

Date _____

Instructor _____

Tooth Numbers

1. _____ 5. _____
2. _____ 6. _____
3. _____ 7. _____
4. _____ 8. _____

Re-evaluation

Instr: _____

Date _____

	S	U	Comments	S	U	Comments
1. Selects appropriate tooth to be sealed.						
2. Cleans and rinses each tooth surface with appropriate agent.						
3. Isolates selected tooth.						
4. Dries tooth surface thoroughly.						
5. Maintains a dry field throughout entire procedure.						
6. Acid-etches surfaces for the appropriate amount of time.						
7. Rinses thoroughly and dries tooth surfaces before applying sealant material.						
8. Fills selected tooth surfaces with the correct amount of material and avoids overfilling pits and grooves.						
9. Light-cures sealant material for the appropriate amount of time.						
10. Checks surfaces for a smooth, consistent appearance.						
11. Checks occlusion with articulating paper.						
12. Correctly adjusts occlusion of sealant, if needed.						

Courtesy of Indiana University Purdue University Fort Wayne Dental Hygiene Program.

173

Chapter 7

Rubber Dam Isolation

Michelle Hurlbutt, RDH, BS and Debi Gerger, RDH, BS, MPH

MediaLink

A companion CD-ROM, included free with each new copy of this book, supplements the procedures presented in each chapter. Insert the CD-ROM to watch video clips and view a large collection of color images that is also included. This multimedia library is designed to help you add a new dimension to your learning.

KEY TERMS

anchor tooth	operating field	rubber dam napkin
inverting instrument	palm grasp	rubber dam punch
isolation	rubber dam clamp	rubber dam stamp or template
key punch hole	rubber dam forceps	septa/septum
ligate	rubber dam frame/holder	
modeling compound	rubber dam material	

LEARNING OBJECTIVES

After reading this chapter, the student will be able to:

- explain the indications and contraindications for use of rubber dam isolation;
- select the armamentarium needed to place and remove a rubber dam;
- demonstrate the proper technique for rubber dam placement and removal;
- discuss the appropriate patient instruction for the use of a rubber dam;
- describe why it is important for the operator to use rubber dam isolation during dental hygiene practice.

I. Introduction

In 1864 a New York City dentist, S.C. Barnum, introduced the rubber dam into dentistry.[1] Designed to isolate one or more teeth, it was originally available as a thin rubber sheet that was purchased by the yard.[2] Today the rubber dam is commonly available in both latex and latex-free precut sheets that are 6″ × 6″ for permanent dentition and 5″ × 5″ for primary dentition. It is also available in a variety of flavors, scents, and colors from light to dark, with darker colors preferred by operators because of the greater contrast between tooth structure and the rubber dam material as well as decreasing glare. The purpose of the rubber dam is to maintain a favorable working environment while protecting the patient and operator during preventive and restorative procedures and to avoid contamination of the operating field by saliva, plaque, blood, and/or crevicular fluid that can diminish the success of the procedure.[3,4,5]

A. In the practice of dental hygiene (based on state regulations), the rubber dam is utilized during application of pit and fissure sealants, desensitizing agents, fluorides; during the treatment of a special needs patients; and during placement and polishing of restorative materials.[6] While the rubber dam may not be utilized as often as other moisture control techniques, the dental hygienist will find it advantageous to successful treatment outcomes.

B. The rubber dam is also a key element in the reduction of bloodborne pathogens or cross-contamination, as well as protecting the patient from ingesting debris.[7]

II. Indications for Use[1]

A. Moisture control. Eliminates or controls excess saliva, water, blood, crevicular fluid, dental materials, infectious contaminants, and tooth fragments from the **operating field.** Treatment outcomes are more favorable if moisture control is maintained throughout the procedure.

B. Improved access and visibility. Access and visibility are greatly improved with the use of the rubber dam because only the isolated teeth are exposed in the operating field. Procedures performed with greater access and visibility will be less prone to postprocedure problems related to contamination. In addition, time saved by working in an area of **isolation** may more than compensate for the time spent applying the rubber dam.[8]

C. Improved properties of dental materials. The four categories of dental materials are metals, ceramics, polymers, and composites. Each material can be described by its physical, mechanical, chemical, and biological properties.
1. These properties can be adversely affected by the presence of oral contaminants including saliva, water, blood, and crevicular fluid.
2. An appropriate oral environment can improve the properties of dental materials, ultimately leading to a high quality preventive or restorative procedure with increased long-term clinical expectancy of restorations.

D. Protection of patient and operator. The rubber dam protects the patient by preventing ingestion and/or aspiration of debris or dental materials as well as protecting the soft tissues. At the same time, the rubber dam protects the operator by reducing transmission of bloodborne pathogens during a dental procedure.

E. Operating efficiency. Using the rubber dam enhances operating efficiency and can lead to increased productivity. Mouth opening is maintained and excessive patient conversation is better managed with the use of a rubber dam. During quadrant procedures, less time may be needed for treatment because it creates an ideal operating field.

F. Special needs patients include those with transient or permanent mental, physical, medical, social, and/or oral needs who may require a modified care plan that could include rubber dam placement. In particular, patients who would benefit from the use of a rubber dam would include those who suffer from difficulty swallowing (dysphagia), limited opening or ability to open, macroglossia, excessive salivation and drooling, resting tremors, involuntary movements, loss of power of voluntary motion (akinesia), partial or complete paralysis, or when sedated or under general anesthesia.

III. Contraindications for Use[1]

A. Malpositioned teeth, partially erupted teeth, and third molars. The ability to place the rubber dam is compromised when teeth are malaligned, not erupted sufficiently to support a clamp, or developmentally malformed or malpositioned third molars. Placement can be accomplished to some degree by modifying where holes are punched in the **rubber dam material.**

B. Latex allergies can be life-threatening and therefore must be avoided in the dental environment. In these cases, treatment will need to be implemented using a latex-free rubber dam.

C. Time consuming. Rubber dam setup, placement, and removal can take as long as 10 minutes and must be considered in patient scheduling.

D. Claustrophobics and asthmatics. People who are claustrophobic, certain asthmatics, and patients who have difficulty breathing through the nose may not be able to tolerate the use of the rubber dam because it may feel too confining.

CLINICAL TIP:

Isolating Your Knowledge: Old rubber dam material will tear more easily because of deterioration. Be sure to use relatively new material with each procedure.

IV. Armamentarium (Figure 7–1)

A. Sterilized basic instrument set-up. Mouth mirror, explorer, and cotton pliers.

B. Rubber dam material. Operator must choose the appropriate size, gauge, and color for the treatment area and the patient.
1. Latex or latex-free (Figure 7–2).
2. Roll of 6′ × 18′ or precut sheets of 5″ × 5″ or 6″ × 6″.
3. Sterile or nonsterile.
4. Gauge (weight/thickness).
   a. Light or thin is 0.15 millimeters.
   b. Medium is 0.20 millimeters.
   c. Heavy is 0.25 millimeters.
   d. Extra heavy is 0.30 millimeters.
   e. Special heavy is 0.35 millimeters; properties include:
      (1) More functional.
      (2) Less likely to tear.
      (3) More effective in tissue retraction.
      (4) More difficult to place.
5. Color.
   a. Dark. Used mainly with adults. Has more contrast and reflects less light; available in gray, green, blue, pink, and purple.
   b. Light. Used mainly with children. Higher patient acceptance; available in ivory, buff, and pastels.

CLINICAL TIP:

Isolating Your Knowledge: Many new rubber dam materials are available to help make placement easier.

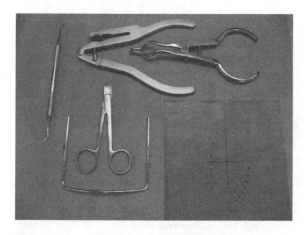

Figure 7–1 Armamentarium for rubber dam placement.

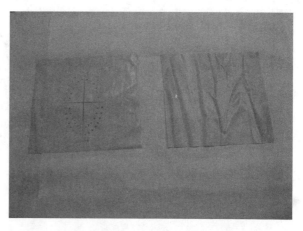

Figure 7–2 Rubber dam material. Latex versus latex-free.

6. Flavors or scents include mint and fruit.

C. **Rubber dam napkin** is placed between the patient's face and rubber dam material; made from paper, gauze, or flannel.

1. Acts as a cushion to increase comfort.
2. Absorbs perspiration, water, and saliva.
3. Acts as a barrier against skin contact with the rubber dam material.

D. Sterile **rubber dam punch** (Figure 7–3). Designed to create holes in the rubber dam material needed for teeth to be isolated and exposed. When operating the punch, select the correct hole size for the treatment tooth/teeth, make a complete puncture with no ragged or leftover material, and punch the correct distance between holes to establish a **septa/septum.** Parts of the rubber dam punch include:

1. Stylus (cutting tip). Working end that is a tapered, sharp pointed plunger; used to create holes rubber dam material (Figure 7–4).
2. Punch plate (wheel table) (see Figure 7–4). A rotating metal disc table with 1 to 6 holes varying in size with 1 being the smallest. Each hole in the punch plate is associated with specific teeth:
   a. Hole 1: Mandibular incisors.
   b. Hole 2: Maxillary incisors.
   c. Hole 3: Premolars and canines.
   d. Holes 4 and 5: Molars.
   e. Hole 6: **Key punch hole** or **anchor tooth** hole.

E. Sterile **rubber dam forceps** (Figure 7–5). Used to place and remove **rubber dam clamp.**

1. Parts.
   a. Beaks: Prongs located at the working end that fit into the holes of the clamp to assist in holding and stretching the clamp into position on the anchor tooth.
   b. Spring: Located between the working end and the handle to allow for opening and closing of the beaks.
   c. Locking bar: Located below between the spring and handle to keep the forceps in a fixed position while the clamp is being positioned.

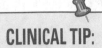

CLINICAL TIP:

Isolating Your Knowledge: The rubber dam napkin provides a convenient method for wiping or drying the patient's lips and face upon removal of the rubber dam.

CLINICAL TIP:

Isolating Your Knowledge: An inappropriately punched rubber dam may occlude the patient's nasal airway. If this happens, fold or cut the superior border of the rubber dam material from under the patient's nose.

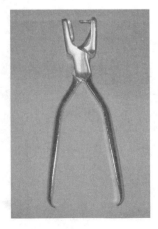

Figure 7–3   Rubber dam punch.

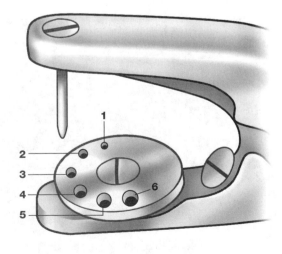

Figure 7–4   Punch plate and stylus.

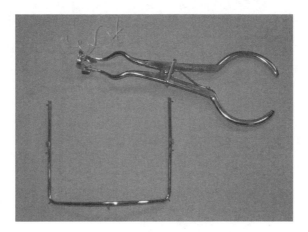

Figure 7–5   Rubber dam forceps and frame/holder.

    d. Handle: Located opposite of the working end and used to open and close the beaks.
2. Grasp.
    a. Underhand **palm grasp.** Use palm-up grasp when placing a maxillary clamp with the beaks oriented in an upright position.
    b. Overhand palm grasp (Figure 7–6). Use palm-down grasp when placing a mandibular clamp with the beaks oriented in a downward position.
3. Operation.
    a. Open forceps: Squeeze handles together to allow spring action to open the beaks of the forceps.
    b. Close and lock forceps: Squeeze handles, allowing the locking bar to slide towards the handles; locking the forceps allows the forceps to remain in a fixed position.
F. Sterile rubber dam clamp/retainer. Made of either chrome or nickel-plated steel. Sterilize between uses. Used to retract gingival tissue and anchor the rubber dam material to the most posterior tooth to be isolated; should have a four-point contact (two on the facial and two on the lingual surface) for stabilization; available in numerous sizes and shapes.

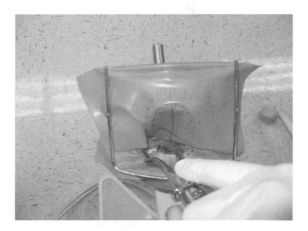

Figure 7–6   Overhand palm grasp.

Figure 7–7   Parts of a rubber dam clamp.

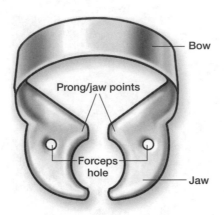

1. Parts (Figure 7–7).
    a. Bow: Rounded portion of the clamp through which the rubber dam material extends.
    b. Forceps hole: Opening where beaks of the forceps are placed.
    c. Jaw: Supports the prongs and may contain wings.
    d. Prong or jaw points: Four prongs that are necessary to stabilize the clamp on the tooth.
2. Designs.
    a. Winged (Figure 7–8). Designed with extra projections for better retention of the dam; marked with an identification number specific for the tooth (i.e., 8).
    b. Wingless (Figure 7–9). Designed without extra projections; marked with a W in front of the identification number (i.e., W8).
    c. Cervical. Designed to be used for Class V, facial restorations.
    d. Posterior.
    e. Anterior.
3. Suggested clamps for anchor teeth.
    a. W7 or 7: Mandibular molar anchor teeth.
    b. W8 or 8: Maxillary molar anchor teeth.
    c. W2 or 2: Premolar anchor teeth.
    d. W9 or 9: Anterior anchor teeth.

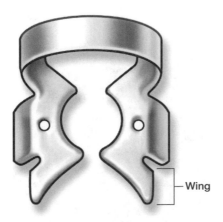

Figure 7–8   Winged clamp.

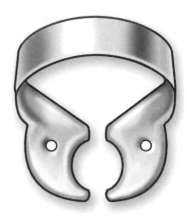

Figure 7–9   Wingless clamp.

G. Sterile or disposable **rubber dam frame/holder** (see Figure 7–5). Made of sterilizable plastic or metal with projections that allow for rubber dam material to be stretched away from the operating field; used to maintain the borders of the rubber dam and to assist in isolating the treatment area; types include:
1. Plastic U-shaped frame. Radiolucent plastic frame placed under the rubber dam material; allows for exposure of radiographs without removal.
2. Young frame. Metal or plastic frame; placed outside or inside of the rubber dam material; may or may not be used with a dam napkin.
3. Ostby frame. Radiolucent plastic frame commonly utilized in endodontics; placed outside of the rubber dam material; allows for exposure of radiographs without removal.
4. Woodbury frame. A frame with attachable elastic straps; positioned behind the patient's head.
    a. Two metal clip arms containing three clips each secure the rubber dam material and retract the cheeks and lips.
    b. Must use a rubber dam napkin.
5. Snap-shut. A plastic frame with a snap-shut design; holds rubber dam material securely in place by two mated frames firmly pressed together.[9]
6. Preframed rubber dam. Rubber dam with a built-in plastic or metal frame, often with prepunched holes; may be sterilizable or disposable.
H. **Rubber dam stamp or template.** Use to properly position the holes on the rubber dam material; various designs are available and include:
1. Template (Figure 7–10). A plastic stencil. Use a pen to mark holes onto the rubber dam material for primary and permanent dentitions.
2. Stamp. Use with an inked pad to mark holes onto the rubber dam material.
3. Study model or wax bite. Use patient's study model or wax bite to locate the proper hole position for severely malposed teeth.
I. Sterile scissors (crown and collar). Use small, straight, or curved scissors to cut a hole for the saliva ejector, a corner portion for retention, or septal portion of rubber dam material during removal phase.
J. Modeling/impression compound. Red or green stick **modeling compound;** utilized to secure the clamp to the tooth to prevent movement during a procedure. However, care must be taken to avoid filling the clamp forceps holes.

CLINICAL TIP:

Isolating Your Knowledge: Rubber dam scissors are available with a hook-shape on one end.

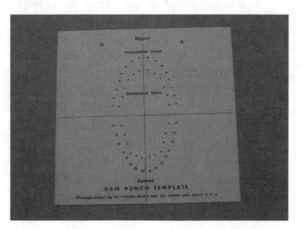

Figure 7–10   Rubber dam template.

Figure 7–11   Rubber dam clamp
ligated with floss.

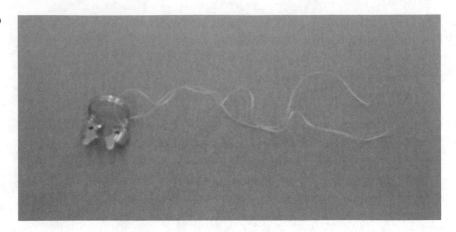

K. Sterile **inverting instrument.** Used to invert or tuck the edges of the dam around the teeth, creating a seal to prevent leakage of saliva or other oral fluids.[10] Use a dull instrument such as a plastic instrument, black spoon, or beavertail burnisher.

L. Floss. Use four 12- to 18-inch strands of waxed floss or dental tape to place rubber dam clamp and material (Figure 7–11).
1. Attach floss to the bow of the rubber dam clamp as a safety ligature, prior to placing in the patient's mouth. If the clamp becomes dislodged or is swallowed during the procedure, pull on the floss to retrieve the clamp.
2. Floss teeth prior to rubber dam placement to test and open the contacts, as well as cleanse the area.
3. Use a floss strand to:
   a. **Ligate** the most anterior tooth in the treatment area. This will wedge the rubber dam material under the contact for stabilization.
   b. Aid in the placement and insertion of the septal portion of the rubber dam material.

M. Lubricant. Use on the patient's lips and the outside and inside of the rubber dam material. Types include:
1. Petroleum jelly. May only be used on patient's lips and corners of the mouth; can degrade latex and may interfere with certain dental materials.
2. Zinc oxide ointment. May be placed on the patient's lips.
3. Cocoa butter. May be placed on the patient's lips and corners of the mouth to prevent irritation.
4. Water-soluble lubricant. Place on both sides of the rubber dam material near the holes to assist in sliding the material over the teeth.

N. Cotton rolls and gauze squares. Use to apply lubricants to lips and rubber dam material; may also use to absorb excess fluid from around the exposed teeth during placement of the rubber dam material; in addition, gauze may be used during the removal process.

V. Isolation Technique

It is important for the operator to prepare for the placement of the rubber dam isolation procedure to ensure a successful treatment outcome. This is accomplished through careful consideration of the patient's tooth/teeth involved, including anomalies, type of procedure planned, and personal product preferences of the operator.

A. Preparation.
1. Evaluate the medical and dental histories for any contraindications or modifications required.
2. Effectively communicate the rubber dam isolation protocol to the patient; answer any concerns or questions.[11]
3. Use a mouth mirror to inspect the treatment area.
4. Floss all teeth within the treatment area.
5. Note the size and shape of the arch prior to punching the material.
6. Choose the correct size holes to punch in accordance with the treatment area.
7. Mark the rubber dam material using the rubber dam stamp or template.
8. Punch the rubber dam material using the correct size punch plate hole; for better access and visibility, the material should be punched two teeth distal to the treatment tooth.
9. Lubricate the outside and inside surfaces of the rubber dam material around the punched holes with a water-soluble lubricant.
10. Select the correct rubber dam clamp for the anchor tooth.
11. Tie floss to the bow of the rubber dam clamp using a slipknot; for additional security, the operator may thread the floss through the forcep's holes in the rubber dam clamp.
12. Insert beaks of forceps into the rubber dam clamp; slide the locking bar into place.
13. Prepare and sequence all other equipment for rubber dam placement.
B. Placement. There are two acceptable techniques of rubber dam placement, a one-step method and a two-step method. The most common technique used is the two-step method, described as follows:
1. Instruct patient to prerinse with an antimicrobial, following the manufacturer's instructions.
2. Position patient appropriately for the area of treatment.
3. Lubricate the patient's lips with selected lubricant.
4. Retrieve rubber dam forceps (beaks already inserted into the clamp).
5. Insert and seat the rubber dam clamp by positioning the lingual jaw, then the facial jaw; stabilize the rubber dam clamp with the nonoperating index finger (Figure 7–12); release rubber dam forceps.
6. Locate the key punch hole in the rubber dam material; stretch over bow and under jaws of the rubber dam clamp.
7. Thread the floss ligature (tie to the bow of the rubber dam clamp) through the key punch hole.

CLINICAL TIP:
Isolating Your Knowledge: Since the patient will be unable to effectively communicate with the rubber dam in place, it is suggested the operator and patient agree on some signs to be used for communication.

CLINICAL TIP:
Isolating Your Knowledge: If using a rubber dam on a fixed bridge, punch holes only for the abutment teeth, not the pontic tooth.

CLINICAL TIP:
Isolating Your Knowledge: Rubber dam material has a shiny and dull side. It is recommended that the powdered dull side be positioned toward the operator to reduce glare.

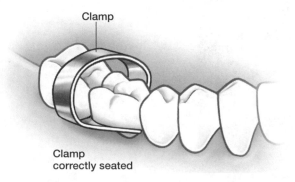
Clamp

Clamp
correctly seated

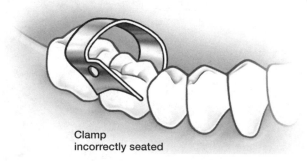
Clamp
incorrectly seated

Figure 7–12   Seating the rubber dam clamp.

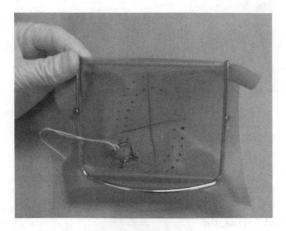

Figure 7–13   Placing the rubber dam frame over the rubber dam material.

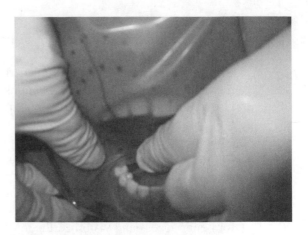

Figure 7–14   Fitting rubber dam material into contact areas.

8. If used, position the rubber dam napkin by carefully pulling the rubber dam material through the opening of the napkin.

9. Position the rubber dam frame over the rubber dam material, hooking the material to the projections as indicated for the type of frame being utilized (Figure 7–13).

10. Fit the last hole, opposite of the key punch hole, over the tooth to stabilize and aid in detecting the remaining holes.

11. Fit the remaining holes into the contact areas using the index fingers of both hands (Figure 7–14).

12. Floss the contacts to further insert the rubber dam material interproximally; if the contacts are extremely tight, a wooden wedge may be used to open the contact (Figure 7–15).

13. Place a floss ligature around the tooth furthest from the anchor tooth or use a rubber dam stop.

14. Invert the rubber dam material by stretching it over the teeth.

15. Using a dull instrument of choice, gently invert the rubber dam material into the sulcular area, working from distal to mesial for each tooth. This will prevent oral fluid seepage. Direct a stream of air into the sulcus while inverting the rubber dam material to create a dry operating field and to prevent the material from slipping out of the sulcus (Figure 7–16).

Figure 7–15   Flossing rubber dam material into contact areas.

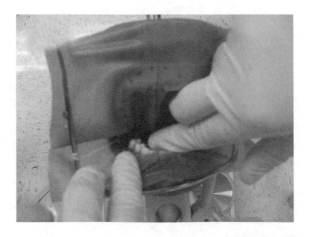

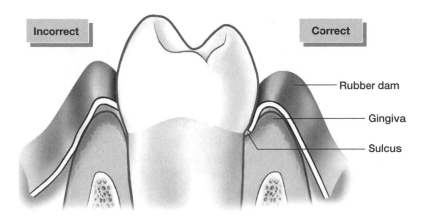

Figure 7–16 Placement of rubber dam material into sulcular area.

16. If needed, modeling compound can be applied to the bow of the rubber dam clamp and tooth to further stabilize.
   a. Soften compound by holding over heat source, such as a butane torch or Bunsen burner until tip bends.
   b. Place the tip of the modeling compound in hot water for 5 seconds.
   c. Twist off approximately 3/8 inch of tip and shape into cone.
   d. Reheat cone of compound in flame.
   e. Place softened compound under bow of clamp (occlusal surface), away from area to be treated.
   f. Repeat procedure for opposite side of the clamp.
   g. At completion of treatment, remove the compound prior to removing the rubber dam clamp and rubber dam material.
17. Place a saliva ejector under the rubber dam material onto the floor of the mouth, opposite the treatment area. An alternative is to cut a small hole in the rubber dam material behind the mandibular incisors and insert the saliva ejector.
18. One-step method alternative. Frequently used method by a novice because it is easier and often involves less time.
   a. Follow preparation steps 1 to 12.
   b. Stretch rubber dam material over the wing or jaw of the rubber dam clamp (see Figure 7–13).
   c. Proceed with preparation step 13.
   d. Replace placement steps 5 and 6 with the following:
      (1) Place rubber dam clamp on the anchor tooth while taking caution to position the clamp supragingivally before releasing forceps.
      (2) Reposition the rubber dam material under the wing or jaw of the rubber dam clamp.
   e. Proceed with placement steps 7 to 14.
C. Removal.
   1. Remove the saliva ejector.
   2. If used, remove modeling compound from rubber dam clamp and tooth by using an explorer or scaler.
   3. Rinse operating field of all debris, using HVE.
   4. Remove floss ligature tie from around tooth.
   5. Use fingers, placed underneath the rubber dam material, to remove inverted material from the sulcus by pulling laterally and toward the occlusal surfaces.

CLINICAL TIP:

Isolating Your Knowledge: For patients who have difficulty breathing only through the nose, an opening in the rubber dam material can be made in the palatal area by pinching the dam with cotton pliers and cutting a small hole.

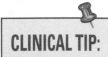

6. Use scissors and cut with one stroke from hole-to-hole on the facial aspect of the rubber dam material; this will create one long opening and decrease the number of rubber dam material remnants; use caution to avoid cutting patient's lip and/or cheek (Figure 7–17).

7. Pull the rubber dam material lingually, freeing the septa material from the interproximal spaces.

8. Remove the rubber dam clamp by placing the beaks of the rubber dam forceps into the holes and squeeze the handle; lift to remove.

9. Remove the rubber dam frame and rubber dam material simultaneously.

10. If placed, remove and use the rubber dam napkin to wipe the patient's lips and mouth to eliminate excess moisture and debris; if not used, a tissue or heated cloth can be used to wipe the lips and mouth.

11. Inspect the rubber dam material to account for any missing material left in the sulcus or oral cavity. If any material is missing, a careful inspection is required; use dental floss or an explorer to remove subgingival remnants.

12. Rinse and evacuate the oral cavity.

13. Inspect the soft tissues for any noticeable trauma.

14. Gently massage gingival tissues in the treatment area.

15. Provide appropriate patient instruction and answer any questions or concerns.

16. Instruct patient to postrinse with an antimicrobial, following the manufacturer's instructions.

17. Process instruments using presoak, ultrasonic cleaning, and sterilization methods. Discard all disposables and disinfect treatment room.

The rubber dam isolation procedure is a favorable technique to control moisture in an operating field, limiting cross contamination, providing benefits to the properties and manipulation of various dental materials, and enhancing patient comfort during care. The application process is relatively painless and can be performed in 3 to 5 minutes in the hands of a skilled operator. It is important to remember that if the rubber dam is left in place for long periods of time or if remnants of the rubber dam material are not completely removed, postoperative pain, gingival irritation, and/or more serious complications may occur. The use of the rubber dam by the dental hygienist can help to ensure successful outcomes for a variety of procedures and should be considered when creating a dental hygiene care plan.

Figure 7–17   Cutting rubber dam material for removal.

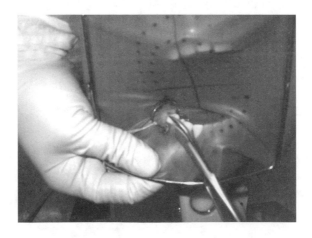

Questions

1. Rubber dam isolation is indicated for moisture control, improved access and visibility, and protection of the patient and operator. A rubber dam may not be indicated for a patient who is claustrophobic or asthmatic.
   a. Both statements are TRUE.
   b. Both statements are FALSE.
   c. The first statement is TRUE. The second statement is FALSE.
   d. The first statement is FALSE. The second statement is TRUE.

2. What is the primary purpose of the rubber dam frame?
   a. To provide a barrier between the patient's face and the rubber dam material.
   b. To anchor the rubber dam material to the rubber dam clamp.
   c. To stretch the rubber dam material away from the operating field.
   d. All of the above are correct.

3. A sterile instrument is used to invert the rubber dam material subgingivally. All of the following instruments can be used for this procedure or step in rubber dam isolation EXCEPT one. Which one is the EXCEPTION?
   a. Black spoon
   b. Plastic instrument
   c. Beavertail burnisher
   d. Sickle scaler

4. During the preparation phase of rubber dam isolation, it is important for the operator to do all of the following EXCEPT one. Which one is the EXCEPTION?

   a. Inform the patient of what the procedure entails and answer any questions.
   b. Lubricate the patient's lips and both sides of the rubber dam material.
   c. Punch the rubber dam material considering any dental anomalies or deviations.
   d. Seat the rubber dam clamp on the anchor tooth using either the one-step or two-step method.

5. After placing the rubber dam clamp, rubber dam napkin, and rubber dam frame, the next step the operator should take is to
   a. pull the floss ligature through the key punch hole.
   b. fit the rubber dam material over the tooth furthest from the anchor tooth.
   c. fit the rubber dam material over the anchor tooth, including the bow and jaws.
   d. insert the septal rubber dam material under each contact using both hands.

6. When removing rubber dam material, it is important to cut each hole slowly and separately to carefully remove the septal material. If the rubber dam material is not completely removed, the tissue may abscess and the involved tooth may be lost.
   a. Both statements are TRUE.
   b. Both statements are FALSE.
   c. The first statement is TRUE. The second statement is FALSE.
   d. The first statement is FALSE. The second statement is TRUE.

References

1. Roberson TM, Heymann HO, Swift EJ Jr, ed. *Sturdevant's Art and Science of Operative Dentistry,* 4th ed., St. Louis, MO: Mosby, 2002.

2. Covington E. *The Efficient Dental Assistant.* St. Louis, MO: Mosby, 1940.

3. Knight GT, Berry TG, Barghi N, Burns TR. Effects of two methods of moisture control on marginal microleakage between resin composite and etched enamel: A clinical study. *International Journal of Prosthodontics,* Vol. 6, 1993, 475–79.

4. Fishelberg G, Hook D. Patient safety during endodontic therapy using current technology: A case report. *Journal of Endodontics,* Vol. 29, 2003, 683–84.

5. Hewlett ER, Cox CF. Clinical considerations in adhesive restorative dentistry—influence of adjunctive procedures. *Journal of the California Dental Association,* Vol. 31, 2003, 477–482.

6. Simonsen RJ. Pit and fissure sealant: Review of the literature. *Pediatric Dentistry,* Vol. 24, 2002, 393–414.

7. Sopena B, Garcia-Caballero L, Diz P, De la Fuente J, Fernandez A, Diaz JA. Unsuspected foreign body aspiration. *Quintessence International,* Vol. 34, 2003, 779–81.

8. Christensen GJ. Using rubber dams to boost quality and quantity of restorative service. *Journal of the American Dental Association,* Vol. 125, 1994, 81–82.

9. Ahlers, MO. A new rubber dam frame design—easier to use with a more secure fit. *Quintessence International,* Vol. 34, 2003, 203–10.

10. Sopena B., Garcia-Caballero L., Diz P., De la Fuente J., Diaz, JA. Unsuspected foreign body aspiration. *Quintessence International,* Vol. 34, 2003, 779–81.

11. Stewardson DA, McHugh ES. Patients' attitudes to rubber dam. *Journal of International Endodontics,* Vol. 35, 2002, 812–19.

Chapter 8

Sutures

Michelle Hurlbutt, RDH, BS and Debi Gerger, RDH, BS, MPH

MediaLink

A companion CD-ROM, included free with each new copy of this book, supplements the procedures presented in each chapter. Insert the CD-ROM to watch video clips and view a large collection of color images that is also included. This multimedia library is designed to help you add a new dimension to your learning.

KEY TERMS

absorbable suture	memory	surgeon's or friction knot
approximate	needle holder	surgical knot tying
bacterial wicking	nonabsorbable suture	suture
dead space	periodontal surgery	tensile strength
elasticity	pliability	throws
hemostasis	primary intention healing	wound
ligate	square knot	

LEARNING OBJECTIVES

After reading this chapter, the student will be able to:

- explain the indications and contraindications for use of a suture;
- discuss the characteristics of an ideal suture;
- describe the criteria for a well-placed suture;
- identify the types of suturing materials and needles available;
- select the armamentarium needed to remove sutures;
- demonstrate the proper technique for removal of sutures;
- discuss the appropriate patient instruction for the use in the removal of sutures;
- describe why it is important for an operator to be able to understand the use and removal of sutures.

I. Introduction

A **suture** is a strand of material used to **ligate** or tie blood vessels and to approximate or sew tissues together until healing has occurred. The use of sutures to aid in the healing process can be traced to ancient Egyptian scrolls dating back to 3000 BC.[1]

Some of the earliest materials used included flax, hair, linen strips, grasses, pig bristles, horse hair, cotton, silk, gut of animals, nylons, polyesters, and metals.[2] The earliest use of gut can be traced back to the ancient Greek physician Galen. The 18th century brought the use of buckskin and silver wire. By the twentieth century, cotton and treated natural materials were the most used materials for suturing.[3] Modern synthetic materials have replaced most of the old suture materials, but a few remain such as silk.

The purpose of the suture is to achieve **primary intention healing** holding tissues together until the **wound** can withstand normal functional stresses. In dentistry, sutures are required to close periodontal surgical wounds as well as secure grafts in place. In addition, sutures are routinely used during oral, implant, orthognathic and **periodontal surgery.** As a competent operator, it remains advantageous for the dental hygienist to be familiar with the basic rules associated with suture placement as well as the types of suture materials available and the technique used to remove sutures.

II. Characteristics of an Ideal Suture

A. Sterile.
   1. Prepackaged with a needle and strand together; needle and strand are coiled in foil, plastic, and cardboard sheaths that are covered by foil or foil and polyethylene tear-open packaging.
   2. After packaging, sutures are sterilized by gamma irradiation or ethylene oxide.
B. High **tensile strength.** Resists deformation and breakage.
C. Easy handling.
   1. Low **memory:** Requires fewer **throws** to secure knot.
   2. Good **elasticity:** Allows for suture to be stretched tight enough to **approximate** tissues but loose enough to prevent tissue necrosis.
   3. High **pliability:** Increases ability to adjust knot security and tension.
D. Holds securely when knotted.
E. Uniform diameter.
F. Tissue biocompatibility.
   1. No tissue reactivity.
   2. Nonallergenic.
   3. Noncarcinogenic.
G. Resistant to infection.
H. Predictable performance.

III. Indications for Use

A. Close a surgical or traumatic wound.
B. Attach grafted gingival tissues or regeneration membranes to recipient sites.
C. Promote primary intention healing.
D. Provide **hemostasis.**
E. Reduce postoperative discomfort.
F. Eliminate **dead space.**
G. Prevent underlying bone exposure.
H. Restore natural anatomic contours.

IV. Contraindications for Use

A. Evidence of infection of the wound.
   1. Reddening of margins of the wound with discharge of pus is a classic sign of infection, and the wound should not be closed until it has been allowed to "clean up," which involves debridement of dead and devitalized tissue, administration of broad-spectrum antibiotic, culture for bacterial infection, and daily evaluation.
   2. Most traumatic wounds are contaminated, and the risk of infection is higher. Persistent fever or toxemia of the patient related to the wound is also an indicator of infection. It is common practice to delay closure in wounds older than 6 hours.

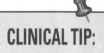

CLINICAL TIP:

Securing Your Knowledge: At the present time, no single suture material can provide all of these characteristics. It is up to the surgeon to select the best material for the procedure.

B. Types of wounds that are typically not sutured.

1. Some large gaping wounds of soft tissue, puncture wounds, and animal bites.

2. Vitality of surrounding tissue is in doubt.

3. Those older than 6 hours may not be sutured because healing has already started.

4. Those better suited for closure with adhesive tapes, liquid tissue adhesives, or staples.

C. Known allergy to suture material. It is important to be aware of the patient's sensitivity to the suture material and, in the case of chromic gut suture, if the patient has a sensitivity to chromium or chromic salts. Although metallic sutures are not commonly used in dentistry, if the patient has a sensitivity to a particular metal, such as nickel, caution should be taken to not use a metallic alloy material that may contain the allergen.

D. Suture material not appropriate for type of wound. The type of material from which the suture is manufactured plays a large role in the effectiveness of the suture. Different tissues have differing requirements for suture support, some needing only a few days while others require weeks or even months. The surgeon must be aware of the differences in the healing rates of various tissues when choosing a suture material. It is also critical the surgeon understand which suture material is appropriate for the clinical site.

V. Classification of Sutures

A. Tissue Behavior

1. **Absorbable suture.**
   a. Made of natural or synthetic material.
   b. Maximum tensile strength lost quickly over time.
   c. Material absorbed via proteolysis or hydrolysis.
   d. Does not need to be removed postsurgery.
   e. Used when extended wound healing is not required.

2. **Nonabsorbable suture.**
   a. Made of natural or synthetic material.
   b. High tensile strength over time.
   c. Does not degrade readily; gradual encapsulation within healed wound by fibrous connective tissue.
   d. Requires removal following primary healing of wound.

B. Structure.

1. Monofilament. Single-stranded or single-filament suture.
   a. Less tissue reactive and resists harboring bacteria (less **bacterial wicking**).
   b. Less tensile strength compared to multifilament suture.
   c. Tends to have significant memory and can be difficult to handle.
   d. Less tissue drag and glides easily through tissue.
   e. Can be placed with less resistance and ties more smoothly than multifilament.
   f. Recommended for regeneration surgery to reduce inflammation.

2. Multifilament. Several suture filaments twisted or braided together to form a strand.
   a. Increased handling and manipulation.
   b. Easy to securely knot but variability in knot strength may arise from technical aspects of manufacturing process.

CLINICAL TIP:

Securing Your Knowledge: Chromic gut suture is plain gut treated with chromic salts to resist enzyme absorption. Generally, this suture causes less tissue irritation and increases tensile strength compared to plain gut.

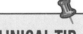

CLINICAL TIP:

Securing Your Knowledge: Proteolysis is a decomposition by natural body enzymes that attack and break down the suture strand. Hydrolysis is a decomposition by water that gradually penetrates the suture strand, breaking it down.

CLINICAL TIP:

Securing Your Knowledge: Encapsulation means to surround, encase, or protect in, or as if in a capsule.

c. Generally has higher tensile strength than monofilament.

d. Increased tissue drag compared to monofilament.

e. Increased bacterial wicking because spaces between filaments can harbor bacteria.[4]

C. Origin

1. Natural: Composed of organic material.

a. Surgical gut. Processed from purified collagen of sheep and bovine intestines; sometimes referred to as cat gut; not recommended for wounds requiring long-term healing and wound security.[2]

(1) Types.

(a) Chromic gut. Plain gut treated with chromic salts to resist enzyme absorption; causes less tissue irritation and increases tensile strength; absorbed in 10 to 14 days.

(b) Plain gut. Weak, easily frayed, and causes moderate tissue reaction; absorbed in 7 to 10 days.

(2) Properties include:

(a) Tensile strength affected by individual patient characteristics.

(b) Can be difficult to handle and knot.

(c) Absorbed via proteolytic enzymatic digestive process; does not require postsurgical removal by the operator.

b. Silk: Processed from raw silk spun by silkworms and by removing natural wax and gums, then impregnated with mixtures of waxes or silicones; choice for most periodontal surgeries[4]; properties include:

(1) High visibility in oral cavity.

(2) Superior handling and easy to knot.

(3) Increased bacterial wicking can be seen; not recommended in areas of infection.

(4) Loses tensile strength when exposed to moisture.

(5) Considered nonabsorbable, but if left in body, will be absorbed by proteolysis and is often undetectable in the wound site even after two years. In dentistry, generally requires postsurgical removal by operator.

c. Surgical cotton: Processed from cotton fibers into long twisted strands; properties include:

(1) Higher tensile strength than gut or silk.

(2) Nonabsorbable and, if left, will become encapsulated within body tissues.

(3) Not routinely used in dentistry.

2. Synthetic: Composed of man-made material.

a. Absorbable.

(1) Polyglactin 910 (Figure 8–1). Copolymer of lactide and glycolide; also known as Vicryl™, Coated Vicryl™, and Vicryl Rapide™.

(a) Retains 70 percent of initial strength at 10 days and 30 percent at 20 days.

(b) Completely absorbed between 60 and 90 days.

(c) Braided multifilament; available in dyed violet or undyed.

(d) Minimal tissue reaction.

(e) Smooth and precise knot placement.

(2) Polyglycolic acid. Homopolymer of glycolic acid; also referred to as PGA, Dexon®; properties include:

(a) In the oral cavity, retained for approximately 16 to 20 days; complete absorption occurs over a period of 60 to 90 days.

CLINICAL TIP:

Securing Your Knowledge: Cat gut is a term used to describe gut suture. It is one of the oldest sutures used, but is unreliably absorbed and loses tensile strength quickly.

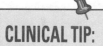

CLINICAL TIP:

Securing Your Knowledge: Raw silk is orange in color and, after processing, is dyed black for increased visibility.

CLINICAL TIP:

Securing Your Knowledge: Due to their limited tissue reaction, synthetic absorbable sutures are often used in periodontal surgical procedures. Despite their absorbability, suture removal is usually performed within 10 days after placement.

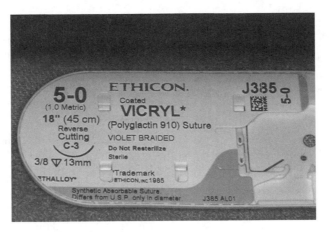

Figure 8–1 Polyglactin 910.

     (b) Braided multifilament.

     (c) Minimal tissue reaction.

  (3) Poliglecaprone 25. Copolymer of glycolide and epsilon-caprolactone; also known as Monocryl™; properties include:

     (a) High tensile strength through two weeks of wound healing and complete absorption in 90 to 120 days.

     (b) Monofilament with high pliability.

     (c) Less tissue reaction than gut.

  (4) Polydioxone. Polymer of paradioxanone; also known as PDS™ and PDS II™; properties include:

     (a) Retains 70 percent of initial strength for approximately 21 days and is reduced to 50 percent at approximately 35 days.

     (b) Absorption usually complete within 180 days.

     (c) Monofilament.

     (d) High memory causes suture to "recoil."

  (5) Polyglyconate. Copolymer of trimethylene carbonate and glycolic acid; also known as Maxon™ and Maxon CV™; properties include:

     (a) Absorption minimal until 30 days with complete absorption seen in 120 days.

     (b) Monofilament; available in clear or dyed green.

     (c) Additional throws needed to secure knot.

b. Nonabsorbable.

  (1) Nylon. Created from polymers of polyamide; available as monofilament or braided filament; generally excellent elasticity; monofilaments also known as Ethilon™, Dermalon®, and braided filaments also known as Nurolon™ and Surgilon®; properties include:

     (a) Monofilament; available in dyed black, blue, or natural, and braided, dyed white or black.

     (b) Excellent elasticity.

     (c) High memory causes suture to "recoil" and requires more throws to secure knot.

     (d) Best used in a wet state.

  (2) Polyester. Created from polyethylene terephthalate polymers; also known as Ethibond™, Ethiflex™, Dacron®, Mersilene™, and Ticron®; properties include:

     (a) Braided; available in dyed green or white.

      (b) Polyester coated with polybutilate (also a polyester) for lubrication to aid in tissue passage; high tissue drag if not coated.

      (c) High tensile strength and does not degrade for up to two years.

      (d) Low tissue reactivity.

(3) Polypropylene. Created from isostatic crystalline stereoisomer of a linear propylene polymer; also known as Prolene™ and Surgilene®; properties include:

      (a) Monofilament; available in radiant blue.

      (b) High tensile strength.

      (c) Biologically inert and elicits little tissue response.

      (d) Holds knots better than other monofilament synthetic materials.

      (e) Useful in contaminated and infected wounds.

(4) Polytetrafluoroethylene. Created from polytetrafluorethylene that has been expanded to produce a porous microstructure that is approximately 50 percent air by volume; also known as Gore-Tex®; properties include:

      (a) Monofilament; undyed with no additives.

      (b) Minimal tissue reaction.

      (c) Tissue attaches to and collagen penetrates suture, making removal difficult.

      (d) Gore-Tex® suture supplied with periodontal guided tissue regeneration (GTC) membranes and guided tissue augmentation material (GTAM).

3. Metallic. Composed of surgical steel (iron-chromium-nickel-molybdenum alloy); also known as Flexon™; properties include:

  a. Available in monofilament or twisted multifilament.

  b. High tensile strength.

  c. Low tissue reactivity.

  d. Holds knot securely but difficult to handle due to kinking; surgeon must be careful of nearby tissues.

  e. Electrolytic reactions in presence of other metals or alloy.

D. Size. United States Pharmacopeia (USP) sets standards and guidelines for the suture industry, including classification of sutures based on their origin. Generally, the surgeon selects the smallest suture that adequately holds the wound edges to promote healing.

1. Size of suture is determined by its diameter.

  a. A number has been assigned to represent diameter ranging in descending order from 10-1 and then 1-0 to 12-0, with 1-0 being the largest and 12-0 being the smallest.

  b. Size is denoted as zeros, with more zeros equaling smaller diameter (i.e., 4-0 or 0000 is larger than 5-0 or 00000)

  c. The smaller the diameter of the suture strand, the less tensile strength of the material.

2. Optimal suture size is generally the smallest size necessary to achieve the desired tension-free closure. Cosmetic procedures, such as grafts, require smaller diameter sutures (5-0, 6-0) versus oral surgery procedures such as extractions of third molars (3-0, 4-0).

VI. Placement of Sutures

Proper suturing technique is needed to ensure good results. Since most sutures today are pre-packaged with a needle and strand together, selection of the needle is as important as the type of suture technique used.

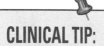

CLINICAL TIP:

Securing Your Knowledge: Twelve-0 suture is smaller in diameter than a human hair. Generally, 3-0 to 6-0 are the most common sizes used in dentistry.

A. Characteristics of an ideal needle.
   1. Sterile and corrosion resistant.
   2. Constructed of high-quality stainless steel.
   3. Penetrates tissue with minimal resistance; always sharp.
   4. Small diameter.
   5. Suture strand permanently attached.
   6. Disposable.
   7. Remains stable in **needle holder.**
B. Needle description. Dozens of needle design choices are available on the market. The primary consideration in selecting a needle is to choose one that will minimize tissue trauma. The needle may be coated with silicon to permit smoother passage through the tissues, thus decreasing tissue trauma. The components of the needle include the swage, body, and point of the needle (Figure 8–2).
   1. Swage (eye). Attachment section of the needle and strand. This creates a single, continuous unit of suture and needle; may be designed as a pop-off to permit easy release of the needle and suture material.
      a. Channel swage. Created in the needle where the suture strand is placed and then crimped over the suture to secure it; diameter is greater than that of the needle body.
      b. Drill swage. Material is removed from the back end of the needle and crimped over the suture strand; diameter is less than that of the needle body.
      c. Non-swaged. Suture strand may be passed through an eye, similar to that found in a sewing needle; eye can be round, oblong, or square; use can result in more tissue trauma; not commonly used in dentistry.
   2. Body (shaft). Midsection of the needle; majority of the needle between the swage to the point. Interacts with the needle holder and helps transmit the penetrating force to the point; grasp at the widest portion of the body (see Figure 8–2).
      a. Body should be as close as possible in diameter as suture strand material.
      b. Curvature or shape of the body is either straight, half-curved, curved, or compound curved; 3/8 curve most effective intraorally (Table 8–1).
      c. Cross-sectional configuration of the body may be round, oval, side-flattened rectangular, triangular, or trapezoid. Oval, side-flattened rectangular, and triangular shapes may be fabricated with longitudinal

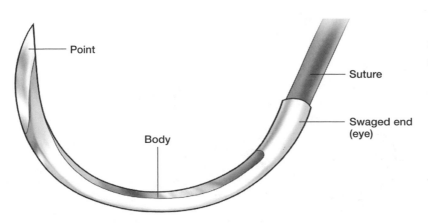

Figure 8–2 Components of the needle include point, body, and swage.

Table 8–1   Shapes of Needle Body

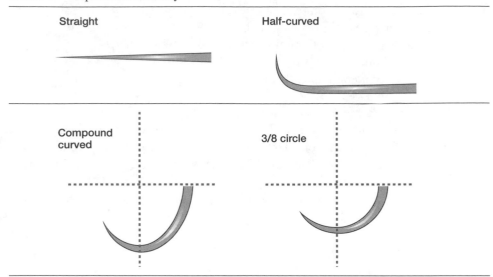

ribs on the inside or outside surfaces; this increases needle stability of the needle holder.

3. Point. Sharpest part of the needle extending from the extreme tip of the needle to the maximum diameter of the body; designed to produce the amount of sharpness needed to penetrate tissues smoothly.

a. Conventional cutting has three cutting edges, two opposing cutting edges, and a third on the inner, concave curvature of the needle directed toward the wound edge (Figure 8–3).

b. Reverse cutting has three cutting edges, with the third edge on the outer convex curvature of the needle, directed away from the wound edge, which reduces the risk of the suture pulling through the tissue (Figure 8–4).

c. Taper-point has no cutting edges, but a sharp tip that flattens to an oval/rectangular shape (Figure 8–5).

C. Suture techniques. The type of suture technique depends on the type and location of the wound, tissue thickness, and the desired end result. Sometimes more than one suture technique is needed. A needle holder is used to grasp the needle at the widest portion of the body, one-half to three-quarters of the distance from the swaged end. Incorrect placement of the needle in the needle holder may result in a bent needle and/or an undesirable angle of entry into the tissue.

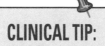

CLINICAL TIP:

Securing Your Knowledge: A reverse cutting needle is the needle of choice for oral mucosa because it is stronger than a conventional cutting needle and designed to cause minimal tissue trauma.

Figure 8–3   Conventional cutting needle.

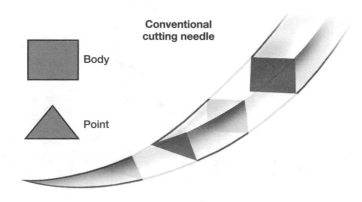

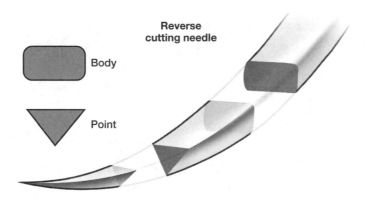

Figure 8–4   Reverse cutting needle.

1. Interrupted.
   a. Most common suture technique used by surgeons and one of the easiest to place.
   b. Less potential for causing wound edema and impaired circulation.
   c. Technique used to close straight-line incisions, vertical incisions, and retromolar areas. It uses a number of strands of suture material to close the wound; also recommended to gain good flap adaptation and tight flap closure.[1]
   d. Allows surgeon to make adjustments in wound adaptation to ensure proper alignment of wound edges.
   e. Requires time and precision to place and there is a greater risk of cross-hatched marks if sutures are removed later rather than earlier in the healing process.
   f. Several variations include circumferential (loop), figure eight, horizontal (Figure 8–6), vertical (Figure 8–7) and cross mattress, interproximal/interpapillary, and interrupted suspensory or sling suture.
2. Continuous uninterrupted.
   a. Uninterrupted or running sutures. Series of interrupted sutures that are tied, not cut, at one or both ends of the wound with one strand of suture material.
   b. Useful for attaching two flaps together and securing multiple interproximal papillae of one flap independently of the other.[4]
   c. There are fewer individual ties and, hence, this technique is quicker than the interrupted suture and generally causes less inflammatory response.
   d. Care must be taken when placing because excessive suture beneath the gingiva can create an environment promoting bacterial wicking.

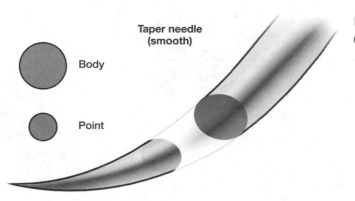

Figure 8–5   Taper needle (smooth).

Figure 8–6   Interrupted horizontal mattress suture technique.

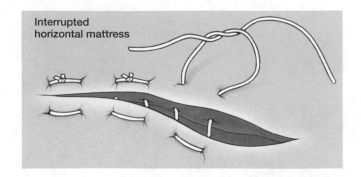
Interrupted horizontal mattress

Figure 8–7   Interrupted vertical mattress suture technique.

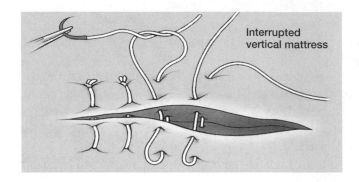
Interrupted vertical mattress

Figure 8–8   Running locked suture.

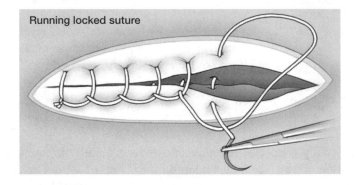
Running locked suture

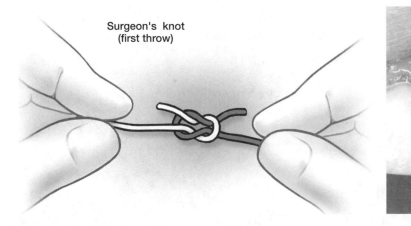
Surgeon's knot (first throw)

Figure 8–9   Square knot.

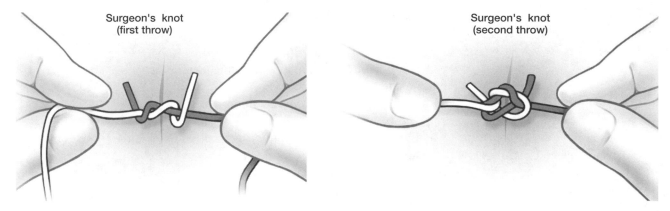

Surgeon's knot
(first throw)

Surgeon's knot
(second throw)

Figure 8–10   Surgeon's knot.

In addition, if a knot is lost or loosened, the approximated edges of the wound can become untied, thus causing potential for poor wound healing.

   e. Types of continuous uninterrupted sutures include running (Figure 8–8), suspensory or sling suture, and continuous lock or blanket suture.

3. **Surgical knot tying.** There are several ways to tie a suture knot; two most common methods are the **square knot** and the **surgeon's or friction knot.**[2]

   a. Square knot (Figure 8–9).

      (1) Easiest and most reliable.

      (2) Can be used with gut, silk, cotton and metallic sutures; if used with synthetic sutures, additional throws may be needed.

      (3) Generally recommended to use two hands with this technique.

      (4) If strands are incorrectly crossed, a granny knot will result, which has a tendency to slip and is not recommended.[2]

   b. Surgeon's or friction knot (Figure 8–10).

      (1) Recommended for use with synthetic sutures.

      (2) Knot security is critical for successful suture placement.

      (3) May be performed with one-handed technique using needle holder.

VII. Removal of Sutures.

A. Armamentarium. Basic setup includes:

   1. Mouth mirror.

   2. Explorer.

   3. Cotton pliers.

   4. Suture removal scissors. Curved sharp scissors with pointed tip.

   5. Sterile 2″ × 2″ gauze.

   6. Topical anesthetic.

   7. Irrigating syringe.

   8. Chlorhexidine gluconate or other antimicrobial agent.

B. Instruct patient to prerinse with antimicrobial agent.

C. Evaluate patient chart for the surgical site and number and type of sutures placed.

D. Patient examination.

   1. Check healing of tissue around sutures; many times sutures and knots are slightly buried in healing tissue.

CLINICAL TIP:

Securing Your Knowledge: A square knot is formed by weaving two strands of suture together with two tight throws in opposite directions (one throw in one direction, and another throw in the opposite direction).

CLINICAL TIP:

Securing Your Knowledge: A surgeon's knot is formed in the same fashion as the square knot, except there are two throws in one direction and another throw in the opposite direction.

CLINICAL TIP:

Securing Your Knowledge: After placing sutures, it is important to document the location, number placed, and type of material used.

2. Assess for signs of infection, deviations in color, shape, and adaptation of tissue or flap.
3. Record any significant findings in chart.
4. Carefully remove periodontal dressing, if present.

E. Remove sutures.
1. Prepare suture site by removing debris.
   a. Rinse.
   b. If needed, use 3 percent hydrogen peroxide on cotton pellet or cotton tip applicator to help debride area.
   c. Gently wipe with gauze sponge.
   d. Rinse again.
   e. Apply topical anesthetic for pain control, if needed.
2. Use cotton pliers, with nondominant hand, to grasp suture knot as close to tissue as possible.
3. Gently pull knot from tissue about 2 millimeters and hold with slight tension.
4. With dominant hand, insert tip of scissor under knot and cut suture in the section that was previously buried in tissue; return scissors to tray; pick up cotton pliers with dominant hand.
5. Gently pull knot end in a vertical direction to allow suture strand on opposite end of cut to be easily removed.
   a. It is important to draw the suture through the tissue slowly.
   b. Never pull the external portion of the suture through the tissue because it could contaminate the healing wound.
6. Place removed suture on a gauze sponge; later count to ensure all sutures placed were removed; move to next suture and continue.
7. Count all sutures and compare with patient record.
8. Using irrigating syringe, rinse area with antimicrobial solution.
9. Gently apply pressure on any bleeding areas with gauze; consult with supervising dentist, if needed; patient may need to gently close on gauze sponge folded against wound site.

F. Evaluate for further treatment needs.

G. Patient information (after suture removal).
1. Oral tissues will be tender. Use gentle pressure and careful plaque control techniques to avoid damaging healing tissues.
2. If bleeding or oozing persists in suture site, contact dentist.

Skillful wound closure, via suturing, requires not only knowledge of proper surgical techniques but also knowledge of the physical characteristics and properties of the suture and the needle. It is important to chart the type, number, and location of sutures at the time of placement. This allows for careful tracking of the treatment in the event that as healing occurs sutures become loosened, lost, or misplaced due to tissue coverage. If the suture needs to be removed, careful charting will assist the operator in knowing the location, number, and type of sutures to be removed. At the time of removal, all sutures should be accounted. Patient instructions are crucial to the successful outcome of suture placement and should be given both verbally and in writing after placement and removal of sutures. Suture removal by the dental hygienist should be considered when creating a dental care plan that includes surgery and is especially important when working in a periodontal practice.

QUESTIONS

1. Characteristics of an ideal suture include all of the following EXCEPT one. Which one is the EXCEPTION?
   a. Sterile
   b. Hemostatic ability
   c. Ease of handling
   d. Tissue biocompatibility

2. If a surgeon required a suture that had the least bacterial wicking and lowest tissue reactivity, he or she would most likely choose a
   a. monofilament natural.
   b. multifilament natural.
   c. monofilament synthetic.
   d. multifilament synthetic.

3. A type of suture that requires the patient to return for suture removal includes
   a. absorbable natural.
   b. absorbable synthetic.
   c. nonabsorbable natural.
   d. absorbable metallic.

4. Chromic gut sutures have higher tensile strength than silk sutures. Most sutures today are prepackaged and disposable.
   a. Both statements are TRUE.
   b. Both statements are FALSE.
   c. The first statement is TRUE. The second statement is FALSE.
   d. The first statement is FALSE. The second statement is TRUE.

5. It is important to never pull the external portion of the suture material through the tissue when performing a suture removal because
   a. after several days of healing, the strand material is weak and could break within tissue, thus becoming more difficult to remove.
   b. this portion of the strand material often holds a knot and would be difficult to pull through the tissue without damage.
   c. this portion of the strand material could contaminate the healing wound.
   d. All of the above.

6. Which of the following techniques creates a suture that is more difficult to remove?
   a. Interrupted suture
   b. Continuous uninterrupted suture
   c. Continuous lock suture
   d. Running suture

7. A patient presents for a suture removal appointment and four interrupted intrapapillary sutures are removed. The chart indicates six were placed. What should the operator do next?
   a. Stop immediately and consult the dentist.
   b. Re-evaluate the area for buried strands and knots that may not be easily visible.
   c. Irrigate with an antimicrobial, chart the discrepancy, and dismiss the patient.
   d. Using cotton pliers, open wound sites to check for remaining sutures.

REFERENCES

1. Macht SD, Krizek TJ. Sutures and suturing: Current concepts. *Journal of Oral Surgery,* Vol. 36, 1978, 710.
2. *Wound Closure Manual.* Somerville, MA: Ethicon, Inc., 1985, pp 1-101.
3. Mackenzie D. The history of sutures. *Medical History (Scottish),* Vol. 17, Number 2, 1973, 158–168.
4. Hutchens, LH. Periodontal suturing: A review of needles, materials, and techniques. *Compendium of Postgraduate Dentistry,* Vol. 2:3, Number 4, 1995.

Chapter 9

Periodontal Dressings

Michelle Hurlbutt, RDH, BS and Debi Gerger, RDH, BS, MPH

MediaLink

A companion CD-ROM, included free with each new copy of this book, supplements the procedures presented in each chapter. Insert the CD-ROM to watch video clips and view a large collection of color images that is also included. This multimedia library is designed to help you add a new dimension to your learning.

KEY TERMS

chemical cure dressing

chlorhexidine gluconate

eugenol

light-cured dressing

periodontal dressing

periodontal surgery

self/auto-cured dressing

suture

LEARNING OBJECTIVES

After reading this chapter, the student will be able to:

- explain the indications and contraindications for use of a periodontal dressing;
- discuss the properties of an ideal periodontal dressing;
- identify the types of periodontal dressings available;
- select the armamentarium needed to place and remove a periodontal dressing;
- demonstrate the proper technique for placement and removal of a periodontal dressing;
- discuss the appropriate patient instructions for the use of a periodontal dressing;
- describe why it is important for an operator to use a periodontal dressing during dental hygiene practice.

I. Introduction

In 1923, Dr. A. W. Ward introduced Ward's WondrPak as a means to protect periodontal surgical sites and increase patient comfort.[1] The original formula contained zinc oxide-eugenol (ZOE), pine oil, asbestos, and alcohol. **Eugenol,** typically present in **periodontal dressings** at a concentration of 40 to 50 percent, has been associated with strong analgesic and antiseptic properties that soothe sensitive dentin and gingival soft tissues.[2] Zinc eugenate is the result of the chemical combination of zinc oxide and eugenol but, unfortunately, as it breaks down, it contributes to gingival irritation, delayed healing, increased inflammation, allergic reaction, and tissue necrosis.[1,2] Because of these reasons, the most commonly used periodontal dressings today do not contain eugenol.[3]

A. Periodontal dressings are available in a variety of forms that include ready-mix, paste-to-paste, and paste-gel preparation. The operator must read and understand the preparation, placement, and removal process for the specific type of material being used. Some of the many considerations include the type of mixing pad, spatula, gloves the operator mixing the materials is wearing or if the system requires a cartridge or syringe setup.

B. The purpose of a periodontal dressing is to cover or protect a site after **periodontal surgery,** control postoperative seepage, minimize infection, aid in shaping and forming new tissue, and aid in retaining tissue. It is not used as often as it was years ago because of improved periodontal surgical procedures that do not require a dressing and the use of antimicrobial mouth rinses such as **chlorhexidine gluconate.**[4] As a competent operator, it remains advantageous for the dental hygienist to understand the preparation, placement, and removal of a periodontal dressing.

II. Characteristics of an Ideal Periodontal Dressing
A. Sets slowly to allow for manipulation and placement.
B. Provides a smooth surface that is nonirritating to tissues.
C. Flexible, yet able to maintain its dimensional stability.
D. Prevents leakage and inhibits bacterial growth.
E. Nonallergenic.
F. Acceptable taste.

III. Indications for Use
A. Protects **sutures** and periodontal surgical site.
  1. Protects against irritation from plaque, smoking, beverages, and food.
  2. Prevents mobilization of soft tissue grafts.
  3. Aids in shaping newly formed tissue.
B. Protects newly exposed root surfaces.
  1. Insulates area from thermal changes.
  2. Protects root surfaces from irritation from plaque.
C. Promotes patient comfort during initial healing phase.
  1. Minimizes postoperative infection.
  2. Protects from surface trauma.
D. Stabilizes mobile teeth during initial healing phase.
E. Helps to control postoperative seepage.

IV. Contraindications for Use
A. Increased irritation and inflammation.
  1. Increased plaque-retention around periodontal dressing.
  2. Decreased ability for patient self-care procedures.
  3. Increased pain.
B. Uncontrolled postoperative bleeding.
C. Unpleasant taste.

V. Criteria for a Well-Placed Periodontal Dressing
Dressing should:
A. Completely cover the wound site.
B. Extend one tooth beyond the end of the incision site.
C. Extend no further than the mucogingival junction.
D. Not interfere with occlusion; use articulating paper to verify.
E. Be of substantial size to resist fracture, but thin enough to adequately contour to the arch.
F. Measure approximately 5 to 6 millimeters in width.
G. Be locked interdentally.

VI. Preparation
Armamentarium includes:
A. Basic setup. Mouth mirror, explorer, and cotton pliers.

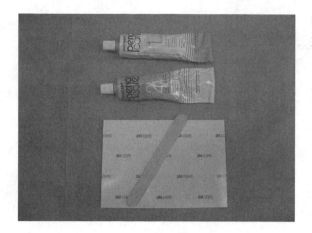

Figure 9–1 Periocare periodontal dressing.

B. Plastic-type filling instrument.
C. Dressing materials include:
1. Zinc oxide with eugenol dressing (Ward's WondrPak).
2. Zinc oxide without eugenol dressing (Coe-Pak Periodontal Dressing, Zone Periodontal Pak, Periocare Periodontal Dressing (Figure 9–1), Peripac Periodontal Pac, Coe-Pak Automix, and Cadpak Automix).
3. **Chemical cure dressing** or **self/auto-cured dressing.**
4. **Light-cured dressing** (Barricaid Visible-Light-Cure Periodontal Dressing, L.C. Peri Gard).
5. Collagen dressing.
6. Cyanoacryltate dressing.[5]
7. Methacrylic dressing.
D. Antibacterial agent.
1. Chlorhexidine gluconate.[6,7]
2. Locally delivered antimicrobials.
E. Mixing spatula with stiff blade.
F. Mixing pad supplied by manufacturer.
G. Wooden tongue blade.
H. Sterile 2″ × 2″ gauze.
I. Cotton tip applicator.
J. Petroleum jelly.
K. Articulating paper.

VII. Placement of Dressing
A. Evaluate the patient's medical history for any contraindications or modifications needed.
B. Effectively communicate the periodontal dressing protocol to the patient and answer any concerns or questions.
C. Appropriately position the patient for the treatment area.
D. Use a mouth mirror to inspect the treatment area; bleeding should be controlled before placing the dressing.
E. Prepare/dispense the periodontal dressing as described by the manufacturer; most commonly used dressings include:
1. Non-eugenol periodontal dressings.
   a. Base and catalyst system to be spatulated on a specific mixing pad.
      (1) Dispense equal amounts of paste (tube 1) and gel (tube 2) onto mixing pad (Figure 9–2).

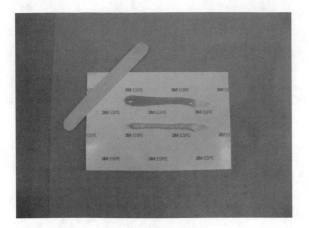

Figure 9–2 Dispense equal amounts of tube 1 (paste) and tube 2 (gel) onto a mixing pad.

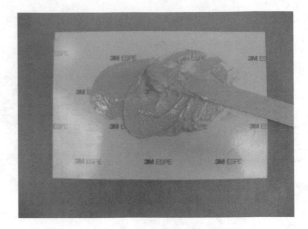

Figure 9–3 Spatulate paste and gel together until a uniform color is reached.

    (2) Using spatula, mix paste and gel together until a uniform color is reached—approximately 30 seconds (Figure 9–3).
    (3) On mixing pad, form mixture into a log with spatula.
    (4) Use moistened finger to test for tackiness.
    (5) Mold into desired shape; material is workable for approximately 15 minutes.
    (6) Clean spatula with orange solvent.
  b. Pre-mixed system to be dispensed from a cartridge.
 2. Light-cured dressings. Single-component, light-activated material supplied in a syringe.
  a. Spatulate the materials as indicated by the directions.
  b. Place wooden tongue blade under warm water to soften and roll periodontal dressing material into a cylindrical shape; cut into two equal length strips.
F. Lubricate gloved fingers with petroleum jelly.
G. Dry surgical area with a 2″ × 2″ gauze.
H. Place one strip along the buccal surface, making certain it contours around the distal surface of the most posterior tooth (Figure 9–4).
I. Move forward, toward the midline, gently pressing the material to conform to the interproximal areas (Figure 9–5).

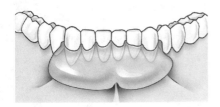

Figure 9–4 Placement of periodontal dressing.

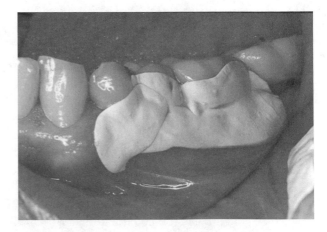

Figure 9–5 Periodontal dressing.

J. Join the lingual strip at the distal surface and bring forward to the midline, using the same technique as for the buccal strip.

K. Join the strips interproximally by applying gentle bi-digital pressure.

L. Use a wet cotton tip applicator to festoon the material, leaving a smooth surface.

M. Material should not extend past the gingival third of the tooth; have the patient close on articulating paper to evaluate occlusal interference.

VIII. Patient Instructions (after periodontal dressing placement)[6]

A. Do *NOT* disturb the dressing; it may take up to two hours for the dressing to harden.

B. Do *NOT* rinse mouth for the first 24 hours.

C. If bleeding occurs, place a gauze, soaked in strong tea, on the dressing for 15 minutes to 1 hour.

D. Drink cold fluids for the first 24 hours to keep the dressing firm; avoid alcohol and carbonated beverages for the first four to five days.

E. Eat foods high in protein for the first three to five days and/or eat foods that are semisolid, such as vegetables, pasta, and fish.

F. Take pain medication and/or antibiotics or an over-the-counter (OTC) analgesic as prescribed, if necessary; additionally, an antimicrobial rinse may be prescribed for use while the material is in place.

G. To minimize swelling, use an ice pack for 15 minutes, then remove for 15 minutes; continue for the first 24 hours.

H. Do not brush the surgical area; however, brush all other areas.

I. Avoid smoking; it delays healing; wait as long as possible before smoking.

J. Although small pieces of the periodontal dressing may break away, contact the office for instruction if the entire dressing breaks away. If the pack comes off after the first postoperative day, minimal damage is done because the pack has already adapted the tissues to the teeth in the first several hours of healing. In some cases, the patient will need to return to the dental office for a new dressing.

K. Schedule patient to return in approximately one week for a postoperative check and to remove or replace periodontal dressing.

IX. Removal

A. Armamentarium.
1. Basic setup. Mouth mirror, explorer, and cotton pliers.
2. Plastic-type filling instrument.
3. Spoon excavator instrument.
4. Sterile 2″ × 2″ gauze.
5. Irrigating syringe.
6. Warm water (saline).
7. Chlorhexidine gluconate or other antimicrobial agent.
8. Dental floss.

B. Evaluate the chart for the periodontal surgical site and number and type of sutures placed.

C. Irrigate the material over the periodontal surgical site with warm water and/or chlorhexidine gluconate.

D. Insert the beaks of cotton pliers or tip of the spoon excavator along the apical margin of the periodontal dressing and exert gentle lateral pressure; do not press or rock periodontal dressing into the wound.

E. Grasp the large pieces with the cotton pliers and place on a 2″ × 2″ gauze.

CLINICAL TIP:

Dressing Up Your Knowledge: If large embrasures exist, small cones of material may be inserted interproximally prior to placing the buccal and lingual strips.

CLINICAL TIP:

Dressing Up Your Knowledge: Advise the postsurgical or post root planing patient to use a dentifrice with sodium fluoride to assist in root caries prevention.

F. Use an explorer and/or dental floss to remove pieces that are remaining on tooth structure and/or interproximal areas.

G. Cleanse the entire area with a syringe of warm water followed by an antimicrobial agent rinse.

H. If sutures are present, remove (see the section on suture removal in the Sutures Chapter).

I. Have dentist evaluate the area and make recommendations accordingly; it is rare to repack the area for an additional week.

X. Patient Information (after periodontal dressing removal)

A. Gingival margin may feel "strange" or different.

B. Tooth/teeth may experience cold sensitivity and/or temporary mobility.

C. Oral tissues may have minor bleeding and will be tender; use gentle pressure and careful plaque control techniques to avoid damaging healing tissues.

The periodontal dressing procedure is considered when protection of a periodontal surgical site is necessary. The material will not only protect the site, it can help to control seepage, minimize infection, aid in shaping and forming newly formed tissue, aid in retaining tissue positioning, and prevent mobilization of grafts. There are many varieties of periodontal dressings being used today with the non-eugenol (base and catalyst or premixed), with the light-cured systems being the most popular. When the periodontal dressing contains the ideal characteristics, the material can be prepared, placed, and removed with ease in the hands of a skilled operator. Care must be taken to follow the manufacturer's instructions as well as the general guidelines for a well-placed periodontal dressing. Patient instructions are vital to a successful outcome and therefore need to be given verbally and in writing after placement and removal of the periodontal dressing. The use of a periodontal dressing by the dental hygienist should be considered when creating a dental care plan and is especially important when working in a periodontal practice.

QUESTIONS

1. All of the following characteristics describe an ideal periodontal dressing EXCEPT one. Which one is the EXCEPTION?
   a. Inhibits bacterial growth.
   b. Sets slowly for easy manipulation.
   c. Has an acceptable taste.
   d. Allergenic.

2. All of the following are criteria for a well-placed periodontal dressing EXCEPT one. Which one is the EXCEPTION?
   a. Extends one tooth past the excision site.
   b. Locks interproximally.
   c. Extends past the mucogingival junction.
   d. Measures 5 to 6 millimeters in width.

3. Currently non-eugenol–type periodontal dressings are not used because they were shown to contribute to gingival irritation, delayed healing, increased inflammation, allergic reactions, and tissue necrosis. When a periodontal dressing is placed, it is important to inform the patient not to rinse for 24 hours, not brush the dressing area, and avoid smoking for as long as possible.
   a. Both statements are TRUE.
   b. Both statements are FALSE.
   c. The first statement is TRUE. The second statement is FALSE.
   d. The first statement is FALSE. The second statement is TRUE.

4. Which of the following protocols should the operator follow during placement of a periodontal dressing?
   a. Keep the surgical area moist for better adhesion of the dressing.
   b. Place the lingual strip of the dressing first, followed by the buccal strip.
   c. Join the buccal and lingual strips of the dressing interproximally.
   d. Extend the dressing past the gingival third of the tooth.

5. When providing instructions following the application of a periodontal dressing, the operator should inform the patient to
a. not disturb the dressing the entire time it is in place.
b. rinse frequently and immediately after placement.
c. use an icepack intermittently for the first 24 hours.
d. keep the area clean with frequent toothbrushing.

REFERENCES

1. Sachs H et al. Oral tissue reactions to suture materials. *International Journal of Periodontal Restorative Dentistry,* Vol. 18, 1998, p. 474.

2. von Fraunhofer J, Argyropoulos D. Properties of periodontal dressings. *Dental Materials,* Vol. 6, 1990, p. 51.

3. Rubinoff CH, Greener EH, Robinson PJ. Physical properties of periodontal dressing materials. *Journal of Oral Rehabilitation,* Vol. 13, 1986, p. 575.

4. Allen D, Caffesse R. Comparison of results following modified Widman flap surgery with and without surgical dressing. *Journal of Periodontology,* Vol. 54, 1983, p. 470.

5. Grisdale, J. The use of cyanoacrylates in periodontal therapy. *Journal of the Canadian Dental Association,* Vol. 64, 1998, p. 623.

6. Checchi L, Trombelli L. Postoperative pain and discomfort with and without periodontal dressing in conjunction with 0.2% chlorhexidine mouthwash after apically positioned flap procedure. *Journal of Periodontology,* Vol. 64, 1993, p. 1238.

7. Thorstensen AE, Duguid R, Lloyd CH. The effects of adding chlorhexidine and polyhexamethylene bisguanide to a light-cured periodontal dressing material. *Journal of Oral Rehabilitation,* Vol. 23, 1996, p. 729.

Chapter 10

Pulp Vitality

Mary D. Cooper, RDH, MSEd

 MediaLink

A companion CD-ROM, included free with each new copy of this book, supplements the procedures presented in each chapter. Insert the CD-ROM to watch video clips and view a large collection of color images that is also included. This multimedia library is designed to help you add a new dimension to your learning.

KEY TERMS

contralateral	irreversible pulpitis	reversible pulpitis
endodontic therapy	ischemic	transient
hyperemia	necrosis	

LEARNING OBJECTIVES

After reading this chapter, the student will be able to:

- explain why pulpal inflammation causes a painful response;
- list the stimuli that can cause an inflammatory response in the pulp;
- differentiate between reversible pulpitis, irreversible pulpitis, and pulp necrosis;
- discuss the purposes of pulp vitality testing;
- discuss the limitations of pulp vitality testing;

- compare the various methods for assessing pulp vitality under the following topics;
  a. purpose of the test
  b. products used
  c. technique
  d. results and their interpretation
- demonstrate competent pulp vitality testing techniques and the appropriate documentation of the findings;
- explain to a patient the pulp test results and the implications of the findings.

I. Introduction

For a pulp to be vital, it must have adequate vascular supply and blood circulation. If either is compromised, the pulp will be affected and the tooth may become symptomatic to the patient. Consequently, the tooth may require **endodontic therapy.**

II. Pulpal Inflammation

A. Process. When exposed to a stimulus, pulpal blood vessels dilate and an inflammatory response occurs.
   1. Edema is typically present with inflammation.
   2. Pulp tissue cannot swell because it is encased within hard, dentinal tissue.
   3. Consequently, the blood vessels become compressed, pressure builds up, and the blood flow becomes restricted, resulting in pain and **ischemic** pulp **necrosis.**

4. Immature permanent teeth are able to tolerate and reverse inflammatory responses better because they have wide apical foramina and relatively strong blood supplies.

B. Stimuli that can trigger an inflammatory response in the pulp due to their location and/or effect on the pulp include:
1. Dental caries.
2. Cracked tooth.
3. Crown fracture.
4. Chemical irritant.
5. Traumatic injury.
6. Thermal changes.
7. Cavity preparation.

C. Categories of pulpal inflammation.
1. **Reversible pulpitis** (pulp **hyperemia**).
    a. Definition. **Transient** inflammatory response in the pulp tissue; patient complains of a short-lived, intermittent pain; dental hygienist must exert caution while providing specific procedures for the patient, since reversible pulpitis may be an iatrogenic condition.
    b. Cause. External stimuli/irritant.
    c. Most common triggers include:
        (1) Too much heat applied to a tooth during rubber cup or amalgam polishing.
        (2) Newly placed restoration(s).
        (3) Exposure to thermal changes, particularly cold temperatures.
    d. Response. An inflamed pulp will form reparative dentin and spontaneously heal (become asymptomatic) if the stimulus causing the inflammatory response is removed.
    e. Pulp test finding (electric/battery operated). Results in an exaggerated, severe, momentary sharp response.
2. **Irreversible pulpitis.** Includes two types, acute and chronic.
    a. Acute pulpitis.
        (1) Definition. An acute inflammatory response of the pulp resulting in pulpal death.
        (2) Causes. Most common include deep carious lesions, large restorations, periapical abscesses, or trauma.
        (3) Patient experiences severe, sharp, unbearable pain that does not abate upon removal of causative factor.
        (4) Unlike reversible pulpitis, the pulp does not have the ability to heal itself when the external stimulus is removed.
        (5) Pulp test finding (electric/battery operated). Results in an over-responsive reaction even to the slightest stimulus—extremely sensitive to the patient.
    b. Chronic pulpitis.
        (1) Definition. A longstanding inflammatory response usually resulting in pulpal death.
        (2) Causes. A deep carious lesion, a large restoration, or periapical inflammation.
        (3) Patient experiences an intermittent, dull, throbbing, bearable pain or no pain at all.
        (4) Pulp test finding (electric/battery operated). Results in an under-responsive reaction, possibly no reaction to stimulus.

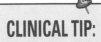

CLINICAL TIP:

Testing Your Knowledge: A swollen body tissue can receive some relief when ice is applied to it, because it decreases the vascularity and slows the blood flow. Some patients receive temporary pain relief from acute pulpitis by applying an ice pack to the painful tooth.

CLINICAL TIP:

Testing Your Knowledge: Blood pressure in the head increases when a person lies down and when bending over; consequently, pulpal pressure and pain are more intense at night when lying in bed.

3. Pulp necrosis.
   a. Definition. Pulpal death due to acute or chronic inflammation.
      (1) Asymptomatic; before it becomes necrotic, some teeth experience pulpal pain and others do not.[1]
      (2) If a periapical abscess is present, the tooth may feel "high" and should not be subjected to percussion testing because it will most likely respond painfully.
   b. Cause. Deep carious lesion or large restoration.
   c. Pulp testing finding (electric/battery operated). Usually there is no response.

III. Pulp Vitality Testing

A. Traditional pulp vitality tests do not directly measure a pulp's vascular supply, but instead indirectly measure the pulp's vitality by testing the nerve response. Tests that rely on nerve response include:
   1. Thermal tests: Cold and heat.
   2. Transillumination: Provides visual assessment only.
   3. Electric pulp tests (EPT).
   4. Percussion: Determines inflammation of the periodontal ligament (PDL) only.
   5. Palpation: Determines presence of periapical involvement only.
   6. Mobility: Determines inflammation of the PDL only.
      Note: Measuring the pulp's vitality through transillumination, percussion, palpation, and mobility require thermal and electric pulp tests for definitive diagnosis of pulpal diseases.

B. Purpose of pulp testing.
   1. Patient may not be able to identify which tooth is the source of pain; in fact, a patient may think one tooth is painful when, in reality, a different tooth is the source of the pulpal inflammation, i.e., referred pain.
   2. Can assist the operator to localize and diagnose the tooth that has pulpal inflammation.

C. Limitations of pulp testing.
   1. Primary teeth and immature permanent teeth. Less responsive to pulp testing because they are not fully innervated with alpha myelinated axons.[2] Additionally, wide open root apices found in immature permanent teeth prevent reliable responses to pulp tests; they are susceptible to false negative readings.
   2. Recently injured tooth. May temporarily experience altered nerve conduction and test nonvital, even though the blood supply and circulation of the injured tooth are intact.
   3. Patient compliance and ability of patient to give subjective feedback regarding the degree of sensation/pain experienced. Traditional pulp testing techniques cannot be used reliably with those who cannot cooperate with the testing procedure, i.e., children and mentally challenged adults.

CLINICAL TIP:

Testing Your Knowledge: Nontraditional pulp tests using pulse oximetry or Doppler flowmetry can be used to reliably test teeth of uncooperative patients and traumatized, primary, and immature permanent teeth.[2]

IV. Methods of Assessing Pulp Vitality in Mature Teeth

A. Thermal tests. Thermal tests, particularly cold tests, are useful assessments in the diagnosis of symptomatic, irreversible pulpitis. Additionally, when a patient cannot isolate which tooth is sensitive, thermal testing may help to identify the offending tooth.
   1. Test preparation.
      a. Instruct patient to raise her or his hand immediately when a sensation is felt.
      b. Isolate tooth/teeth.

CLINICAL TIP:

Testing Your Knowledge: Dry teeth with gauze and not with the air/water syringe; the air may be too uncomfortable for the patient.

   c. Dry tooth/teeth with gauze.
   d. Apply the testing agent to the middle third of the facial crown for 5 seconds, or until the patient feels a sensation.
   e. Before testing a suspected tooth, test the **contralateral** tooth first; this is done to:
     (1) Let the patient get comfortable with the procedure.
     (2) Determine the "normal" reaction of a similar tooth.
2. Types of tests.
   a. Cold tests.
     (1) Refrigerant spray (Endo Ice®—Hygienic Co.), a popular and frequently used product.[3]
       (a) Characteristics.
         i. Clear, colorless, liquefied gas at $-26.2°C$.
         ii. Usually penetrates castings, although occasional false negative readings can occur with some that have porcelain fused-to-metal crowns or significantly calcified pulps.
       (b) Technique.
         i. Hold a large cotton pellet with forceps.
         ii. Spray Endo Ice® onto the pellet until saturated.
         iii. Wait for it to crystallize—approximately 1 second.
         iv. Apply to the dried, facial, middle third of the tooth surface.
       Caution: Material should not be sprayed directly onto tooth because it can cause craze lines in the enamel.[4]
     (2) Ice pencil.
       (a) Made by freezing water in a plastic needle sheath or in an anesthetic cartridge that is drained of its solution.
       (b) Not used frequently, because they are not nearly as cold as refrigerant spray or dry ice sticks; the ice pencil stick melts relatively quickly, dripping water onto the gingiva, which results in false positive readings.
     (3) Carbon dioxide (CO_2) ice/snow.[3]
       (a) Characteristics.
         i. Requires a dry ice cylinder to create a CO_2 dry ice stick.
         ii. Due to the CO_2 stick's extremely cold temperature ($-98°C$), it is one of the most effective tests for hard-to-diagnose teeth, i.e., those with old, calcified pulps and porcelain fused-to-metal crowns.
       (b) Technique.
         i. Pressing CO_2 stick on a hard-to-diagnose tooth for approximately 20 to 30 seconds can often elicit a response where the refrigerant spray did not.
         ii. Compared to water ice sticks, false positives are minimized, because there is no dripping of water onto the gingival tissues.
       Caution: When using a CO_2 stick, its extremely cold temperature can cause enamel crazing.[5]
     (4) Cold bath. Although more time consuming to perform, it is one of the most accurate thermal testing methods because the entire tooth crown is exposed to the temperature change instead of one tooth surface.[5,6] This method is effective with a tooth that has full crown coverage.

      (a) Characteristics. More time consuming than the other methods, because the suspected tooth must be isolated with a rubber dam; requires no anesthesia.

      (b) Technique. Once the tooth is isolated:

         i. Fill a disposable syringe with ice water.

        ii. Spray water on the tooth until the entire crown is bathed in the cold water.

       iii. Wait 10 to 15 seconds for the patient's response.

       iv. Use high-volume evacuation (HVE) to remove the water.

  b. Heat tests. Heat tests are usually unnecessary and rarely used. If an operator chooses to conduct a heat test, applying heated gutta percha to the tooth surface is discouraged. Hot gutta percha adheres to enamel, resulting in a prolonged and often painful episode for the patient. An alternative method to use is a warm water bath, which is reliable for diagnosing irreversible pulpitis. Use the following procedure:

    (1) Isolate the tooth with a rubber dam.

    (2) Fill a disposable syringe with warm/hot water; have HVE available.

    (3) Spray the water onto the isolated tooth until the tooth is bathed in the water.

3. Interpretation of thermal tests. The duration of the response and the type of discomfort—i.e., throbbing versus sharp—are important factors to consider in the interpretation of a thermal test.

  a. No response. Indicates a necrotic, nonvital pulp or a false positive reading due to immature tooth with a wide apex, older tooth with a calcified pulp, or a tooth that has experienced recent trauma.

  b. Mild-to-moderate pain that goes away a few seconds after the thermal stimulus is removed from the tooth surface. Considered a "normal" response, the type found with a healthy tooth.

  c. Severe, momentary, sharp pain that goes away almost immediately after the thermal stimulus is removed from the tooth surface signifies reversible pulpitis.

  d. Moderate-to-strong, throbbing, painful response that does not go away after the thermal stimulus is removed from the tooth surface; throbbing pain tends to linger for a few minutes, signifies irreversible pulpitis.

B. Transillumination. Intraoral camera can be used as a fiberoptic transilluminator; useful to diagnose cracks in a tooth; a necrotic pulp may appear dark.

C. Electric pulp test. The electric pulp tester, digital or analog (wireless version is battery operated), is one of the most frequently used methods for pulp testing.

1. Limitations.

  a. Does not provide any information about the blood supply or circulation within the pulp.

  b. Cannot be used to diagnose stages of pulpitis.

  c. Numbers displayed are of no true value beyond the assessment of vital/nonvital—the numbers do not give the operator any information about the condition of the pulp.

  d. If a patient presents with symptomatic pulpitis, the EPT is of no value.

2. Factors that may affect the EPT reading.

  a. False positive reading. Patient feels a sensation, yet the pulp is nonvital; this can occur when a(n):

CLINICAL TIP:

Testing Your Knowledge: Applying heat to a symptomatic tooth will result in an intense response. It is advisable to have refrigerant spray available in case the patient needs quick relief.

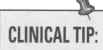

CLINICAL TIP:

Testing Your Knowledge: To assess if the tooth is nonvital, the EPT must be used alone. It is imperative to conduct thermal testing as well.

(1) Metallic restoration is in contact with the gingiva. Electric current spreads to the gingiva or PDL and the patient feels a sensation.

(2) EPT tip is placed directly on a metallic crown/restoration resulting in the metal conducting the sensation.

(3) Tooth is covered with saliva, which acts as a conductor, and the PDL is stimulated.

(4) EPT tip inadvertently touches the gingiva.

b. False negative reading. Patient does not feel any sensation, yet the pulp is vital; this can occur when a(n):

(1) Pulp is calcified.

(2) Tooth has significant secondary dentin formation, highly resistant enamel.

(3) Apex is open/immature.

(4) Tooth has a porcelain crown or composite—ceramics and resins are nonconducting.

(5) Tooth has been recently traumatized.

(6) EPT does not produce enough current when the electrode tip does not make good contact with the tooth surface.

3. Armamentarium (Figure 10–1).

a. Vitalometer.

b. Insert tips, short and long.

c. Ground clip.

d. Toothpaste.

e. Cotton rolls.

4. Technique.

a. Orient patient to procedure.

b. Instruct patient to raise a hand when a tingling sensation is felt.

Figure 10–1   Pulp vitality tester.

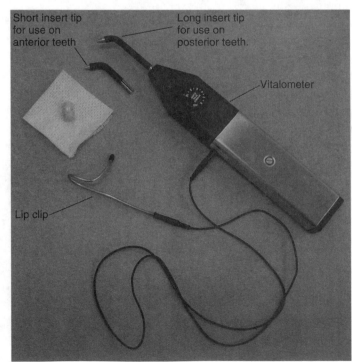

Short insert tip for use on anterior teeth

Long insert tip for use on posterior teeth.

Vitalometer

Lip clip

   c. Identify and isolate the teeth to be tested with cotton rolls—test tooth and comparison tooth.

   d. Select and insert a probe tip (see Figure 10–1).

     (1) Short tip for anterior teeth.

     (2) Long tip for posterior teeth.

   e. Set the pulp tester on the lowest setting and depress button to establish if the current is working.

   f. Rest ground clip over patient's lip into mucobuccal fold—completes the circuit by providing a ground.

   g. Dry teeth and surrounding gingiva with gauze.

   h. Apply toothpaste to the probe tip—improves contact and acts as a conductor between the tooth and the electrode.

   i. Establish a finger rest.

   j. On the contralateral vital tooth, apply the probe tip to the middle of the facial or lingual surface of the tooth (Figure 10–2).

   k. If using an analog unit, turn the output control knob clockwise to activate the unit and slowly increase the control knob; if using a digital unit, the pulsating stimulus will automatically increase at a preset rate.

   l. When the patient feels a tingling sensation, remove the probe tip and record the reading.

   m. Repeat the procedure to determine reliability of vitality.

   n. Average the readings and record with the tooth number in the patient's chart.

   o. Repeat the procedure on the suspicious tooth.

   p. Repeat procedure a few times to be sure of the reading.

   q. Average the readings and record with the tooth number in the patient's chart.

   r. Remove cotton rolls and rinse toothpaste from the patient's mouth using water and saliva ejector.

   s. Prepare equipment for disinfection/autoclaving according to manufacturer's directions.

     Contraindication: Do not use with a patient who has an unshielded cardiac pacemaker, which is uncommon today.

D. Percussion. Percussion is an important endodontic test. It consists of lightly tapping the crown of a tooth with the handle end of a single-ended instrument to determine if the apical portion of the PDL is inflamed.

   1. Percussion-sensitive tooth. Indicates the PDL is inflamed; however, it does not give any definitive information on the tooth's pulp vitality.

CLINICAL TIP:

Testing Your Knowledge: Digital pulp testers are gentle, painless, and less jolting than analog testers. The reason for this is that a digital unit produces a pulsed stimulus—the stimulus is perceived by the patient well before it crosses the patient's pain threshold.

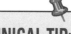

CLINICAL TIP:

Testing Your Knowledge: Electric pulp testers should be cleaned and disinfected with a cloth containing disinfectant. The probe tips are removed, washed with soapy water, and autoclaved between uses.

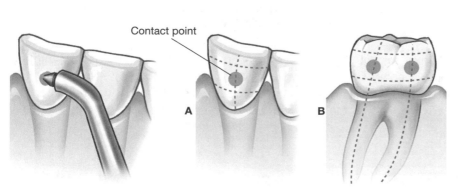

Figure 10–2 Position of pulp tester: (A) Place pulp tester in middle third of tooth; (B) Placement of pulp tester on multirooted tooth.

2. Thermal testing must also be completed to assess the tooth's vitality.
3. Patient complaint. Pain when chewing/biting.
4. Procedure.
    a. Before performing a percussion test on a suspicious tooth, test a healthy tooth so the patient gets a sense of what "normal" feels like.
    b. Tap a few teeth, including the suspicious tooth, randomly—this method of testing will improve the reliability of the test by preventing the patient from knowing when the suspicious tooth is being tested.
    c. Tap each tooth from all accessible surfaces—facial, lingual, mesial, and distal. If the patient feels pain, the degree of pain should be recorded as + = mild, ++ = moderate, and +++ = severe pain.

E. Palpation. Operator gently palpates (presses) an index finger against the alveolar bone and surrounding soft tissue to detect any swelling, which indicates pulpal necrosis has led to periapical involvement.

F. Mobility. If a tooth's pulp is inflamed, the PDL will most likely become inflamed; an acute periapical abscess may cause some transient mobility of a tooth.[4]

V. Assessing Pulp Vitality in Immature Teeth

A. Pulse oximetry. A noninvasive, effective technique for assessing the vitality of young teeth; a reliable test used to differentiate between vital and nonvital primary and/or immature permanent teeth.[2,7]
    1. Procedure. Place a modified probe on the crown of the suspected tooth and objectively assess a tooth's vascularity by measuring its arterial blood oxygen saturation level.[2]
    2. Recommendation for use.
        a. Use on primary teeth and permanent incisors and premolars.
        b. Caution: Teeth with thicker hard tissue surrounding the pulp—i.e., older teeth with significant secondary dentin formation/pulpal obliteration and molars and canines—cannot have their pulpal circulations detected with a pulse oximeter.

B. Laser Doppler blood flow monitor. Laser Doppler Flowmetry (LDF) is capable of recording blood flow signals from vital tooth pulps.
    1. Most effective in assessing the pulpal status of traumatized anterior teeth.[8] LDF can be used to monitor revascularization of immature incisors following severe trauma.
    2. When other methods of pulp testing are recording no vitality, LDF can determine if revascularization and vitality is occurring.[8]
    3. Test is technique sensitive, requiring the use of rubber dam isolation to improve its validity and reliability.[9,10]
    4. Use of LDF is controversial, up to 80 percent of the LDF from an intact tooth without rubber dam is of nonpulp origin, coming from other tissues outside of the pulp, i.e., periodontal tissues; but in a recent study only 43 percent of the LDF was of pulp origin.[10]

Pulp vitality testing provides the operator a method to assess the vitality of a suspected nonvital tooth. However, note that an accurate assessment of the pulp can at times be difficult. Communication between the operator and patient is vital in order to make as close a definitive diagnosis as possible.

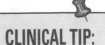

CLINICAL TIP:

Testing Your Knowledge: Causes of periodontal ligament inflammation include rapid orthodontic movement, a lateral periodontal abscess, a newly placed restoration with an occlusal discrepancy, occlusal trauma, and late stage irreversible pulpitis/early pulpal necrosis.

QUESTIONS

1. All of the following stimuli can trigger an inflammatory response in the pulp EXCEPT one. Which one is the EXCEPTION?
   a. Dental caries
   b. Trauma
   c. Crown fracture
   d. Recession

2. Of the following choices, the MOST likely cause of reversible pulp is
   a. exposure to cold temperatures.
   b. a deep, carious lesion.
   c. a periapical abscess.
   d. trauma.

3. One of the MOST effective cold tests to use to assist in diagnosing the vitality of the pulp is
   a. refrigerant spray.
   b. an ice pencil.
   c. carbon dioxide ice/snow.
   d. a cold bath.

4. Heat tests are available to test the vitality of the pulp. However, applying heated gutta percha to the tooth surface is not recommended.
   a. Both statements are TRUE.
   b. Both statements are FALSE.

   c. The first statement is TRUE. The second statement is FALSE.
   d. The first statement is FALSE. The second statement is TRUE.

5. All of the following factors may affect the electronic pulp test (EPT) in giving the operator a false positive reading EXCEPT one. Which one is the EXCEPTION?
   a. EPT touches the gingiva.
   b. Metallic restoration is in contact with the gingiva.
   c. Tooth has been recently traumatized.
   d. Tooth is covered with saliva.

6. Using percussion is an important endodontic test. A percussion-sensitive tooth indicates a tooth's pulp vitality.
   a. Both statements are TRUE.
   b. Both statements are FALSE.
   c. The first statement is TRUE. The second statement is FALSE.
   d. The first statement is FALSE. The second statement is TRUE.

REFERENCES

1. Michaelson PL, Holland GR. Is pulpitis painful? *Journal of International Endodontics,* Vol. 35, Number 10, 2002, October, 829–32.

2. Goho C. Pulse oximetry evaluation of vitality in primary and immature permanent teeth. *Pediatric Dentistry,* Vol. 21, Number 2, 1999, 125–27.

3. Jones VR, Rivera EM, Walton RE. Comparison of carbon dioxide versus refrigerant spray to determine pulpal responsiveness. *Journal of Endodontics,* Vol. 28, Number 7, 2002, July, 531–33.

4. Jones DM. Effect of the type of carrier used on the results of dichlorodifluoromethane application to teeth. *Journal of Endodontics,* Vol. 25, Number 10, 1999, October, 692–94.

5. Cohen S, Burns RC., eds. *Pathways of the Pulp,* 8th ed. St. Louis, MO: Mosby, 2002.

6. Schwartz S, Cohen S. The difficult differential diagnosis. *Dental Clinics of North America,* Vol. 36, Number 2, 1992, April, 279–92.

7. Radhakrishnan S, Munshi AK, Hegde AM. Pulse oximetry: A diagnostic instrument in pulpal vitality testing. *Journal of Clinical Pediatric Dentistry,* Vol. 26, Number 2, 2002, Winter, 141–45.

8. Lee JY, Kallaya Yanpiset, Asgeir Sigurdsson, William F. Vann Jr. Laser Doppler flowmetry for monitoring traumatized teeth. *Dental Traumatology,* Vol. 17, Number 5, 2001, October, 231–35.

9. Evans D, J. Reid, R. Strang, and D. Stirrups. A comparison of laser Doppler flowmetry with other methods of assessing the vitality of traumatized anterior teeth. *Endodontics and Dental Traumatology,* Vol. 15, Number 6, 1999, December, 284–90.

10. Soo-ampon S, N. Vongsavan, M. Soo-ampon, S. Chuckpaiwong, and B. Matthews. The sources of laser Doppler blood-flow signals recorded from human teeth. *Archives of Oral Biology,* Vol. 48, Number 5, 2003, May, 353–60.

ELECTRONIC PULP VITALITY PERFORMANCE COMPETENCY

Student _____

Date _____

Instructor _____

Re-evaluation

Instr: _____

Date _____

	S	U	Comments	S	U	Comments
1. Assembles the proper armamentarium: • cotton rolls, toothpaste, vitalometer, tips, ground clip.						
2. Depresses switch button making sure there is current.						
3. Allows display to return to zero.						
4. Orients patient to the procedure.						
5. Gives instructions on how to respond to sensations.						
6. Identifies test tooth, comparison tooth, and sites of contact.						
7. Attaches ground wire into the vitalometer.						
8. Selects correct tip for teeth selected (short for anterior; long for posterior).						
9. Isolates teeth with cotton rolls, making sure cotton rolls don't touch the teeth.						
10. Slides ground clip over patient's lip into the mucobuccal fold.						
11. Dries tooth surfaces and surrounding gingiva.						
12. Applies a small amount of toothpaste to probe tip.						
13. Establishes a finger rest.						
14. Touches probe to the contact site on the tooth *adjacent* to the test tooth 3 mm from gingiva.						
15. Keeps tip in continuous contact with tooth.						
16. Depresses button for a digital readout.						
17. Releases button as soon as patient responds.						
18. Records first reading at ____.						
19. Repeats procedure on the *contralateral tooth* and records reading at ____.						
20. Repeats procedure on the *test tooth* and records reading at ____.						
21. Removes cotton rolls and rinses toothpaste from patient's mouth.						
22. Prepares equipment for disinfection/autoclaving and puts other materials away.						

Courtesy of Indiana University Purdue University Fort Wayne Dental Hygiene Program.

Chapter 11

Taking Alginate Impressions and Trimming Study Models

Mary D. Cooper, RDH, MSEd and Deb Stuart, CDA, EFDA, MS

MediaLink

A companion CD-ROM, included free with each new copy of this book, supplements the procedures presented in each chapter. Insert the CD-ROM to watch video clips and view a large collection of color images that is also included. This multimedia library is designed to help you add a new dimension to your learning.

KEY TERMS

alginate	gypsum	sol
cast	hydrocolloid	study model
elastic	hydrophilicity	syneresis
gel	imbibition	thermoplastic
gelation	inelastic	utility wax
gelation time	retarder	

LEARNING OBJECTIVES

After reading this chapter, the student will be able to:

- identify the purposes for taking alginate impressions;
- list each ingredient in alginate powder and describe each ingredient's function;
- discuss the factors that influence the properties of an alginate impression;
- differentiate between fast set and regular set alginate;
- describe the setting mechanism of alginate impression material and discuss how the setting time can be modified;
- explain how alginate impressions are susceptible to dimensional instability;
- list the armamentaria needed to take a set of alginate impressions for a patient;
- differentiate between the various types of impression trays and explain how to select a tray with the proper fit;

- explain how alginate impressions are disinfected and the importance of properly disinfecting them;
- describe the clinical technique for the appropriate mixing and taking of alginate impressions;
- competently take accurate alginate impressions for patients;
- assess the quality of alginate impressions;
- compare and contrast the uses and properties of different dental impression materials;
- explain how diagnostic study models are poured and trimmed;
- explain how to take a wax bite registration;
- state the differences between stone and plaster;
- competently pour and trim study models.

I. Introduction

Impression materials are used to create accurate replicas of teeth and their supporting structures, such as gingiva, alveolar ridge, hard and soft palates, and frena. An impression can be taken to create a negative reproduction of a single tooth, a quadrant, or full arch. Dental hygienists often take impressions of maxillary and mandibular arches for the purpose of fabricating study models or casts, often for the making of bleaching trays.[1] Models replicate the tissues for study, while casts are used for fabrication of restorations since they produce accurate replica of tissues.

II. Dental Alginate

Dental **alginate** is an elastic irreversible **hydrocolloid** that cannot transform its physical property once it is set. It is the most widely used impression material in dentistry.

A. Uses. Making **study models** and **casts,** since it cannot reproduce the fine surface detail of the teeth necessary for crown and bridge accuracy.

B. Properties. Consists of **elastic,** hydrocolloid material that sets chemically and irreversibly; moisture and humidity affect the material.[1,2,3,4]

   1. Accuracy. Poor.
   2. Long-term stability. Poor.
   3. Elastic recovery. Poor (poorest of all the elastic materials).
   4. Tear resistance. Good.
   5. **Hydrophilicity.** Excellent.
   6. Dimensional stability. Poor.

C. Composition of alginate powder.[2,3,4]

   1. Inert silica fillers such as diatomaceous earth or zinc oxide; reinforcing fillers added to increase the strength and stiffness of the material.
   2. Sodium or potassium alginate. Carbohydrate polymer that dissolves in water forming a **sol.**
   3. **Retarders,** such as trisodium phosphate or sodium carbonate. Used to delay the alginate's setting reaction so the impression material can be adequately mixed with water, loaded into a tray, and carried to the patient's mouth before setting.
   4. Calcium sulfate dehydrate. A reactor that produces the chemical reaction.
   5. Antimicrobial agent. May be added to powder to help reduce microbial content of powder.

D. Types of alginates.[1,2,3,4]

   1. Fast set (Type I) alginate.

Figure 11–1   Regular set alginate material, spatula, and rubber bowl.

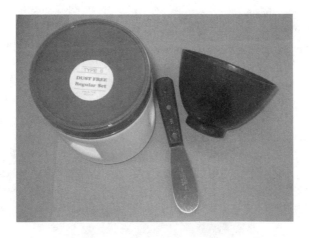

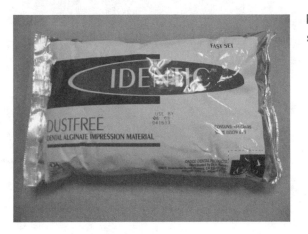

Figure 11–2   Preweighed, sealed alginate material.

     a. Typically gels (sets) within one to two minutes with a mixing time of 45 seconds.

     b. Recommended for experienced operators who can mix and prepare the material and place in the patient's mouth in a short amount of time.

  2. Regular set (Type II) alginate (Figure 11–1).

     a. Gels within 2 to 4 minutes with a mixing time of 1 minute.

     b. Recommended to be used by operators when first learning so there is enough working time to thoroughly mix the material and place in the patient's mouth before **gelation** occurs.

E. Packaging and storage.

  1. Purchased in bulk containers or in preweighed, sealed individual packets (Figure 11–2).

  2. Storage. Store in a cool, dry area for no longer than one year.

III. Process of Obtaining Dental Impressions

A. Equipment and materials.

  1. Personal protective equipment (PPE). Wear gloves, protective eye wear, mask, and disposable gown or lab coat.

  2. Mouthrinse. Place in plastic cup; instruct patient to rinse prior to taking impression.

  3. Rubber bowl (Figure 11–3). Use a clean, smooth, and flexible rubber bowl to aid when stroping material. Disposable bowls are available for infection control.

  4. Spatula. Use a reasonably stiff, wide-blade metal spatula (see Figure 11–1).

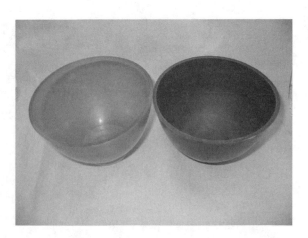

Figure 11–3   Rubber mixing bowls.

Figure 11–4 Measuring devices include water cylinder and powder scoop.

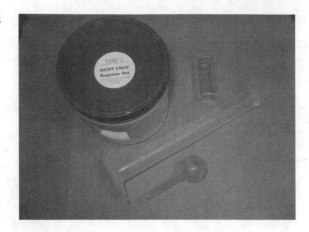

5. Measuring devices. Include a plastic water cylinder and powder scoop, which are generally supplied with the product (Figure 11–4).
6. **Utility wax.** Use when stock tray needs to be modified slightly to improve impression tray fit.
7. Base plate wax. Use to take a wax bite registration for the patient.
8. Disinfectant. Appropriate disinfectants for alginate impressions include iodophors and bleach.
9. Plastic sandwich bag or headrest cover.
10. Impression trays.
   a. Types of impression trays. Include reusable metal and disposable, plastic trays.
      (1) Plastic tray. Requires use of a tray adhesive on the inside prior to loading with alginate to improve the retention of the set alginate impression in the tray during removal from the patient's teeth.
      (2) Solid metal tray. Retains alginate material when loading tray or removing from patient's mouth through the use of rim-locks, which are designed as overhangs on the edge (rim) of the tray.
      (3) Perforated tray (Figure 11–5). Perforations (holes) are designed to improve the mechanical, locking retention of the alginate material in the tray, preventing material from separating from the tray during removal from the patient's teeth.

Figure 11–5 Metal perforated impression trays.

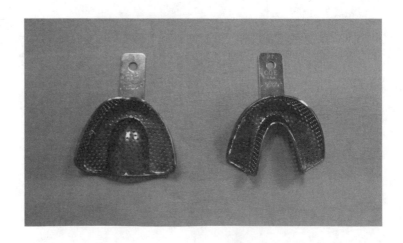

b. Sizes of impression trays. Impression trays have letters, such as S, M, L for small, medium, and large, or numbers on their handles referring to the size of the tray—the lower number, the larger the tray (i.e., #1=large).

    (1) Small.

        (a) Maxillary #7

        (b) Mandibular #22

    (2) Medium.

        (a) Maxillary #4 and #5 (narrower)

        (b) Mandibular #21

    (3) Large.

        (a) Maxillary #1

        (b) Mandibular #20

B. Preparation for taking an impression.

1. Seat the patient in an upright position with the head well supported by the headrest;[1] for comfort, the patient's shoulder should be at the same height as the elbow of the standing operator.

2. Explain the procedure to the patient and the reason for taking the impression(s).[1]

3. Instruct patient to remove any removable appliance(s).

4. Ask the patient to rinse with antimicrobial mouthrinse to reduce the microbial count.

5. Examine the oral cavity for any factors that may influence the procedure, such as tori, height, width, and length of the palatal vault, and malpositioned teeth.

6. Select the correct size(s) impression trays by trying them in the oral cavity.

    a. When placing the mandibular impression tray, the operator should stand in front of the patient (i.e., 8:00 position for right-handed; 4:00 position for left-handed).

    b. When placing the maxillary impression tray, operator should stand behind the patient (i.e., 11:00 position for right-handed; 1:00 position for left-handed).

    c. Length of tray. Adequate length is needed to cover the tuberosity (maxillary arch) or retromolar pad area (mandibular arch).

    d. Width of tray. Must provide adequate width—should not touch any buccal gingiva of the arch. Borders should be approximately ¼″ away from soft tissues. Ideally, thickness of the alginate gel between the tray and the tissues should be approximately 3 millimeters.

    e. There should be no encroachment on the soft tissues of the vestibule or tongue attachment.

7. Ways to modify a stock tray to improve the fit include:

    a. Bending buccal flanges out to accommodate second/third molars (use a metal tray).

    b. Adding utility wax (⅜ inches wide) to posterior edge of the tray to prevent alginate material from slipping out of the tray (Figure 11–6).

    c. Covering edges that are uncomfortable on the soft tissues with utility wax.

    d. Elongating length of tray to cover the tuberosity or retromolar area using utility wax.

8. Run a square of baseplate wax under hot water to soften the material. Place the wax in the patient's mouth and have him or her bite hard enough to imprint an occlusal registration into the wax.

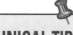

CLINICAL TIP:

Modeling Your Knowledge: Saliva on the teeth and soft tissues may cause insufficient detail in the impression and surface changes in the alginate resulting in rough study models/casts. If a patient has excessively thick saliva, it may be necessary to wipe the teeth and tissues with a 2″ × 2″ gauze square before using an antimicrobial rinse.

Figure 11–6   Utility wax added to the flange edges of impression trays.

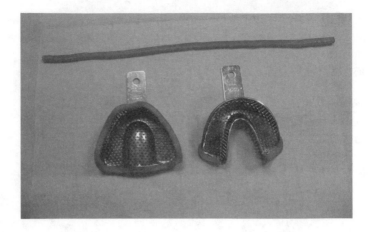

CLINICAL TIP:

Modeling Your Knowledge:
Always follow manufacturer's recommended directions for measuring, dispensing, and mixing any dental material.

CLINICAL TIP.

Modeling Your Knowledge:
The best method for controlling the setting (gelation) time of alginate impression material is to alter the temperature of the water in the mix. If you want the impression to set quickly use warm water; if you want to slow down the setting time, use cold water. Also, it is not advisable to vary the setting time of an alginate impression by altering the amount of water in the mix. Increasing or decreasing the amount of water in the mix will weaken the final gel strength.

CLINICAL TIP:

Modeling Your Knowledge:
Another method of mixing alginate includes using an alginator or a ziplock bag.

C. Measuring, dispensing, and mixing.
   1. Measuring. The following directions are most often recommended for measuring the powder and water; however, always follow the directions provided by the manufacturer. The operator should wear a mask when measuring alginate powder to prevent breathing silica particles.
      a. Powder.
         (1) Mandibular impression (all sizes): 2 scoops of powder.
         (2) Maxillary impression (large tray): 3 scoops of powder.
         (3) Maxillary impression (medium tray): 2 scoops of powder.
      b. Water. Note the markings on the cylinder provided by the manufacturer: The three marks indicate the amount of water to be added.
   2. Dispensing.
      a. Measure the appropriate amount of room temperature or slightly cool tap water and pour into the rubber bowl.
      b. Tumble the canister of powder upside down a few times to "fluff" the powder; this action disrupts the settled particles and permits accurate measurement.
      c. Slowly remove the lid to minimize the fine particles from being distributed around the room.
      d. Lightly dip the scoop into the powder; slightly overfill the powder scoop without compacting and tap the scoop lightly with the spatula to fill large voids.
      e. Use the blade of the spatula to scrape the excess powder away and achieve a level scoop; add the scoop of powder to the mixing bowl.
      f. Repeat for additional scoops.
      g. After dispensing the powder from a bulk container, firmly replace the container's lid as soon as possible to prevent exposure to moisture and humidity, which affects the material.
   3. Mixing.
      a. Begin by slowly stirring powder and water with spatula until the particles are moist; alginate should not drip off the spatula.
      b. Then begin to mix more quickly by using a stroping action (squeeze the material between the spatula and the side of the bowl to work out air bubbles and lumps); turn the bowl while stroping (Figure 11–7).
      c. Continue mixing until the consistency is smooth and creamy.
D. Factors in dispensing and mixing alginate that influence its properties.[2,3,4]
   1. Water temperature. **Gelation time** is affected by the temperature of the water; it is recommended to use room temperature, tepid water; using

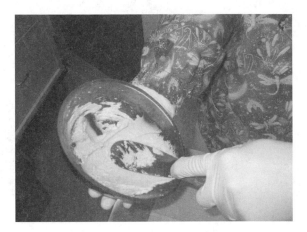

Figure 11–7   Thoroughly mix the powder and water using a stroping motion.

warm water decreases the working and setting; using cold water increases the working and setting time.

2. If tap water is used, the operator must be aware that warm and extremely hard water accelerates the total working and setting times.
3. Even spatulation yields a smooth mix with minimum air incorporation, creating a strong gel that does not drip off the spatula; excess air weakens the gel.
4. Undermixing. If an insufficient amount of time is used for mixing, the strength of the final **gel** will be reduced; insufficient spatulation results in the failure of the powder ingredients to dissolve enough in the water to permit the chemical reaction to proceed uniformly throughout the mix.
5. Overmixing. Results in shortening the setting time; produces poor results because the gel is broken up as it forms during prolonged spatulation, impairing the strength.

E. Loading the tray.
   1. Mandibular tray. Use the spatula to load the tray from the lingual side of the tray.
      a. Overload the tray with impression material.
      b. Once alginate is placed in tray, wet and smooth material using a moist finger to create a surface with fewer air bubbles.
   2. Maxillary tray. Load the tray from the posterior edge in one big mass and then shape to the outer edges of the tray; again, wet and smooth material using a moist finger (Figures 11–8, 11–9, and 11–10).

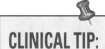

CLINICAL TIP:

Modeling Your Knowledge: Although different manufacturers have slight variations in the time required for the setting of alginates, most require 1 minute for mixing and 1 minute for loading the tray.

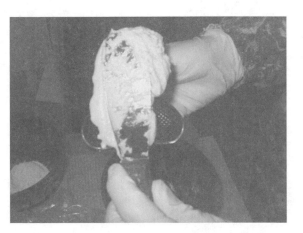

Figure 11–8   Load the maxillary tray from the posterior edge in one big mass.

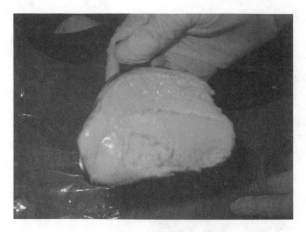

Figure 11–9   Shape the material to the outer edges of the tray.

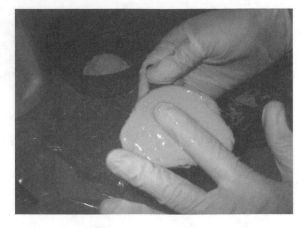

Figure 11–10   Wet and smooth the material with a moist finger before placing the tray in the patient's mouth.

CLINICAL TIP:

Modeling Your Knowledge: It is recommended that the mandibular impression be taken first to introduce the patient to the procedure. The mandibular impression usually encounters little difficulty and is easier for the patient, such as decreasing the chance of gagging.

CLINICAL TIP:

Modeling Your Knowledge: Hold impression material in place until initial set occurs—material is no longer sticky. Then release hold. Leave the impression in the mouth for another 2 minutes to maximize strength and tear resistance of the set alginate and detail of the alginate impression.

3. Try to have less alginate in the posterior than the anterior part of the tray—this reduces the amount of alginate that will flow out of the back end of the tray and therefore minimize patient gagging.

F. Seating the tray.[1]

Instruct patient to breathe through the nose during the procedure and lean slightly forward to prevent gagging.

1. Mandibular tray.
   a. Instruct patient to open.
   b. Retract one side of the lips/cheek; rotate the heel of one side of the tray through the opening.
   c. Rotate the tray so the opposite heel enters the mouth.
   d. Suspend the tray directly over the teeth, centering the handle of the tray with the midline of the arch.
   e. Slowly seat the tray so the heels are gently pressed over most of the posterior teeth.
   f. Lower the tray over the anterior teeth; avoid pressing the tray down too hard; occlusal/incisal surfaces of the teeth should lightly touch the tray.
   g. With the free hand and gauze square, pull out the cheeks and lower lip to allow excess alginate to spill into the vestibule.
   h. Instruct patient to raise the tongue to the roof of the mouth and then stick the tongue out to muscle mold the lingual side of the impression; have the patient make an "O" with lips to muscle mold the facial side of the impression.
   i. Stabilize each side of the tray with fingers from one hand until the alginate has set—avoid removing this stabilization, otherwise the patient's tongue or cheek movements may dislodge the tray.

2. Maxillary tray.
   a. Introduce the tray into the mouth similarly to the mandibular tray; seat the posterior part of the tray first to minimize the amount of material that will extrude distally.
   b. While seating the tray on the teeth, align handle of tray with midline of the face; tip the patient's head slightly forward and keep the patient in that position until the material sets.

c. Instruct patient to make an "O" with the lips to muscle mold the facial side of the impression (Figure 11–11).

d. Stabilize each side of the tray with fingers from one hand until the alginate has set—avoid removing this stabilization, otherwise the patient's tongue or cheek movements may dislodge the tray.

G. Suggestions to control gagging.

Gagging occurs when the soft palate is stimulated. The gag reflex can be controlled through diversion and positive suggestion.

1. Avoid saying the impression may cause gagging.

2. Try to divert the patient's thinking while the impression material is setting. This can be done by asking the patient to breathe deeply through the nose; lift the right leg, lower the leg, and repeat with the left arm, or hum a tune.

3. Topical anesthetic can be applied to the palate and tongue.

4. For severe gagging, nitrous oxide can be used to significantly reduce the gag reflex.

H. Removing the impression tray.

1. Before removing the impression tray, check the remaining material in the bowl for tackiness (gelation)—approximately 2 to 3 minutes.

2. Breaking the seal. A significant vacuum seal occurs when impressions are taken, so a quick forceful snap is necessary to break the seal. An alternate method of breaking the seal is to loosen/lift the distal buccal corner edge the tray with an index finger.

3. To avoid distorting and tearing the alginate during removal, remove the tray in one direct movement from the teeth; straight down in the case of the maxillary, straight up with mandibular. Avoid twisting or rocking the tray during its removal (Figure 11–12).

4. Protect the opposite arch by inserting your fingers against the handle portion of the tray.

I. Cleaning and disinfecting the impression[5–9] (Figure 11–13).

1. Rinse the impression under cool running tap water to remove saliva and debris.

2. Shake off the excess water and spray with a disinfectant (iodophor or bleach).

3. Place in a closed plastic sandwich bag for a minimum of 10 minutes.

4. Upon removal of impression, rinse, and then use gentle blasts of air to remove excess moisture.

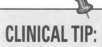

CLINICAL TIP:

Modeling Your Knowledge: When removing the impression tray, pull cheeks and lips away before snapping handle in proper direction.

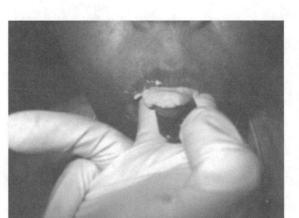

Figure 11–11   After placing the maxillary tray into the mouth, instruct the patient to make an "O" with the lips to muscle mold the facial side of the impression.

Figure 11–12   Remove the tray in one direct movement from the teeth to avoid distorting and tearing the alginate material during removal.

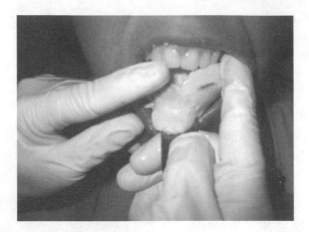

J. Factors that cause dimensional change. Dimensional changes can produce an inaccurate impression in the resultant study model or cast. Causes of dimensional change include:

1. Tearing. When separating an alginate impression from the patient's teeth, there is less chance of the impression tearing (permanently deforming) if the impression is removed rapidly with a sharp thrust or "snap."

2. Shrinking. Leaving an alginate impression in air results in its loss of water, with resulting shrinkage, causing an evaporation process called **syneresis.**[1,2,3,4]

3. Swelling. An alginate impression stored in or in contact with water will absorb the additional water and swell, a process known as **imbibition.**[1,2,3,4]

K. Preserving dimensional accuracy.

1. Pour alginate impression in **gypsum**—stone or plaster—as soon as possible after disinfecting impression to prevent dimensional change.

2. If time does not permit pouring of an alginate impression immediately after it is disinfected, shake off excess disinfectant and wrap impression in a wet paper towel.

   a. Place impression into a plastic sandwich bag.

   b. Seal bag to ensure storage at 100 percent humidity.

   c. Store alginate impressions for as short a period as possible to prevent dimensional changes.

   d. To prevent imbibition never store in water.

CLINICAL TIP:

Modeling Your Knowledge: An alginate impression will slowly shrink even under 100 percent humidity. Avoid storing for longer than one hour.

Figure 11–13   Disinfect and place impression in a closed baggy for a minimum of 10 minutes before pouring.

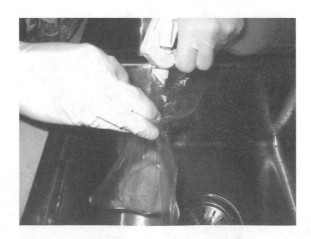

L. Making a tongue for mandibular impressions. Before pouring alginate impressions, the tongue area of the mandibular impression must be filled.
  1. Purpose.
      a. Eliminates excessive carving of plaster material once model is poured.
      b. Impression does not become "buried" into the model.
  2. Technique.
      a. Measurement. Use 1 scoop powder to ⅓ measure of water; mix.
      b. Formation.
          (1) Use two fingers to mold into impression tray and add alginate evenly to border of tray.
          (2) Hold until material is set—approximately 2 to 3 minutes.
M. Assessing the quality of the impression. A good impression will accurately reproduce the teeth and the surrounding anatomical structures without voids or tears; peripheral rolls should be smooth and continuous; midline should be centered.
N. Cleaning and disinfecting the armamentarium.
  1. Autoclave spatulas and metal trays.
  2. Use a surface disinfectant on the plastic water measure cylinder, powder scoop, and rubber bowl(s).

IV. Other Impression Materials

A. Elastic impression materials. Flexible and rubbery when set (see Figure 11–14 for an example of elastic vs. inelastic impression material). Types include:
  1. Hydrocolloids.[10] Known for their accuracy, reliability, and relatively inexpensive cost. Agar (reversible, demonstrates **thermoplastic** properties), a seaweed derivative that has been replaced by newer, elastomeric materials, requires a water bath to heat and temper the sol and water-cooled impression trays to cool the material so it will reach gelation temperature in the mouth.
      a. Uses. Final impressions for crowns, bridges, partial and full dentures.
      b. Properties.
          (1) Accuracy. Excellent.
          (2) Long-term stability. Good.

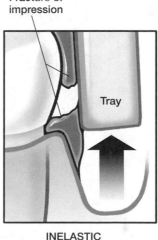

CLINICAL TIP:

Modeling Your Knowledge: Elastic materials can be removed from undercuts without undergoing any permanent shape distortion (Figure 11–14). An undercut is an area that has enough of a curve to make it difficult for a rigid material to tear upon removal.

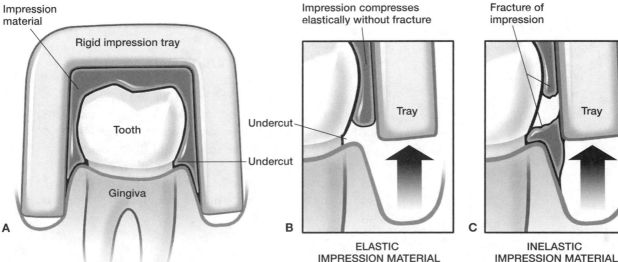

Figure 11–14   (A) Making an impression. (B) Removing elastic impression material. (C) Removing inelastic impression material.

CLINICAL TIP:

Modeling Your Knowledge: Automix guns are available for several materials.

(3) Elastic recovery. Good.
(4) Tear resistance. Good.
(5) Hydrophilicity. Excellent.
(6) Dimensional change. Poor.

2. Elastomers. Include rubber impression materials; most available as two-paste systems; contain a catalyst and base; require less material in trays than hydrocolloids.

a. Uses. Final impression for crowns, bridges, and dentures.

b. Properties.
   (1) Provide excellent surface detail reproduction.
   (2) Set chemically.
   (3) Working and setting times are shortened by increases in temperature and humidity.
   (4) More stable in air.
   (5) Viscosity varies from high (thick, putty-like) to low (light body material).

c. Types.
   (1) Polysulfide rubber. Oldest elastomeric impression material; more accurate than alginate material, but not as accurate as other elastomers.
      (a) Used for bridges, crowns, and inlays.
      (b) Dispensed as two pastes—a base and an accelerator; dispense both pastes in equal amounts.
      (c) Properties.
         i. Accuracy. Better than alginate, but not as accurate as other nonaqueous elastomeric materials.
         ii. Long-term stability. Good.
         iii. Elastic recovery. Excellent.
         iv. Tear resistance. Good.
         v. Hydrophilicity. Fair.
         vi. Dimensional stability. Fair.
         vii. Long setting time. 12 to 15 minutes.
         viii. Humidity and heat accelerate setting.
         ix. Must be poured immediately because the curing reaction results in a by-product of water and a great deal of shrinkage.
      (d) Characteristics.
         i. Difficult to mix due to viscosity.
         ii. Easily stains clothing.
         iii. Unpleasant taste and smell due to sulfur.
   (2) Polyether.[10] Stiffest of the elastomers, which makes it suitable for a disposable triple tray; sets quickly (Figure 11–15).
      (a) Used for construction of final full dentures and partial dentures, as well as bridge, crown, or inlay.
      (b) Dispensed as two pastes, a base and catalyst; use equal lengths and mix according to manufacturer's directions.
      (c) Properties include:
         i. Accuracy. Excellent.
         ii. Long-term stability. Good.
         iii. Elastic recovery. Good.
         iv. Tear resistance. Poor.
         v. Hydrophilicity. Good to excellent.

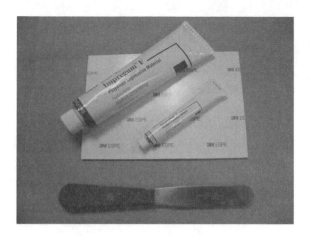

Figure 11–15   Polyether impression material.

      vi. Dimensional change. Poor.

     vii. Working and setting times are shorter than with polysulfide rubber.

(d) Characteristics. Unpleasant taste.

(3) Condensation silicone.

(a) Used for final impressions for permanent restorations, temporary crowns, and bridge fabrication.

(b) Dispensed in varying viscosities and a putty-base with a catalyst; mix according to manufacturer's directions.

(c) Properties include:

       i. Accuracy. Good.

      ii. Long-term stability. Good.

     iii. Elastic recovery. Good.

     iv. Tear resistance. Good.

      v. Hydrophilicity. Poor; not compatible with gypsum; difficult to pour model without voids and bubbles.

      vi. Dimensional change. Poor.

     vii. Polymerization occurs by a condensation reaction producing a by-product of ethyl alcohol; relatively high polymerization shrinkage.

    viii. Must pour immediately.

(d) Characteristic. Cleaner material to use.

(4) Addition silicone (polyvinyl silicone).[10] Most popular of the rubber impression materials.

(a) Used for crown and bridge impressions.

(b) Dispensed as two pastes and mixed or in automix gun (gun and cartridge system) (Figure 11–16). Materials (two pastes) are mixed and dispensed through the tip.

(c) Properties include:

       i. Accuracy. Excellent.

      ii. Long-term stability. Excellent.

     iii. Elastic recovery. Excellent.

     iv. Tear resistance. Good to excellent.

      v. Hydrophilicity. Fair.

      vi. Dimensional change. Excellent.

     vii. Wearing latex gloves to mix putty material can prevent setting.

Figure 11–16   Automix gun.

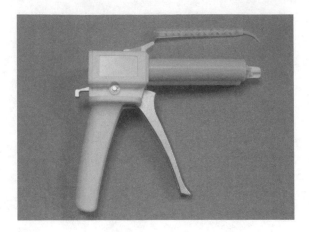

B. **Inelastic** impression materials. Used in areas where there are no undercuts;
when removed from the mouth, they are rigid.
   1. Types.
      a. Dental impression compound. A thermoplastic material used to take
         an impression of a prepared tooth or an edentulous ridge.
         (1) Uses. Bite registration, single crown preparation with no under-
             cuts, or spacer impressions.
         (2) Dispensed as sticks or cakes and melted in a water bath.
         (3) Properties. Not flexible, rigid, and difficult to remove.
      b. Zinc oxide-eugenol (ZOE) impression material (paste).
         (1) Uses. Impressions of edentulous ridges.
         (2) Dispensed as two pastes and mixed.
         (3) Properties. Not flexible, produces poor detail, and sets chemi-
             cally with water as a by-product.
         (4) Characteristics. Smells like cloves.

V. Pouring Diagnostic Cast or Study Models

A. Armamentarium.
   1. Rubber bowl.
   2. Spatula.
   3. Vibrator (Figure 11–17).
   4. Scale (Figure 11–18).
   5. Impressions.
   6. Wax bite registration.
   7. Glass or acrylic slab.
   8. Stone or plaster.
B. Gypsum products.
   1. Model stone. Usually buff in color.
      a. Properties.
         (1) Moderate strength, low setting expansion, moderate working
             time and a long setting time.
         (2) Provides excellent detail.
      b. Dispensing. Available in bulk or in preweighed single-use packages.
         Ratio of stone to water is 100 grams to 30 milliliters respectively;
         use scale for weighing stone.

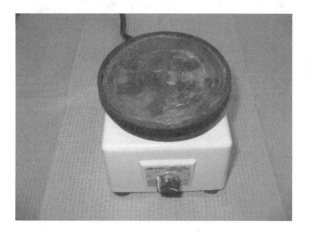

Figure 11–17   Vibrator. Used to reduce the number of bubbles produced during the mixing process.

2. Plaster. Usually white in color.
   a. Properties.
      (1) First gypsum material available to dentistry.
      (2) Used when strength is not a critical requirement.
      (3) Detail not as good as stone.
   b. Dispensing. Ratio of plaster to water is 100 grams to 50 milliliters respectively; use scale for weighing plaster.
C. Procedures. Double-pour technique.
   1. Impression. First stage pour:
      a. Measure the water into a rubber bowl and then sift the dental stone into the water to produce a smoother mix.
      b. Mix the stone and water with a spatula until the mix is thick and creamy.
      c. After the initial mix, press the bowl of stone on a vibrator to bring air bubbles to the surface, collapsing bowl when turning. The total mixing time should not exceed 1 minute.
      d. Place the impression on the vibrator and slowly add stone beginning with molar area and vibrate anteriorly into teeth imprints.
      e. Once the teeth are filled with stone, fill the entire impression tray on vibrator.
   2. Base. Second stage pour. Using the remainder of the stone, make a base the shape of the impression tray; place on acrylic or glass slab.

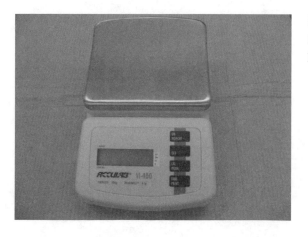

Figure 11–18   Scale. Weighs gypsum material used when pouring casts.

a. Invert the impression onto the base.

b. Assure the occlusal plane is parallel to the tabletop; avoid applying pressure to the impression material.

c. Smooth the sides with the spatula, removing as much excess as possible while holding the handle of the tray.

d. To facilitate separating the impression tray from the model, avoid covering the edge of the impression tray with stone.

(1) Allow 45 minutes before separating cast from impression—exothermic reaction occurs, giving off heat during setting process. Once the material is completely cooled, the material is set.

(2) Using laboratory knife, place on the edges of the impression tray and slightly twist to release the alginate from the gypsum material.

(3) Once margins are free, pull upward—this helps with separation.

(4) Wet strength versus dry strength. When models are first poured, excess water is present, which causes the material to have poor wet strength. After 24 hours, the excess water has evaporated, creating a material that is two to three times stronger than a newly poured model—dry strength.

D. Perform proper disinfection/sterilization of armamentarium.

VI. Trimming Diagnostic Study Models

A. Armamentarium (Figure 11–19).

1. Pencil.
2. Small ruler.
3. Clear protractor.
4. Level.
5. Lab knife.
6. Paintbrush.
7. Sandpaper/sanding block.
8. Glass or acrylic slab.
9. Model trimmer (Figure 11–20). Follow manufacturer's directions; some model trimmers require water for trimming, while newer models do not.

a. Adjust the water supply so a small amount of water is sprayed on the grinding wheel. To avoid clogging and promote proper functioning never use the model trimmer without water.

b. Avoid exerting too much pressure against the trimming wheel during procedure—the wheel will cut faster, resulting in a more rapid removal of stone from model.

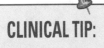
CLINICAL TIP:

Modeling Your Knowledge: If the tray does not freely release from the cast, determine the location of the obstruction. Use a laboratory knife to remove the obstruction.

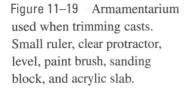
CLINICAL TIP:

Modeling Your Knowledge: Always remember to make sure the model trimmer is level before using.

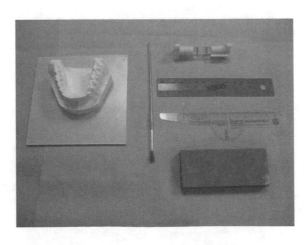

Figure 11–19   Armamentarium used when trimming casts. Small ruler, clear protractor, level, paint brush, sanding block, and acrylic slab.

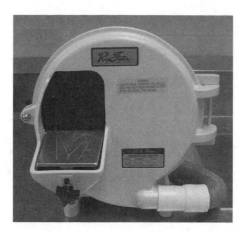

Figure 11-20   Model trimmer.

      c. After model trimming is complete, clean the wheel of the stone by letting the motor run, with water on, for at least 1 minute before turning off the machine.

B. Preparation. Soak the study models in water for 5 minutes—using wet models will prolong the life of the trimming wheel.

C. Trimming the mandible.
  1. Base.
     a. Place model on a flat surface with occlusal surface down; make sure model is resting on occlusal surfaces of teeth only—excess material may need to be removed from retromolar area (Figure 11–21).
     b. Locate the lowest level at the predetermined height ($1\frac{1}{4}''$ to $1\frac{1}{2}''$).
     c. Mark with a pencil all around the model at the same level.
     d. Trim the model to the marked line, checking height and parallelism throughout—base should be parallel to occlusal plane.
  2. Sides. Trim the right and left sides parallel to an imaginary line through the central fossae of the posterior teeth, from canine to last molar—approximately 5 to 6 millimeters from alveolar ridge
  3. Anterior border. Trim a semi-circular curve from canine to canine—again approximately 5 to 6 millimeters from alveolar ridge (Figure 11–22).

D. Trimming the maxilla.
  1. Base.
     a. Place the maxillary and mandibular models in occlusion with wax bite in place.

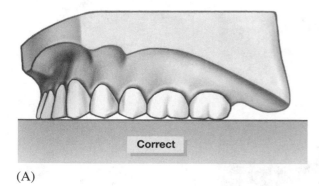

(A)

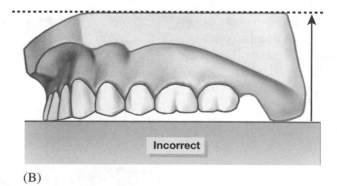

(B)

Figure 11–21   When trimming mandibular model, place on a flat surface with occlusal surface down. (A) Correct. (B) Incorrect.

Figure 11–22   Trim the anterior border of the mandible in a semi-circular curve from canine to canine.

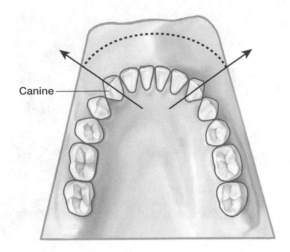

Canine

b. Rest models on finished base of mandibular model.
c. Locate the lowest desired level (2½ inches to 3 inches) and mark with a pencil all around the model at the same level.
d. Trim maxillary model, by itself, to marked line.
e. Evaluate with both models together; bases need to be parallel to tabletop.

2. Sides. Trim the right and left sides parallel to an imaginary line through the central fossae of the posterior teeth, from canine to last molar—approximately 5 to 6 millimeters from alveolar ridge (Figure 11–23).

3. Anterior border. Trim a straight cut from each canine to the midline in a V-shape, again approximately 5 to 6 millimeters from alveolar ridge (Figure 11–24).

E. Trimming posterior borders. Trim the posterior borders with the models occluded to create a flat surface.
1. Using a pencil and a small ruler, draw a line from the incisive papilla to the back (posterior) of maxillary model, following the mid-palatine suture (Figure 11–25).
2. Using a clear protractor, draw a line across the back perpendicular to the midline (see Figure 11–25).
3. Place maxillary and mandibular models in occlusion to insure no portions of the posterior teeth will be trimmed. If needed, move line back.
4. Trim maxillary model, by itself, to marked line.

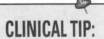

CLINICAL TIP:

Modeling Your Knowledge: Depending on the patient's occlusion, the narrowest arch may need to be trimmed first. It is recommended to trim the sides with models occluded to create a flat surface.

Figure 11–23   Trim the sides parallel to an imaginary line through the central fossae of the posterior teeth—from canine to the last molar.

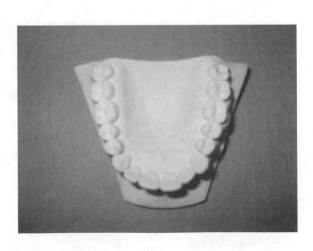

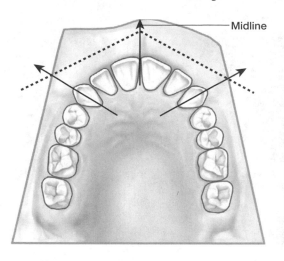

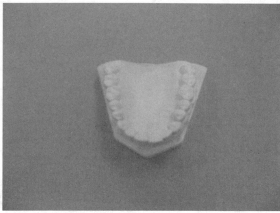

Figure 11–24   For the maxillary anterior border cut, trim a straight cut from canine to canine in a V-shape.

5. Again, place models in occlusion, without the wax bite; trim the back of the mandibular model to match the maxillary model; once backs are placed on flat surface, they should not rock.

F. Trimming posterior corners (heels). Trim heels of both models parallel to the side cut of the opposite side; cuts should be no wider than ½ inch (Figure 11–26).

G. Completed model. When complete, the occluded models should sit on the posterior base in centric occlusion and laterally on their sides.

H. Finishing.

1. Using a lab knife, smooth any excess plaster from the front and side; cut peripheral borders to eliminate an "overhanging ledge" appearance.

2. Remove all positive bubbles from hard and soft tissues.

3. Fill in small air bubbles/voids by wetting the void with water and filling in with a small mix of slurry stone, which is a thin mix of water and stone using a brush or small spatula; use a wax knife to trim any raised blebs.

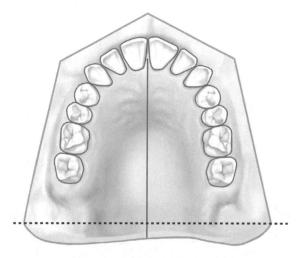

Figure 11–25   Using a pencil and a small ruler, draw a line from the incisive papilla to back of model.

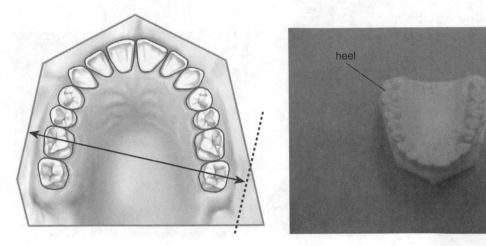

Figure 11–26   Trim the heels parallel to the side cut of the opposite side.

4. Use sandpaper to smooth model.
5. Soak in model soap for 30 minutes and then polish with a soft cloth.
6. Place patient's name and date on both casts.

Dental impressions are taken for many reasons, including the making of bleaching trays. This is an additional duty the dental hygienist can perform and therefore adds to the vital role as a health care professional.

QUESTIONS

1. All of the following are positive properties of dental alginate EXCEPT one. Which one is the EXCEPTION?
   a. Tear resistant
   b. Accuracy
   c. Long-term stability
   d. Hydrophilicity

2. Syneresis is a dimensional change that can occur with an alginate impression. It involves swelling of the alginate material.
   a. Both statements are TRUE.
   b. Both statements are FALSE.
   c. The first statement is TRUE. The second statement is FALSE.
   d. The first statement is FALSE. The second statement is TRUE.

3. All of the following factors should be considered when selecting an impression tray EXCEPT one. Which one is the EXCEPTION?
   a. Length of mandibular tray should cover tuberosity.

b. Borders should be approximately ¼ inch away from soft tissues.
   c. Width should be wide enough not to touch any buccal gingiva.
   d. Thickness of alginate between the tray and tissues should be approximately 3 millimeters.

4. When placing the mandibular impression tray, the operator should stand behind the patient. When placing the maxillary impression tray, the operator should stand in front of the patient.
   a. Both statements are TRUE.
   b. Both statements are FALSE.
   c. The first statement is TRUE. The second statement is FALSE.
   d. The first statement is FALSE. The second statement is TRUE.

5. When mixing alginate impression material, which of the following should be practiced?
   a. The alginate should be mixed slowly, yet thoroughly.

b. The alginate should drip off the spatula once properly mixed.

c. The water should be added to the powder.

d. The manufacturer's directions should be followed.

6. Which of the following impression materials cannot be used with undercuts?

a. Alginate

b. Agar

c. Polysulfide rubber

d. Zinc oxide-eugenol

7. Polysulfide rubber is the oldest elastomeric impression material. Although it is more accurate than alginate material, it is not as accurate as other elastomers.

a. Both statements are TRUE.

b. Both statements are FALSE.

c. The first statement is TRUE. The second statement is FALSE.

d. The first statement is FALSE. The second statement is TRUE.

8. All of the following impression materials can be used when taking an impression for the purpose of permanent restorations EXCEPT one. Which one is the EXCEPTION?

a. Agar

b. Dental alginate

c. Polysulfide rubber

d. Polyether

9. When trimming diagnostic study models, the sides of the models should be trimmed parallel to an imaginary line through the central fossae of the posterior teeth. The heels (posterior corners) should also be trimmed parallel to the side cut on the same side.

a. Both statements are TRUE.

b. Both statements are FALSE.

c. The first statement is TRUE. The second statement is FALSE.

d. The first statement is FALSE. The second statement is TRUE.

10. Which of the following is an inelastic impression material?

a. Alginate

b. ZOE impression paste

c. Polysulfide rubber

d. Addition silicone

REFERENCES

1. Nathe C. Taking an alginate impression. *The Journal of Practical Hygiene,* Vol. 12, Number 1, 2003, 28–29.

2. Ferracane JL. *Material in Dentistry: Principles and Applications,* 2nd ed. Philadelphia: Lippincott, Williams, and Wilkins, 2001.

3. Gladwin M, Bagby M. *Clinical Aspects of Dental Materials.* Philadelphia: Lippincott, Williams, and Wilkins, 2000.

4. Phillips RW, Moore BK. *Elements of Dental Materials for Dental Hygienists and Dental Assistants,* 5th ed. Philadelphia: W.B. Saunders Co., 1994.

5. Matyas J, Dao N, Caputo AA, Lucatorto FM. Effects of disinfectants on dimensional accuracy of impression material. *Journal of Prosthetic Dentistry,* Vol. 64, Number 1, 1990, 25–31.

6. Ralph WJ, Gin SS, Cheadle DA, Harcourt JK. The effects of disinfectants on the dimensional stability of alginate impres-sion materials. *Australian Dental Journal,* Vol. 35, Number 6, 1990, 514–17.

7. Bergman B, Bergman M, Olsson S. Alginate impression materials. Dimensional stability and surface detail sharpness following treatment with disinfectant solutions. *Swedish Dental Journal,* Vol. 9, 1985, 255–62.

8. Herrera S, Merchant V. Dimensional stability of dental impressions after immersion disinfection. *Journal of the American Dental Association,* Vol. 113, 1986, 419–22.

9. Andrieu, SC, Springstead, MC, Cline MV. Disinfection procedures for alginate impressions and study casts in the dental office. *The Journal of Practical Hygiene,* Vol. 2, Number 1, 1993, 19–21.

10. Christensen, GJ. What category of impression material is best for your practice? *Journal of the American Dental Association,* Vol. 128, 1997, 1026–27.

DENTAL IMPRESSIONS PERFORMANCE CHECK-OFF

Student ______________________

Date ______________________

Instructor ______________________

Patient ______________________

Re-evaluation

Date ______________________ Date ______________________

Instructor ______________________ Instructor ______________________

Patient ______________________ Patient ______________________

	S	U	Comments	S	U	Comments	S	U	Comments
1. Impressions are treatment planned appropriately.									
2. Trays fit in length (adequate coverage of retromolar areas and tuberosities) and width.									
3. Explains procedure to patient and coaches patient when necessary.									
4. Uses utility wax when indicated.									
5. Demonstrates correct mixing of material (smooth mix).									
6. Demonstrates correct loading of trays with adequate material in all areas.									
7. Correctly places trays in mouth before material sets and removes when set.									
8. Impression—results with no voids, smooth peripheral rolls, no occlusal surfaces hitting trays, and all anatomy is present.									
9. Uses appropriate infection control procedures.									

STUDY CASTS PERFORMANCE CHECK-OFF

Student _____

Date _____

Instructor _____

Patient _____

Re-evaluation

Date _____

Instructor _____

Patient _____

	S	U	Comments	S	U	Comments
1. Produces a model free of air bubbles, voids, and defects on anatomic portion.						
2. Produces a smooth tongue space on mandible.						
3. Retromolar/tuberosity areas are present.						
4. Produces an adequate base thickness.						
5. Lateral borders trimmed parallel to central grooves of posterior teeth.						
6. Trims all borders to be symmetrical.						
7. Trims maxillary anterior to a point at midline; trims mandibular anterior rounded from canine to canine.						
8. Study casts remain occluded when placed on lateral and posterior borders.						
9. Places patient's name and date on both casts.						
10. All anatomy is present (i.e., frena, vestibule, teeth).						

243

Chapter 12

Marginating, Finishing, and Polishing Dental Amalgam Restorations

Mary D. Cooper, RDH, MSEd

MediaLink

A companion CD-ROM, included free with each new copy of this book, supplements the procedures presented in each chapter. Insert the CD-ROM to watch video clips and view a large collection of color images that is also included. This multimedia library is designed to help you add a new dimension to your learning.

KEY TERMS

articulating paper	finishing bur	overhang
cavosurface	flash	polishing
cleoid-discoid carver	green stone	pumice
contra angle	linen abrasive strip	slurry
corrosion	mandrel	spoon excavator
disc	margination	tarnish
ditching	open margin	tin oxide
finishing		

LEARNING OBJECTIVES

After reading this chapter, the student will be able to:

- explain the rationale and goals for amalgam margination, finishing, and polishing;
- discuss the indications and contraindications for amalgam finishing and polishing;
- differentiate between amalgam finishing and polishing;
- explain the steps involved in finishing an amalgam;
- explain how the SHOFU® system is used to polish an amalgam;

- explain how the pumice/tin oxide system is used to polish an amalgam;
- assess an amalgam restoration and determine whether it needs replacement, margination, finishing, and/or polishing;
- competently marginate, finish, and polish amalgam restorations in both laboratory and clinical settings.

I. Introduction

The primary purpose of marginating, **finishing,** and **polishing** a dental amalgam restoration is to produce smooth surfaces.[1] Smooth surfaces do not easily retain plaque, are easy to keep clean by the patient, contribute to localized periodontal health in the adjacent area, and are less prone to recurrent decay.

Figure 12–1 Margination. A restorative surface that is flush with the existing tooth surface.

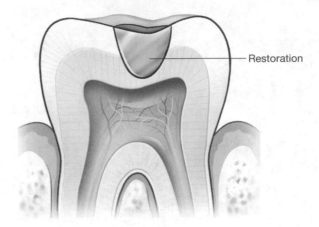

Restoration

Finishing procedures should be done after a dental amalgam has completely set and has gained high strength, usually 24 hours after placement.[2]

II. Margination

Margination is the process of using instruments and various abrasives on an overcontoured dental amalgam surface to produce a restorative surface that is flush with the existing tooth surface (Figure 12–1).

A. Indications for use.
   1. Excess interproximal material (i.e., **overhang,** such as a Class II amalgam restoration); affects:[1,3]
      a. Gingival tissues appearing inflamed in the area.
      b. Localized vertical bone loss radiographically or when probing.
      c. Dental floss often fraying.
   2. Overcontoured amalgam surface, i.e., Class V restoration, may present with gingival inflammation adjacent to the surface.
B. Benefits of margination include:
   1. Removes excess amalgam.
   2. Facilitates plaque control.
   3. Promotes healthier periodontal tissues.
   4. Recreates functional anatomy to the restored tooth surface.
C. Armamentarium for margination.[1]
   1. Finishing knives. Amalgam or gold knife (Figure 12–2).
      a. Excellent for removing moderate-to-large overhangs and contouring bulky restorations.
      b. Available in a variety of sizes and blade shapes. Single, sharp cutting edges may be straight or curved.

Figure 12–2 Finishing knife, cleoid discoid, and finishing strips.

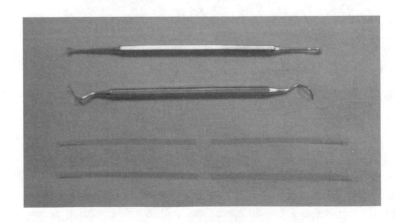

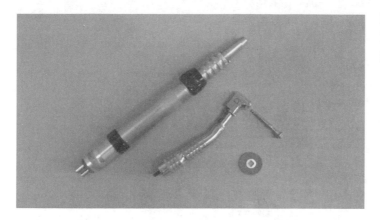

Figure 12–3   Slowspeed handpiece, **contra-angle,** mandrel, and disc.

    c. Offset shanks. Provide good access to posterior surfaces.

2. Files. Used to remove slight to bulky overhangs and overcontoured surfaces at gingival margins.

    a. Types.

        (1) Multiple cutting edges, varying in coarseness.

        (2) Straight blades, may not adapt well to rounded tooth surfaces.

    b. Application.

        (1) Begin with coarsest file and work through progressively finer files as amalgam is removed.

        (2) Use short, multidirectional strokes.

        (3) Create small grooves on the amalgam surface.

        (4) Finish with a curette/scaler or an amalgam/gold knife to remove the grooves.

3. Scalers, curettes, **spoon excavators,** and **cleoid-discoid carvers** (see Figure 12–2). May be used alone to remove slight overhangs of amalgam; generally not first instrument of choice because they are not rigid or strong enough to reduce a bulky, large overhang.

4. Ultrasonic scaler.

    a. Standard ultrasonic inserts. Those used for moderate-to-heavy calculus deposit removal, such as the chisel, straight or straight triple bend, are ideal for margination.

    b. An insert designed for fine debridement and deplaquing is too thin and weak to be used for margination and will be damaged.

5. Finishing **discs** on **mandrel** (Figures 12–3 and 12–4).

    a. Available in various abrasive grits and sizes.

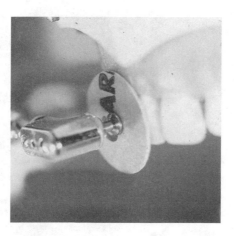

Figure 12–4   Finishing disc on mandrel.

Figure 12–5   Overhang.

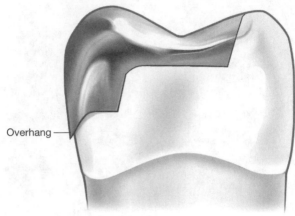

Overhang —

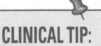

CLINICAL TIP:

Polishing Your Knowledge: Abrasives are always used in succession from most coarse to least coarse.

CLINICAL TIP:

Polishing Your Knowledge: Avoid using an amalgam knife like a scaler. Remove calculus by getting beneath the most apical portion of the deposit and breaking it off in a large piece. If an amalgam overhang is removed in this way, the amalgam restoration will most likely fracture.

b. Application.
   (1) Use a slow-speed handpiece.
   (2) Snap a small flexible disc impregnated with coarse abrasives (i.e., fine garnet) onto the mandrel.
   (3) Adapt disc using short, overlapping strokes from amalgam to tooth surface—this action will prevent **ditching** of the **cavo-surface** margin.
   (4) Use additional discs with finer abrasives (i.e., cuttle) to achieve a smooth surface.
6. Finishing/polishing strips (see Figure 12–2).
   a. Description. Thin, flexible strip of metal (lightening strip), **linen abrasive strip,** or plastic impregnated with abrasive particles on one side.
      (1) Plastic strips. In the middle of the strip the abrasive is separated by a smooth space that is useful for "flossing" through the interproximal contact without abrading the contact.
      (2) Available in varying grits, i.e. extra fine to coarse.
   b. Purpose. Used to smooth interproximal restorative surfaces.
D. Technique to remove a large overhang.[1,3]
   1. Assess the overhang (Figure 12–5).
      a. Use an explorer; if large enough, it can be viewed on a radiograph (Figure 12–6).
      b. Assess the condition of the adjacent gingival tissue to determine ease of access to overhang.

Figure 12–6   Radiograph showing overhang.

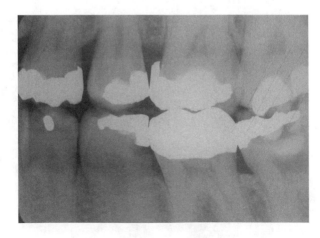

c. Select instruments based on the size of the overhang and ease of sub-gingival access.

2. Initial margination.[1,3]

a. Use a sharp amalgam or gold knife or an appropriate ultrasonic scaler insert.

b. Secure a fulcrum.

c. Insert the blade/insert into the sulcus with the tip of the blade/insert against the apical margin of the restoration.

d. Angulate the blade/insert so only a small portion of the amalgam will be removed.

e. Use short, overlapping, shaving strokes.

f. Avoid removing too much of the overhang with one stroke, because this could potentially cause ditching.

g. Work strokes from the buccal to the midpoint interproximally and from the lingual to the midpoint interproximally.

h. If using a gold knife, use moderate lateral pressure to shave the amalgam. As amalgam shavings come off, the pressure should be decreased (similar to root planing) until the amalgam surface is flush and the anatomy is correct.

3. Select the appropriate curette, modified sickle scaler, spoon excavator, or cleoid-discoid carver for the area.

a. Engage the blade at an angle between 45 degrees and 90 degrees.

b. Use oblique strokes to shave off excess material.

c. Position the cutting edge so it lies against both the restoration and the adjacent tooth whenever possible—this method will reduce ditching or undercontouring the restoration.

4. Finish with an abrasive strip.

a. With the abrasive side facing the amalgam, enter with the nonabrasive section of the strip to avoid disrupting the contact; use a sawing motion to "floss" the strip under the contact.

b. Press the strip against the surface requiring polishing.

c. Pull the strip back and forth (buccal-lingually) and up and down a few times.

d. To remove the strip, pull it toward the buccal and slide it out from the embrasure.

CLINICAL TIP:

Polishing Your Knowledge: Avoid using a curette or scaler with a working end that has been oversharpened. The lateral pressure needed to shave off the amalgam will likely break the working end of the instrument.

CLINICAL TIP:

Polishing Your Knowledge: If a dental amalgam restoration is under-contoured, has **open margins** or an open contact, there are no techniques the dental hygienist can use to restore functional anatomy (Figure 12–7). The restoration should be replaced.

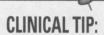

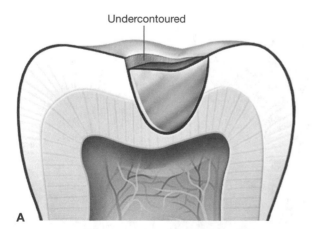
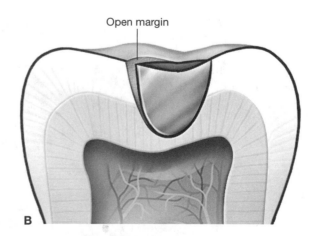

Figure 12–7   Results of poor carving. (A) Undercontoured. (B) Open margin.

Figure 12–8   Use explorer to evaluate cavosurface margin.

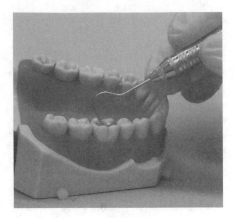

5. Evaluate end-product.
   a. Cavosurface margins should be flush.
   b. Amalgam surface should be smooth.
   c. Anatomical contour is restored and contact is present.
   d. No evidence of tissue trauma in adjacent soft tissues.
   e. Expose bitewing radiographs for remaining overhang.

III. Finishing and Polishing[1,3]

A. Benefits of finishing and polishing.
   1. Removes **flash** from the cavosurface, producing smooth margins.
   2. Improves overall surface smoothness and luster of the restoration.
   3. Reduces surface **tarnish** and **corrosion.**
   4. Facilitates plaque control; since the surface is smooth and homogenous, it is easier to clean.
   5. Decreases plaque retention.
   6. Increases life of the restoration.
   7. Improves esthetics of the restoration.
   8. Reduces the number of decisions to replace old amalgam restorations.
   9. Removes slight overcontours of the amalgam, flash, and small irregularities and scratches from the amalgam surface.

B. Evaluate restoration.
   1. Use explorer to evaluate cavosurface margins (Figure 12–8).
   2. Use **articulating paper** to evaluate patient's occlusion; if premature contacts (high spots), darker spots from articulating paper will be evident (Figure 12–9).
   3. Adjust accordingly.

Figure 12–9   Use articulating paper to evaluate patient's occlusion.

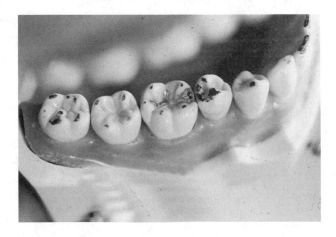

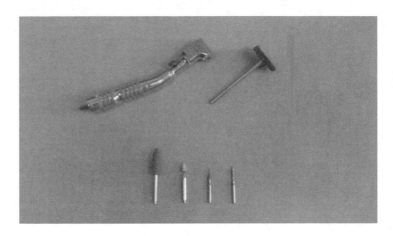

Figure 12–10   Armamentarium. Contra-angle, Robinson's brush, green polishing stone, white polishing stone, interproximal bur, and flame-shaped bur.

C. Explain finishing procedure and rationale to patient.
D. Armamentarium for finishing a dental amalgam.
   1. Slow-speed handpiece with a contra-angle attachment and/or prophy angle.
   2. Stones and burs. Use to remove excess material and irregularities from occlusal surface, grooves, and cavosurface margin.
      a. Stones[1,3] (Figure 12–10).
         (1) **Green stones.** Coarse abrasive stones.
            (a) Purpose. Use to reduce high spots on an amalgam surface and redefine anatomy and remove deep scratches; use articulating paper to assess high spots.
            (b) Available in a variety of shapes and sizes.
               i. Occlusal surfaces: Use a tapered or round shape to redefine anatomy and remove deep scratches.
               ii. Smooth surfaces, such as proximal, buccal, and lingual: Use tapered shape if area is accessible.
            (c) Application (Figure 12–11). Place the side of the stone in the center of the restoration and work the bur toward the cavosurface margin with light, overlapping, short strokes;

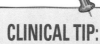

CLINICAL TIP:

Polishing Your Knowledge: Whenever a slow-speed handpiece and a contra-angle bur or stone are used, it is important to maintain a wet field (to reduce the risk of thermal injury to the pulp) and to run the handpiece at a speed of 20,000 rpm. A wet field can simply be produced with water.

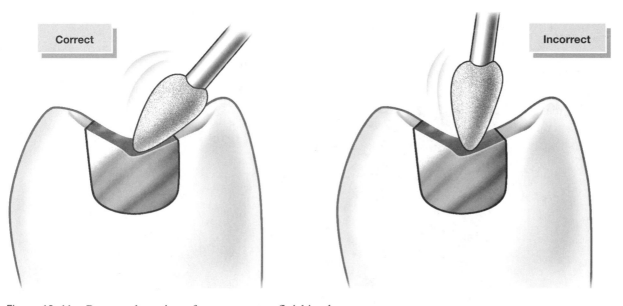

Figure 12–11   Proper adaptation of green stone or finishing bur.

Figure 12–12   Place green stone on cavosurface margin.

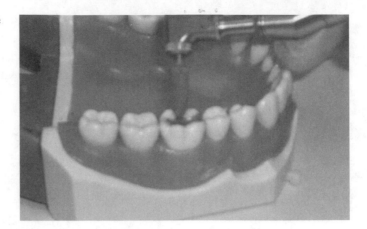

CLINICAL TIP:

Polishing Your Knowledge: Small burs are used for defining the pits and grooves on the occlusal surfaces, especially if the amalgam is small. Larger burs are used first on a large amalgam. Then proceed to smaller burs to define anatomy.

CLINICAL TIP:

Polishing Your Knowledge: Do not use carbide burs with few flutes (i.e., 3 to 5). These burs are used for cutting cavity preparations and must not be used for finishing procedures. To do so would cause significant removal and destruction of the restoration. Finishing burs have many flutes, typically 12 or more.

always move the stone from the amalgam to the tooth to avoid fracturing the amalgam margin (Figure 12–12).
(2) White stones (see Figure 12–10). Use on tarnished and pitted areas.
b. **Finishing burs.** Contain more flutes, "cutting edges" versus "cutting burs"; available in a variety of shapes and sizes, i.e., round, flame, and pear.
(1) Purpose. To reduce high spots and smooth the amalgam surface.
(2) Application (see Figure 12–11).
(a) Select the largest finishing bur and shape that will best adapt to the surface.
(b) Place the side of the bur in the center of the restoration and work the bur toward the cavosurface margin with light, overlapping, short strokes; always move the bur from the amalgam to the tooth to avoid fracturing the amalgam margin (Figure 12–13).
(c) Proximal surfaces.
 i. Use a flame-shaped finishing bur (see Figure 12–10) or finishing discs when area is accessible.
 ii. Move bur from tooth to amalgam to avoid ditching.
 iii. Use caution near gingival margins.
c. Finishing discs.
(1) Select appropriate size and grits; always use coarser discs first and follow with fine grits.

Figure 12–13   Place side of bur in the center of the restoration when beginning to polish.

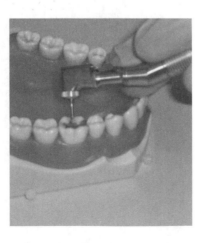

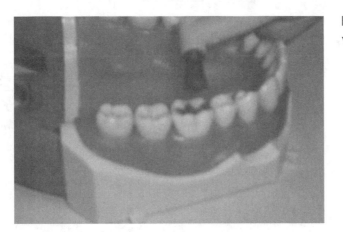

Figure 12–14   Apply pumice with a flexible rubber cup.

(2) Use short, overlapping strokes and move diagonally across the cavosurface margins.

E. Armamentarium for polishing dental amalgams.

Polished restorations have superior surface texture and are less prone to surface discoloration.[2] Polishing is the final step in the finishing/polishing procedure and is used to remove fine surface scratches. It creates an amalgam surface that is smooth and lustrous. Polishing can be achieved in one of two ways, using an abrasive **slurry** or abrasive cups and mini-points.

1. Abrasive slurries. Apply using light, intermittent pressure to prevent overheating of the restoration and the tooth's pulp; technique involves using:

   a. Flour of **pumice.** To create a thin slurry, mix with water in a dappen dish.

      (1) Apply to the amalgam with a clean, flexible, webless, rubber cup and/or a bristle brush. Pumice does the polishing (Figure 12–14).

      (2) Rinse the pumice slurry from the restoration with water and high volume evacuation (HVE). Amalgam surface will be smooth and have a semi-gloss, satin finish.

      (3) Polish proximal surface(s) with medium and fine finishing/polishing strips.

   b. **Tin oxide.** Use following flour of pumice; mix with water (or alcohol) to create a thin slurry.

      (1) Apply with a clean, webless rubber cup or brush.

      (2) Rinse the tin oxide slurry from the restoration with water and HVE. Amalgam surface will be mirror-like and shiny.

2. Abrasive cups and points (SHOFU®) (Figure 12–15). Some operators choose to use abrasive cups and points to polish amalgams. Silicone polishers impregnated with polishing abrasives are used to create brilliant, reflective surfaces.

   a. Types include Brownie®, Greenie®, Super greenie®.

      (1) Brownies are the coarsest of the three abrasives and are used as prepolishers; they create smooth, dull luster surfaces.

      (2) Greenies are finer abrasives; they create lustrous sheens.

      (3) Super greenies (green with a yellow-banded shank) are the finest of the abrasives. Used for the final step, they create super polish shines.

   b. Availability. All three abrasives are available as cups for proximal surface polishing and as mini-points for occlusal surface polishing.

CLINICAL TIP:

Polishing Your Knowledge: The operator can use a brush in a straight handpiece with tin oxide to polish an amalgam. Polish until the tin oxide begins to dry and a high luster is achieved.

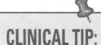

CLINICAL TIP:

Polishing Your Knowledge: All rotary instruments create heat. Therefore, always use light, intermittent pressure when polishing.

CLINICAL TIP:

Polishing Your Knowledge: When using SHOFU® cups and points, the slowspeed handpiece is used at the same slow speed that is used when polishing teeth with prophy paste, i.e., 5,000 rpm. Finishing burs and stones require much higher speeds, i.e., 20,000 rpm.

Figure 12–15   SHOFU® points and cups.

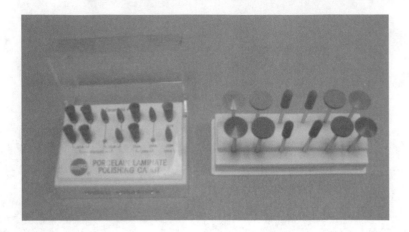

CLINICAL TIP:

Polishing Your Knowledge: It is important to rinse the amalgam thoroughly with water after each abrasive is used, i.e., Brownie, Greenie, Super greenie. The coarser abrasive particles must be washed away or else they will scratch the restoration when the next, finer abrasive cup and/or point is used.

Manufacturer recommends using a slowspeed handpiece at 5,000 rpm to 7,000 rpm when polishing with any of the three abrasives.

c. Technique.
   (1) Select a cup or point appropriate for the surface. Order of use is Brownies → Greenies → Super greenies.
   (2) Mount cup or point in contra-angle slowspeed handpiece.
   (3) Spray water on the cup/point and use light, intermittent strokes under wet conditions.
   (4) Rinse with water and HVE after each colored abrasive.
   (5) Evaluate after each colored abrasive is used.
   (6) Evaluate the end-product with mouth mirror and explorer.
d. Evaluation criteria for amalgam polishing.
   (1) Amalgam is smooth, free of scratches, with a lustrous shine.
   (2) All cavosurface margins are flush with the enamel surfaces.
   (3) Adjacent soft tissue is not traumatized.

Dental hygienists can use the recall appointment as an opportunity to evaluate the patient's amalgam and possibly accomplish the task of finishing and polishing if time permits. Polished amalgams can increase the longevity of the amalgam and should be part of the maintenance appointment for patients.

QUESTIONS

1. All of the following are benefits of margination EXCEPT one. Which one is the EXCEPTION?
   a. Removes excess amalgam.
   b. Promotes healthier periodontal tissues.
   c. Facilitates plaque control.
   d. Improves luster of restoration.

2. The purpose of using a finishing bur is to
   a. smooth interproximal restorative surfaces.
   b. smooth amalgam surface.
   c. cut amalgam.
   d. prevent ditching of the cavosurface margin.

3. Which of the following abrasives is the coarsest?
   a. Brownies

   b. Greenies
   c. Super greenies
   d. All are equally abrasive.

4. Polishing is used to remove fine surface scratches. It can be achieved by using finishing knives.
   a. Both statements are TRUE.
   b. Both statements are FALSE.
   c. The first statement is TRUE. The second statement is FALSE.
   d. The first statement is FALSE. The second statement is TRUE.

5. Finishing burs are used to remove high spots. When using, move the bur from the amalgam to the tooth.
   a. Both statements are TRUE.
   b. Both statements are FALSE.
   c. The first statement is TRUE. The second statement is FALSE.
   d. The first statement is FALSE. The second statement is TRUE.

REFERENCES

1. Paarmann C. Finishing, recontouring, and polishing amalgam restoration. *The Journal of Practical Hygiene,* Vol. 2, Number 1, 1993, 9–15.
2. Bryant RW, Collins CJ. Finishing techniques for amalgam restorations: Clinical assessment at three years. *Australian Dental Journal,* Vol. 37, Number 5, 1992, October, 333–39.
3. Rogo EJ. Overhang removal: Improving periodontal health adjacent to Class II amalgam restorations. *The Journal of Practical Hygiene,* Vol. 4, Number 3, 1995, 15–23.

Chapter 13

Temporary Restorations

Shirley Gutkowski, RDH, BSDH

 MediaLink

A companion CD-ROM, included free with each new copy of this book, supplements the procedures presented in each chapter. Insert the CD-ROM to watch video clips and view a large collection of color images that is also included. This multimedia library is designed to help you add a new dimension to your learning.

KEY TERMS

Atraumatic Restorative Treatment (ART)	mixing pad	temporary
	recement	triturator
eugenol	resin	
glass ionomer		

LEARNING OBJECTIVES

After reading this chapter, the student will be able to:

- place temporary fillings in certain circumstances;
- recall the different dental materials available;
- recall how to cement crowns temporarily;
- know how to prepare the tooth and the provisional crown;

- state the procedures for cementing crowns;
- state the procedures for placing a temporary restoration;
- understand the process of Atraumatic Restorative Treatments (ART).

I. Introduction

The scope of practice for dental hygienists is increasing. More procedures can be performed for patients than in the past, including services that had once only been legally performed by dentists. One such category of procedures is the **temporary** cementation of a crown, inlay, or onlay. It is not uncommon for a crown to come off during the prophylaxis appointment. A dental hygienist who can temporarily recement the crown, then reschedule the patient for definitive treatment, is a valuable member of the dental team. A second procedure that can be performed is the placement of temporary restorations, which is an expanded function in the practice acts of some states.

II. Temporary Restorations

These restorations are designed to fill a need for a short time; the patient may present to the office as an emergency or a situation may present itself during a routine dental hygiene appointment. Examples include:

A. Temporary crowns.
1. Individualized by dentist.
   a. There are different types of temporary or provisional crowns; each dentist may have a preference for one type over another.
   b. Made to protect the tooth and provide comfort during the period of time following the first visit of the crown procedure and the final visit when the crown is permanently placed.
2. Most often temporary crowns are created by the dentist and placed by a qualified dental auxiliary as defined by the state practice act.
   a. After the tooth is prepared, the temporary crown is placed and cemented with a material that will hold temporarily for a few weeks.
   b. In most states, dental hygienists can also cement temporary crowns, although it may be impractical because the dental hygienist must leave the patient who is there for dental hygiene treatment to perform a procedure that can be delegated to another qualified dental team member.
3. Procedure to **recement** temporary crowns. Recementing a temporary or provisional crown implies the patient already had the crown cemented once and needs to have the crown recemented. Often, this appointment is short and the procedure is performed accordingly.
   a. Armamentarium includes:
      (1) Mouth mirror. Aids in visualization and provides reflected light.
      (2) Explorer. Use to remove excess cement material after recementation of the crown.
      (3) Forceps. Helps manipulate cotton rolls.
      (4) Cotton rolls. Need four to six in number to isolate tooth.
      (5) Cotton pellets. Use to dry tooth prior to recementing the crown.
      (6) Floss. Use approximately 12 inches to evaluate the contact and ensure it is open.
      (7) **Mixing pad.** Use for mixing cement material with a spatula or to place premixed or capsulated material.
      (8) Spatula. Use for mixing materials, if not already premixed, and to deliver material into the crown.
      (9) Large diameter ultrasonic tip. Use to remove remaining cement from crown before recementing.
      (10) Scaler. Use to remove excess cement material from around the crown or interproximal areas after recementation.
   b. Remove old cement from the crown by using a large diameter ultrasonic insert.
      (1) Set power to high on ultrasonic unit. The water setting is inconsequential to remove cement.
      (2) Work over the sink to contain the water from the ultrasonic handpiece; it is recommended to place a paper towel over the drain in case the crown slips from fingers.
      (3) Place tip of the insert at the edge of the cement to begin the removal process; the cement will start to break apart.
      (4) As with any ultrasonic procedure, use light pressure.
      (5) Continue process until the majority of the cement is removed.
   c. Isolate the tooth with cotton rolls. Place one each on the buccal and lingual of the tooth needing the crown recemented. If the tooth is on the maxillary arch, place only one cotton roll on the buccal side. This will help hold the cheek out of the way as well as absorb any saliva.

d. Place a 2″ × 2″ gauze square toward the back of the mouth to catch the crown should it slip from the fingers.
e. Place the crown on the prepared tooth.
  (1) Note anatomy on the crown to determine its orientation.
  (2) Have patient close to determine occlusion and if it seats properly.
  (3) Mark the buccal of the crown with disclosing solution.
  (4) Remove the crown.
f. Mix temporary cement as directed by the manufacturer; there are several types of cement. The mixing should be accomplished on an oil-resistant mixing pad to a luting (putty-like) consistency.
g. Dry the tooth with cotton pellets.
h. Place a small amount of temporary material, enough to coat the sides without overfilling, into the crown using a dental spatula. Remove all of the cement displaced after placement—the less excess cement, the better. However, there should be enough in the crown to creep out ensuring a good cementation.
i. Place the crown on the prepared tooth.
j. Instruct the patient to close on a cotton roll placed on top of the crown to seat it. Keep in place during the setting time.
k. After the initial set time, as indicated by the manufacturer, remove the cotton roll on which the patient is biting.
l. Gently remove excess cement from around the crown by using a:
  (1) Scaler for the majority of the cement.
  (2) 204S or explorer for removal of interproximal cement; use caution to avoid inadvertently removing the newly cemented crown.
  (3) Floss to evaluate that the contact is open.
    (a) Use a double strand and tie a knot in the center.
    (b) Wrap the floss around the middle finger, or the usual anchor finger.
    (c) Carefully and gently press the floss down through the contact into the embrasure.
    (d) Avoid bringing the floss back through the contact, because it can dislodge the crown.
      i. Floss using an in and out motion.
      ii. Using the knot, dislodge the excess material.
      iii. Unwrap one of the anchor fingers and drag the floss out from between the teeth.
m. Inform patient this is a temporary remedy and reschedule an appointment for permanent cementation of the crown as soon as possible.

III. Permanent Crowns

Permanent crowns can also dislodge; a number of situations can cause this including recurrent caries, improperly fitting crown, poorly cemented crown, or just an occurrence.
A. Recementing a permanent crown. Implies the patient already had a crown cemented.
  1. Armamentarium includes:
    a. Mouth mirror. Aids in visualization and provides reflected light.
    b. Explorer. Use to remove excess cement material after recementation of the crown.
    c. Forceps. Helps manipulate cotton rolls.
    d. Cotton rolls. Need four to six in number to isolate tooth.

CLINICAL TIP:
Maintaining Your Knowledge: Under ideal circumstances, using a rubber dam is the best way to isolate the tooth during this procedure. If cementation is at the time of preparation, the tooth may already have a rubber dam in place.

CLINICAL TIP:
Maintaining Your Knowledge: Other cautions to practice are to remove the floss by pulling through between the teeth and instructing the patient not to eat on the side with the temporary filling for a few hours until the material is fully set.

e. Cotton pellets. Use to dry tooth prior to rementing the crown.
f. Floss. Use approximately 12 inches to evaluate the contact and ensure it is open.
g. Mixing pad. Use to mix cement material with a spatula or to place premixed or capsulated material.
h. Spatula. Use to mix materials, if not already premixed, and to deliver material into the crown.
i. Large diameter ultrasonic tip. Use to remove cement remaining before recementing the crown.
j. Scaler. Use to remove excess cement material from around the crown or interproximal areas after recementation.

2. Remove old cement from the crown by using a large diameter ultrasonic insert.
   a. Set power to high on ultrasonic unit. The water setting is inconsequential to remove cement.
   b. Work over the sink to contain the water from the ultrasonic handpiece; it is recommended to place a paper towel over the drain in case the crown slips.
   c. Place tip of the insert at the edge of the cement to begin the removal process; the cement will start to break apart.
   d. As with any ultrasonic procedure, use light pressure.
   e. Continue process until the majority of the cement is removed.

3. Isolate the tooth with cotton rolls. Place one each on the buccal and lingual of the tooth needing the crown recemented. If the tooth is on the maxillary arch, place only one cotton roll on the buccal side. This will help hold the cheek out of the way as well as absorb any saliva.

4. Place a 2″ × 2″ gauze square toward the back of the mouth to catch the crown should it slip from the fingers.

5. Place the crown on the prepared tooth.
   a. Note anatomy on the crown to determine its orientation.
   b. Instruct patient to close to determine occlusion and if it seats properly.
   c. Mark the buccal of the crown with disclosing solution.
   d. Remove the crown.

6. Mix cement as directed by the manufacturer. There are several types of cement. The mixing should be accomplished on an oil-resistant mixing pad to a luting (putty-like) consistency.

7. Dry the prepared tooth with cotton pellets.

8. Place a small amount of cement, enough to coat the sides without overfilling, into the crown using a dental spatula. Remove all of the cement displaced after placement—the less excess cement, the better. However, there should be enough in the crown to creep out ensuring a good cementation.

9. Place the crown on the prepared tooth.

10. Instruct the patient to close on a cotton roll to seat the crown and have patient bite on something such as a cotton roll during the setting time.

11. After the initial set time, as indicated by the manufacturer, remove cotton roll on which the patient is biting.

12. Gently remove excess cement from around the crown by using a:
    a. Scaler for the majority of the cement.
    b. 204S or explorer for removal of interproximal cement. Use caution to avoid inadvertently removing the newly cemented crown.
    c. Floss to evaluate that the contact is open.

(1) Use a double strand and tie a knot in the center.
(2) Wrap the floss around the middle finger, or the usual anchor finger.
(3) Carefully and gently press the floss down through the contact into the embrasure.
(4) Avoid bringing the floss back through the contact, because it can dislodge the crown.
   (a) Floss using an in and out motion.
   (b) Using the knot, dislodge the excess material.
   (c) Wrap one of the anchor fingers and drag the floss out from between the teeth.

IV. Temporary Fillings

Temporary fillings may be placed in most states by dental hygienists. Often, a tooth has been prepared and restored and then the restoration is lost. Another example is restoring a tooth with a temporary filling until a permanent restoration can be placed.

A. Armamentarium includes:
1. Mouth mirror. Aids in visualization and provides reflected light.
2. Explorer. Use to remove excess cement material.
3. Forceps. Helps manipulate cotton rolls.
4. Cotton rolls. Need four to six in number to isolate tooth.
5. Cotton pellets. Use to dry tooth prior to placing material.
6. Floss. Use approximately 12 inches to evaluate the contact and ensure it is open.
7. Mixing pad. Use for mixing filling material with a spatula or for placing premixed or capsulated material.
8. Spatula. Use for mixing materials, if not already premixed, and for delivering material.

B. Remove broken bits of restorative material if they are present and easily removed; use hand instruments and high-volume evacuation (HVE).

C. Clean the preparation as well as possible using hand instruments; rinse and dry. If the lesion is already prepared, remove the loose old restorative material.

D. Place temporary material into the preparation (Figure 13–1). Depending on lesion location, may need to place a matrix band. Some materials may

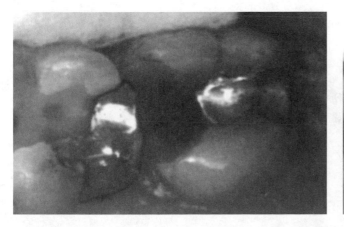
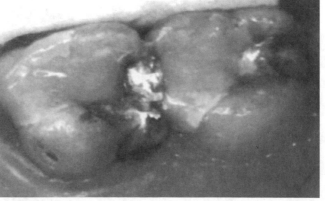

Figure 13–1   Glass ionomer temporary filling in minimally prepared teeth. *Photos courtesy of Geoff Knight.*

Figure 13–2   Powder and liquid mixed together.

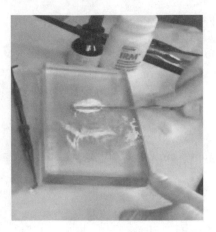

come in two bottles, one powder and the other a liquid (Figure 13–2), or in a capsule that must be triturated (Figure 13–3). Other materials are available; always read and follow manufacturer's directions.

E. Instruct patient not to eat on the side with the temporary restoration for a few hours to allow the material to fully cure.

F. Reschedule patient for definitive treatment.

V. Atraumatic Restorative Technique (ART)

ART is a technique used to restore teeth with minimal instrumentation. It is performed without anesthetic, making it an ideal technique for patients who are very young and/or phobic about dental care.[1-9]

A. History (Figure 13–14).
1. ART was developed for use in villages where no electricity was available.
2. It is also useful in public health settings or third-world conditions.

B. **Glass ionomer** (Figure 13–5). Material of choice for the ART technique.
1. Highly dynamic dental material that releases fluoride and recharges with fluoride from the environment.
2. Benefit, aside from arresting the decay process, is that it bonds directly to the tooth, decreasing the need for a preparation other than removing gross decay. More discussion on glass ionomers is covered in further detail in Chapter 6, Dental Sealants.

C. Patient case selection for ART include those:

Figure 13–3   Capsule in the **triturator.**

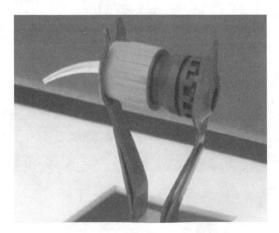

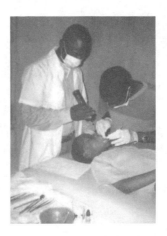

Figure 13–4   ART in action in South Africa. *Photo from http://www.whocollab.od.mah .se/expl/artsa.html. Courtesy of the Liberian Community Oral Health Workers Association (LICOHWA).*

1. With rampant decay.
2. Who have difficulty getting an appointment for a permanent procedure due to office hours or finances.
3. With sensitive teeth due to decay. The cavitated lesions will be filled, decreasing sensitivity.
4. Who are young in age.
5. Who have fearful parent(s).

D. Armamentarium includes:
1. Mouth mirror. Aids in visualization and provides reflected light.
2. Explorer. Use to remove excess material.
3. Forceps. Helps manipulate cotton rolls.
4. Cotton rolls. Need four to six in number to isolate tooth.
5. Cotton pellets. Use to dry tooth.
6. Triturator. Use to mix materials that come pre-measured.
7. Material in capsule form.
8. Floss. Use approximately 12 inches to evaluate the contact and ensure it is open.
9. Mixing pad. Use to mix material with a spatula if the premixed capsules are not used.
10. Spatula. Use to mix the two-part glass ionomer material.
11. Timer. Use to time the mixing of the two-part material.
12. Spoon excavator or curette (Figure 13–6). Use to remove decayed material from tooth.

CLINICAL TIP:

Maintaining Your Knowledge: This procedure, which requires no anesthetic to perform, is atraumatic to the tooth and causes little discomfort. Therefore, this technique is recommended for fearful patients or young children.

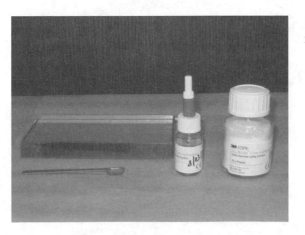

Figure 13–5   Glass ionomer materials.

Figure 13–6   Spoon excavators—small and large.

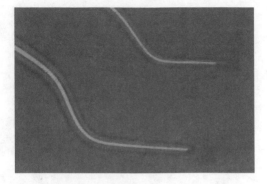

13. Carver.
14. Saliva ejector.

E. Procedure.

1. Remove decayed tooth material with curette or dental spoon excavator; use light strokes (Figure 13–7).
2. Isolate tooth with cotton rolls to keep the soft tissue from interfering with the process and to keep excess saliva from the site.
3. Mix glass ionomer as directed by the manufacturer; either the capsule in a triturator or the powder/liquid material on a mixing pad with a spatula.
4. Fill decayed area of tooth with the material; depending on the location of the decay, it may be necessary to use a matrix band.
   a. If the capsule is used, place it into the applier and extrude the material directly into the prepared area of the tooth.
   b. If the two-part system is used, the spoon excavator can be employed to transport the material from the mixing pad to the tooth until the void is filled with material.
   c. Material sets quickly and, immediately after mixing, can be flowable. It is advisable to wait a few seconds until the material is more workable before trying to place it into the tooth.
5. After 45 to 90 seconds, instruct patient to close together to adjust occlusion naturally. Material is rather soft and no adjustments will need to be made if the occlusion is set before the material hardens fully.
6. After 90 to 120 seconds, remove the excess material with hand instruments such as a scaler, explorer, or a curette.

Figure 13–7   Remove soft decayed portion with a spoon excavator.

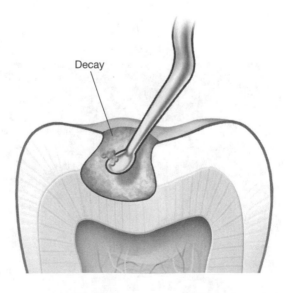

Decay

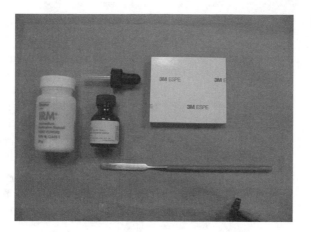

Figure 13–8 IRM materials.

VI. Temporary Materials

Use of these materials is determined by the dentist and can include:

A. Zinc oxide eugenol (ZOE) cement or IRM (Dentsply) (Figure 13–8).

1. Benefits
   a. Contains **eugenol,** which is derived from clove oil and cinnamon leaf, for analgesic effects.
   b. Long history. Has been used safely for decades.
   c. Inexpensive. Materials that have been around a long time are less expensive than newer materials. Requires no light cure since it is a self-curing material of chemical reaction.
   d. Removes cleanly. The nature of a temporary filling is that it is not intended to be in service for a long time. To place a permanent filling, the temporary material must be removed cleanly.
   e. Sets in 5 minutes.
   f. Lasts for up to one year. This is not the ideal amount of time for this type of temporary filling material to be in place; on occasion it may be necessary that it last that long.
   g. Provides sedative qualities. If the decay is near the pulp of the tooth, the dentist may request a temporary material that has sedative qualities before placing a permanent restoration to allow for easy access should the tooth need root canal therapy.
   h. Ease of manipulation.

2. Types of ZOE.
   a. Powder/liquid components.
      (1) Armamentarium includes:
         (a) Mixing pad. Use to mix the components.
         (b) Spatula. Use to mix the components.
         (c) Timer. Use to time the actual mixing.
         (d) Materials to mix.
      (2) Mixing. Use mixing pad and spatula to mix; follow manufacturer's directions (i.e., IRM).
         (a) Fluff powder before dispensing to ensure uniform density of contents.
         (b) Use powder measuring scoop provided and fill to excess.
            i. Avoid packing powder.
            ii. Level scoop with spatula.
         (c) Place powder on pad.
         (d) Dispense 1 drop of liquid for each level scoop of powder used. Immediately replace dropper cap to prevent evaporation.

(e) Keep liquid and powder separated until spatulation.

(f) When ready to mix, add 50 percent of powder to liquid and spatulate.

(g) Add remaining powder into mix in two to three increments. Spatulate thoroughly; mix will appear stiff.

(h) Strope (spatulate vigorously) for 5 to 10 seconds to create a smooth and adaptable working consistency.

b. Capsulated. Preloaded capsules contain the precise proportions of all elements of the finished material. Inside the capsule are the ingredients separated by a membrane that must be broken to allow the components to mix. The capsule may have an application tip, allowing for direct placement of the material and one-time use of the capsule.

(1) Benefits.

(a) Premeasured. There is no error in measuring the ingredients.

(b) No mixing difficulties and uniform mix. Proportions are always accurate, and the triturator will mix to a perfect consistency.

(c) Ensures less mess. No chance for spilling the ingredients.

(2) Proper mixing. Follow directions in the package, with photographs, to handle the material for mixing.

(a) Hold the bottom half of the capsule.

(b) Twist the top half of the capsule until a snap is heard, indicating the membrane separating the ingredients is ruptured, then continue turning until the top cannot go further.

(c) Immediately insert capsule into triturator.

(d) Set the amalgamator to HIGH and mix for 10 to 30 seconds (see package insert for times associated with specific machines). If mixed improperly, for too long or short a time, the material will not be workable in one or more dimension.

(e) Insert capsule into applier; remove press cap to access material (Figure 13–9).

(3) Placement.

(a) Isolate the tooth with cotton rolls. This will help keep the tooth dry and the tongue out of the way.

(b) Dry the tooth lightly with compressed air.

(c) Extrude the material out of the capsule onto a mixing pad or into a gloved hand; use enough material to fill the preparation.

(d) Form mixed material into a ball. The ball shape will allow for easy packing into the prepared tooth.

CLINICAL TIP:

Maintaining Your Knowledge: The triturator is a mixing machine originally used to rapidly mix amalgam capsules. Evolution of dental materials has employed the triturator, also known as amalgamator, to mix other dental materials as well.

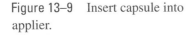

CLINICAL TIP:

Maintaining Your Knowledge: ZOE is also used as a surgical dressing. The eugenol is a potent healing promoter.

Figure 13–9   Insert capsule into applier.

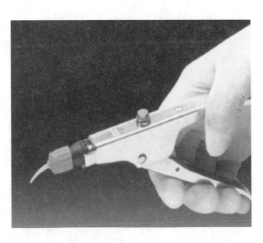

(e) Fill preparation with the material, pressing into the space and forming it with any dental instrument—many use a small condenser. This is a temporary filling—the life span of the material is short.

(f) Instruct patient to close teeth together before material sets to settle occlusion; this only takes 1 or 2 seconds.

(g) Remove excess material with a scaler before it becomes totally set; this material has a long working time.

B. Cavit (3M ESPE). Self-curing, radiopaque temporary restorative material with an extreme surface hardness.

1. Benefits.
   a. Contains no eugenol. Not every circumstance warrants a material with sedative properties; some research shows that eugenol remaining on the prepared surfaces can interfere with the adhesion of the permanent cement.[10]
   b. Inexpensive. Cavit has been available for decades, and is cost effective.
   c. Easy to use. No mixing is required.

2. Armamentarium includes:
   a. Mouth mirror. Aids in visualization and provides reflected light.
   b. Explorer. Use to remove excess material.
   c. Forceps. Helps manipulate cotton rolls.
   d. Cotton rolls. Need four to six in number to isolate tooth.
   e. Cotton pellets. Use to dry tooth.
   f. Floss. Use approximately 12 inches to evaluate the contact and ensure it is open before the material sets.
   g. Mixing pad. Use to place material from tube.
   h. Spatula. Use to manipulate material on mixing pad.

3. Procedure (as provided by manufacturer's recommendations).
   a. Squeeze a small amount of material onto a mixing pad, enough to fill the void in question.
   b. Isolate the tooth with cotton rolls to keep the soft tissue out of the way and aid in visibility to the area.
   c. Dry the preparation with compressed air or cotton pellets. Area should remain glistening moist, not desiccated—material needs some moisture for the chemical reaction to proceed.
   d. Place enough material into the prepared area to fill the void. Shape the filling and remove excess material. Patient should keep teeth apart during the initial phase of the chemical adhesion process.
   e. After 5 minutes, instruct patient to close together to mark occlusion—this step will impress the opposing teeth into the soft temporary filling material.
   f. Remove any excess material with a scaler.
   g. Advise caution about eating hot or hard foods, which may dislodge the material.
   h. Reappoint patient to return as soon as possible for definitive treatment.

C. Glass ionomer. Material that bonds with the tooth and releases fluoride, arresting decay.

1. Benefits.
   a. Provides a fluoride reservoir. The chemical complexities of this material allow fluoride to be released into the surrounding tissue. Fluoride is not a structural component of the material, so when fluoride is

available in the vicinity, such as with fluoride toothpaste, the material readily absorbs it for release later.

b. Color adds urgency to have definitive treatment completed.

c. Flowable. Material flows easily. For preparations with complex anatomy, the flowability of this material increases the chance of the material getting into all the parts of the preparation.

d. Well tested in ART applications.[1-9]

e. Remains in place as a single surface restoration for three to five years,[9] which is long for most temporary fillings. In young children who are not good candidates for traditional fillings, a glass ionomer temporary filling can be serviceable until the child is older.

f. Chemically bonds to tooth structure so no intermediate bonding step with dentinal bonding agents is needed; this also improves the margin between the material and the tooth.[11,12]

2. Disadvantage. Weak in comparison to composite **resin.**

3. Procedure.

a. Remove soft enamel with spoon excavator or curette (see Figure 13–7).

b. Isolate tooth with cotton rolls to create easy visualization of the tooth, as well as isolation from copious amounts of saliva.

c. Use compressed air or cotton pellet to remove moisture. Do not desiccate the tooth; some moisture facilitates the bond of the material with the tooth.

d. Mix the material as recommended by the manufacturer.

   (1) Powder/liquid components (hand mixing technique). Use mixing pad or glass slab to mix.

      (a) Fluff powder by tipping the container upside down three or four times before dispensing.

      (b) Use powder measuring scoop provided and fill to excess.
         i. Avoid packing powder.
         ii. Level powder.

      (c) Place powder on pad or glass slab.

      (d) Dispense two drops of liquid.

      (e) Use metallic or plastic cement spatula to mix.

      (f) Add powder to liquid in one portion; continue to mix until a viscid consistency is reached—material should almost drip from spatula.

   (2) Capsulated.

      (a) Tap capsule against the counter to loosen the powder in the capsule.

      (b) Push the black end of the capsule against the counter into the capsule—this breaks the membrane between the powder and liquid.

      (c) Put capsule into applier. Click once to fully penetrate the separating membrane; allow the powder and liquid to mix.

      (d) Remove capsule from applier and place into triturator (amalgamator). Glass ionomers have a short working time; mixing quickly after puncturing the membrane assures a good mixture and working time.

      (e) Triturate for 10 seconds on HIGH as per the manufacturer's directions.

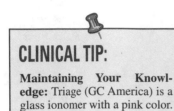

CLINICAL TIP:

Maintaining Your Knowledge: Triage (GC America) is a glass ionomer with a pink color.

(f) Replace capsule into applier and click until material becomes visible in cannula—the clear tip (see Figure 13–9).

(g) Extrude material directly into void in the tooth until the void is filled.

(h) Wait 45 to 60 seconds, then start forming restoration with the spoon excavator attempting to form some occlusal anatomy. Once the material has set for approximately 15 more seconds, use floss to ensure contact is open.

(i) At 90 seconds, instruct patient to close to adjust occlusion.

(j) At 120 seconds, remove excess material with a scaler.

VII. Aftercare

Aftercare for a temporary restoration differs from that for a permanent restoration. Because the material has a low compressive strength and is not intended to stay in the mouth for a long time, certain precautions are advised.

A. Keep the tooth clean with toothbrushing and flossing. A temporary filling usually has little anatomy and is less self-cleansing than non-restored teeth.

B. Use caution with eating; avoid foods that are:
1. Hot. May soften some materials.
2. Hard. May prematurely wear, chip, or break the restoration.
3. Sticky. May cause loosening or premature removal.

C. Pain control may be necessary if the patient presents with tooth discomfort. If the tooth is broken, it may cause:
1. Soft tissue laceration, such as the tongue or buccal mucosa. If so, use:
   a. Warm salt water rinses. Mix one teaspoon of salt with one-half cup of warm water.
   b. Over-the-counter (OTC) pain medications. Dental hygienists should not recommend medications of any kind. It is best to mention that the patient will get relief from the OTC pain medication taken for other pain.
2. Cold sensitivity. Instruct patient to avoid cold foods and beverages until permanent restoration is placed.

D. Reschedule patient for definitive treatment as soon as possible.

> **CLINICAL TIP:**
>
> **Maintaining Your Knowledge:** Cold sensitivity rarely occurs when using a glass ionomer.

Temporary restorations are in the realm of practice for the dental hygienist. Some restorative materials are more temporary than others. Glass ionomers for instance can be serviceable for years, and in a primary tooth may easily last until the tooth is exfoliated. ART technique is a process that is slowly finding its way into public health settings and private clinical settings.

QUESTIONS

1. What is the BEST way to remove cement from the inside of the crown before recementation?
   a. Use a large-diameter ultrasonic insert.
   b. Use a scaler.
   c. Use a chemical bath in the ultrasonic cleaner.
   d. It is impossible to remove cement from the inside of a crown; therefore, the crown should be remade.

2. Can glass ionomers be used on the primary dentition?
   a. Yes, any primary tooth can benefit from glass ionomers as a sealant and temporary restoration.
   b. Yes, only those teeth with decay.
   c. Yes, when the tooth is loose and about to be exfoliated.
   d. No, they are too caustic.

3. To ensure powder measurements are accurate, what can the operator do first?
   a. Fluff the powder.
   b. Pack powder tightly.
   c. Tap the cartridge to loosen powder.
   d. There is nothing the operator can do to ensure powder measurements are accurate.

4. The reason to first tap the capsule before placing into a triturator is to
   a. break the membrane between the powder and liquid.
   b. loosen the powder.
   c. mix the powder and liquid.
   d. make sure that there is material in the capsule.

5. The cannula is
   a. part of the capsule that keeps the powder separated from the liquid.
   b. the container where the capsules are stored.
   c. the portion of the spatula that mixes the cement.

d. the part of the capsule from where the material can be extruded.

6. What are the criteria when treatment planning ART?
   a. Fearfulness of patient, longevity of tooth, and pain.
   b. Degree of decay, age of patient, and tooth sensitivity.
   c. Color of material, amount of material to mix, and the size of the excavator.
   d. Level of pain, age of patient, and color of the material.

7. When will a dental hygienist most likely place a temporary crown?
   a. When the patient is in the hygiene operatory for a prophylaxis appointment.
   b. When the dentist asks for the service.
   c. When the assistant is out ill.
   d. Never.

8. How much cement should be placed into the crown before seating it onto the tooth?
   a. Enough to fill the crown.
   b. Enough to flow over the sides.
   c. Enough so there is no excess to remove once it is placed.
   d. Enough so there is some excess to remove once it is placed.

REFERENCES

1. Frencken J, Phantumvanit P, Pilot T, Songpaisan Y, van Amerongen E. *Manual for the Atraumatic Restorative Treatment Approach to Control Dental Caries.* WHO: Groningen, 1997.

2. Honkala E, Behbehani J, Ibricevic H, Kerosuo E, Al-Jame G. The atraumatic restorative treatment (ART) approach to restoring primary teeth in a standard dental clinic. *International Journal of Pediatric Dentistry,* Vol. 13, 2003, 172–79.

3. Croll T, Nicholon J. Glass ionomer cements in pediatric dentistry: Review of the literature. *Pediatric Dentistry,* Vol. 24, Number 5, 2002, 423–29.

4. Berg J, Farrell J, Brown L. Class II glass ionomer/silver cement restorations and their effect on interproximal growth of mutans streptococci. *Pediatric Dentistry,* Vol. 12, Number 1, 1990, 20–23.

5. Frencken J, Kakoni F, Sithole W. Atraumatic Restorative Treatment and glass-ionomer sealants. *Caries Research,* Vol. 30, 1996, 428–33.

6. Rutar J, McAllan L, Tyas J. Three-year clinical performance of glass ionomer cement in primary molars. *International Journal of Paediatric Dentistry,* Vol. 12, Number 2, 2002, 146–47.

7. Ewoldsen N, Covey D, Lavin M. The physical and adhesive properties of dental cements used for atraumatic restorative treatment. *Special Care Dentistry,* Vol. 17, Number 1, 1997, 19–24.

8. Qvist V, Manscher E, Teglers PT. Resin-modified and conventional glass ionomer restorations in primary teeth: 8 year results. *Journal of Dentistry,* Vol. 32, 2004, 285–94.

9. Mandari G, Frencken, van't Hof M. Six-year success rates of occlusal amalgam and glass ionomer restorations placed using three minimal intervention approaches. *Caries Research,* Vol. 37, 2003, 246–53.

10. Bayindir F, Akyil MS, Bayindir YZ. Effect of eugenol and non-eugenol containing temporary cement on permanent cement retention and microhardness of cured composite resin. *Dental Materials Journal,* Vol. 22, Number 4, 2003, December, 592–99.

11. Mount G. *An Atlas of Glass-ionomer Cements: A Clinicians' Guide* (3rd ed.). London: Dunitz, 2002.

12. Katsuyama S, Ishikawa T, Fujii B. *Glass Ionomer Dental Cement: The Materials and Their Clinical Use.* St. Louis, MO: Ishiyaku EuroAmerica, 1993.

Chapter 14

Medical and Dental Emergencies

Mary D. Cooper, RDH, MSEd

MediaLink

A companion CD-ROM, included free with each new copy of this book, supplements the procedures presented in each chapter. Insert the CD-ROM to watch video clips and view a large collection of color images that is also included. This multimedia library is designed to help you add a new dimension to your learning.

KEY TERMS

allergen	cyanosis	orthopnea
anaphylactic shock	diaphoresis	polydipsia
angina pectoris	dyspnea	polyphagia
angioedema	hyperventilation	polyuria
antibody	hypocapnia	pruritus
antigen	hypoxia	tachycardia
anxiolytic	idiopathic	tachypnea
apnea	ketoacidosis	thrombosis
asphyxia	ketones	tonic-clonic seizure
atopic	Kussmaul's respirations	urticaria
bradycardia	Levine sign	
bronchospasm		

LEARNING OBJECTIVES

After reading this chapter, the student will be able to:

- list steps that should be taken to provide supportive care during an emergency;
- predict, prevent, recognize, and manage medical emergencies;
- compare and contrast the American Society of Anesthesiologists (ASA) classifications;
- list the medications and equipment likely to be used in an emergency in the dental office;
- describe the pathophysiology of syncope;
- differentiate between the causes of vasovagal and orthostatic hypotension;
- identify the signs and symptoms of presyncope and syncope;

- differentiate between the symptoms of partial and complete airway obstruction;
- assist a choking patient;
- recognize the symptoms of respiratory failure and hyperventilation;
- manage a hyperventilating patient;
- compare and contrast bronchoconstriction and bronchospasm associated with asthma;
- list common allergens (triggers) of asthma;
- differentiate between the causes of intrinsic and extrinsic asthma;
- manage a patient experiencing a panic attack;
- recognize signs and symptoms of heart failure;

- recall the most prevalent cause of emphysema;
- manage an emphysemic emergency;
- compare and contrast type 1 to type 2 diabetes mellitus;
- list the signs and symptoms of hyperglycemia;
- manage a patient experiencing hypoglycemia;
- identify oral manifestations associated with diabetes mellitus;
- recognize the symptoms of a cerebrovascular accident (CVA) and recall how to manage a patient experiencing a CVA;
- compare and contrast hyperthyroidism and hypothyroidism;
- recognize and manage seizure disorders;

- differentiate between stable and unstable angina; recall how to manage a patient experiencing an episode of angina;
- recognize the symptoms of myocardial infarction (MI); recall how to manage a patient experiencing MI;
- identify clinical manifestations of allergies; recall how to manage a patient experiencing an allergic reaction;
- list common allergies experienced in dentistry;
- identify the most important drug in the treatment of an allergy;
- identify the four commonly used categories of drugs with significant overdose potential.

To prevent medical emergencies in a dental setting, a comprehensive health history, with baseline vital signs, must be taken. It is essential for the healthcare provider to obtain this information prior to performing any dental treatment. The information provided through the health history will help determine the risk status of patients and how treatment may need to be altered, as well as identify the potential for certain emergencies. In turn, healthcare providers should obtain the basic knowledge to recognize, assess, and manage a potentially life-threatening situation until further medical assistance is provided. Although medical emergencies are not highly prevalent in a dental setting, a survey revealed there is an incidence of 7.5 emergencies per dentist over a ten-year period.[1]

I. Emergency Preparedness

It is essential for the dental team to have an established protocol for emergency situations. Each member of the team should be responsible for his or her role in the "plan of attack" when an emergency situation arises. It is advisable to frequently practice emergency drills and conduct simulated emergency events. In addition, all members of the dental team should be certified in basic life support (BLS) to assist in an emergency dealing with cardiac arrest.[2] Since most states require dental healthcare professionals to be certified in BLS, only a brief description will be addressed.

A. Cardiopulmonary resuscitation (CPR).
   1. Sequence of CPR.
      a. Assess the problem.
      b. Activate Emergency Medical Service (EMS). Call 911.
      c. Perform the ABCDs of CPR. Airway, breathing, circulation, and defibrillation (automatic external defibrillator [AED]).
   2. Adult two-rescuer CPR.
      a. Establish unresponsiveness.
      b. First rescuer.
         (1) Open airway. Tilt head, lift chin, or thrust jaw.
         (2) Check breathing. Look, listen, and feel.
         (3) If breathing is absent or inadequate, give two slow breaths (2 seconds per breath).

(4) Ensure effective chest rise.

(5) Check carotid pulse for sign of circulation.

(6) If no sign of circulation or breathing, provide rescue breathing—one breath every 5 seconds (approximately ten to twelve breaths per minute).

  c. Second rescuer.

    (1) If no signs of circulation are present, give 15 compressions, followed by 2 slow breaths, given by rescuer 1.

    (2) After four cycles of compressions and breaths, rescuer 1 provides 2 rescue breaths and rechecks for signs of circulation.

    (3) If no signs of circulation are present, continue 15:2 cycles of compressions and ventilations until EMS arrives.

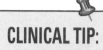

CLINICAL TIP:

Protecting Your Knowledge: Use a defibrillator, if available.

B. Vital signs. It is essential to measure the baseline vital signs—blood pressure (B.P.), respiration rate (R.R.), and heart (pulse) rate (H.R.)—for patients (see Table 14–1). This information provides normal values and can be compared to readings obtained during an emergency. All information should be recorded on the medical/dental history.

C. American Society of Anesthesiologists (ASA) Classifications.[3] It is vital to estimate the medical risk of the patient who is receiving dental care; this information can possibly prevent the risk of a medical emergency occurring in the dental office. Classification include:

1. ASA I: Normal, healthy patient with no apparent systemic disease.

2. ASA II: Patient with a mild systemic disease. Examples include those with:

  a. Well-controlled type 2 diabetes.

  b. Healthy pregnant women.

  c. Healthy patients with allergies, especially to drugs.

  d. Healthy patients with extreme dental fears.

3. ASA III: Patient with a severe, but not incapacitating systemic disease. Includes those with:

  a. Stable **angina pectoris.**

  b. Well-controlled type 1 diabetes.

  c. Emphysema.

  d. Status post-cardiovascular accident (CVA) and postmyocardial infarction more than one month.

4. ASA IV: Patient with a life-threatening, incapacitating systemic disease. Includes those with:

  a. Unstable angina pectoris.

  b. CVA within the past month.

  c. Severe chronic obstructive pulmonary disease or congestive heart failure.

Table 14–1 Vital Signs[3]

Vital Signs	0–1 year	1–6 years	6–11 years	11–16 years	Adult	Elderly
				Age		
Temperature (°F)	96–99.5	98.5–99.5	98.5–99.6	98.6–100.6	98.6–100.6	97.2–99.6
Pulse (beats per minute)	80–160	70–120	70–120	60–100	60–100	60–100
Respirations (per minute)	40–60	25–40	18–25	16–25	16–18	12–25
Blood pressure (mm Hg)						
Systolic	74–100	80–122	84–120	94–120	90–140	100–150
Diastolic	50–70	50–80	54–80	62–88	60–90	60–90

Table 14–2   Emergency Kit for the Dental Office[1,4,5]

Drug/Equipment	Treatment/Condition
Albuterol	Acute asthmatic attack or respiratory distress
Epinephrine (EpiPen)	Cardiac arrest, anaphylaxis, or acute asthmatic attack
Benadryl	Allergic reactions
Oxygen	Respiratory distress
Oral glucose (i.e. cake frosting)	Manage hypoglycemia
Diazepam	Convulsions
Ammonia spirits	Syncope
Methoxamine	Hypotension
Nitroglycerine	Angina
Atropine	Bradycardia
Hydrocortisone	Adrenocortical insufficiency and severe allergic reaction

5. ASA V: Patient *not* expected to survive 24 hours (not applicable to dentistry). Includes those with end stage of:
   a. Cancer.
   b. Infectious disease.
   c. Renal disease.
   d. Respiratory disease.
6. If an emergency situation exists, add an *E* before the ASA classification.
D. Emergency kit for the dental office (Table 14–2). The dental office should be equipped with emergency equipment and medications likely to be used in an emergency, along with an oxygen source and resuscitation mask or face shield. Each team member should be aware of the drugs and their purposes in an emergency situation. It is essential to always keep emergency office equipment in working condition and medications updated and readily available.

II. Unconsciousness

A. Syncope (Vasovagal/Vasodepressor) = fainting. Most common form of unconsciousness; transient loss of consciousness (fainting) caused from a decreased circulation of blood to the brain.[6,7,8]
1. *Most common medical emergency experienced in the dental office.* It affects individuals of all ages, although it is more common in young adults and not common in children, because they are more likely to show emotions.[6]
2. Precipitating factors include stress—emotional or physical.[6]
   a. Psychogenic (psychological) factors include fear, emotional stress, pain, and the sight of blood, to name a few.
   b. Nonpsychogenic (physical) factors include hunger, exhaustion, and hot, humid, crowded environments.
3. Pathophysiology.
   a. When fear is initiated, adrenaline (epinephrine/norepinephrine) is released into the bloodstream in preparation for physical activity—"fight-or-flight" response.
   b. When the patient does not fight or flee, blood pools in the muscles, resulting in a drop of circulating blood, including blood going to the brain.
   c. This decreased flow of blood returning to the heart and brain causes a decrease in pulse and B.P.; therefore,
   d. Cerebral ischemia results, causing fainting.
4. Signs and symptoms.
   a. Presyncope: Results when the body is affected by inadequate circulation of blood and oxygen.[6]

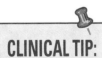

CLINICAL TIP:

Protecting Your Knowledge: Since emotional stress is a precipitating factor in causing syncope, the outward showing of emotions decreases the risk of fainting.

(1) Skin. Ashen in color, moist and/or cool— **diaphoresis** (cold sweat), and goose bumps.
(2) Patient feels warmth in head and neck, lightheadedness or dizziness, and numbness or tingling in toes and fingers.
(3) **Tachycardia** and increase in B.P.
   b. Syncope: Period when patient loses consciousness.[6]
(1) Irregular breathing, can be either jerky and gasping, quiet and shallow, or it may cease entirely—**apnea.**
(2) Possibly convulsions with muscular twitching.
(3) **Bradycardia** and decrease in B.P., which causes the transient loss of consciousness.
   c. Postsyncope: Period when patient returns to consciousness and heart (pulse) rate and returns to normal.
5. Dental emergency management.
   a. Place patient in supine position (Figure 14–1) to facilitate blood return to the brain. Place pregnant patient on left side before elevating her feet. If the patient is able, have him or her move legs vigorously.
   b. Assess ABCDs.
   c. Administer oxygen, which may assist in recovery.
   d. Place crushed aromatic ammonia capsule under patient's nose, if patient is breathing and has a pulse—stimulates breathing and muscle movement.
   e. Monitor vital signs. H.R., R.R., and B.P.
   f. Activate EMS only if patient's condition is or becomes unstable; vital signs are not within baseline limits for the patient.
   g. Suspend dental treatment for the day since a second episode is possible; have escort take patient home.
6. Prevention. Identify factors that may predispose patient to syncope.
   a. Take a thorough medical history and evaluate any conditions that may trigger a syncope episode.
   b. Use stress-reduction protocol. Always try to calm and reassure patient.
   c. Encourage patient to verbalize apprehension and/or fear.
B. Postural (orthostatic) hypotension. Disorder of the autonomic nervous system (ANS) in which fainting is related to positioning. Results from a rapid fall in B.P. when moving from a supine to an upright position. A greater

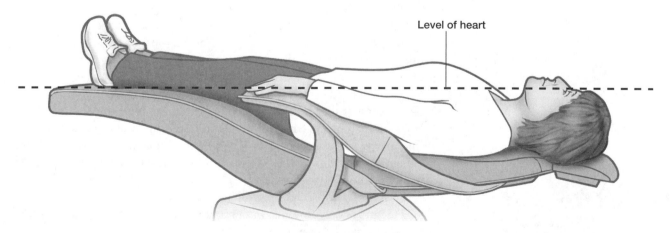

Figure 14–1   Supine position. Place patient so head is level with the heart.

than 20 mm Hg drop in systolic pressure or a greater than 10 mm Hg drop in diastolic pressure.

1. Precipitating factors include:
   a. Prolonged recumbency or convalescence for a week or longer or a long dental appointment—one- to three-hour treatment sessions.
   b. Pregnancy. Usually in the first trimester (reason unknown) or late in the third trimester due to uterus compressing the inferior vena cava, which decreases the venous return from the legs.
   c. Age (elderly), due to a change in B.P.
   d. Varicose veins from excess blood pooling in legs.
   e. Side effects from some medications, such as antihypertensives, some tranquilizers and antidepressants, narcotics, and antiparkinson drugs.[6]

2. Pathophysiology. Reaction of the ANS when patient assumes an upright position; blood needs to go upward from the heart (opposite gravity) to provide oxygen to the brain and glucose needed for consciousness.

3. Signs and symptoms. Similar to those with vasodepressor syncope, but associated with positioning; therefore, elevate chair slowly to an upright position—two or three positional changes over a period of 1 to 2 minutes. Make sure the patient is stable once in a standing position.

4. Dental treatment and management.
   a. Assess consciousness.
   b. Place patient in supine position.
   c. Assess ABCDs.
   d. Administer oxygen.
   e. Monitor vital signs to determine if they are within the baseline limits for the patient.
   f. Slowly elevate patient.
   g. If patient has no history of orthostatic hypotension, have escort drive patient home. If patient has a history of chronic orthostatic hypotension, he or she may be allowed to drive home when fully recovered.

III. Respiratory Distress

Since dental treatment is conducted in or around the proximity of the oral cavity, compromising the upper respiratory airway may occur. Respiratory emergencies are among the most common problems encountered in dental practice.[9] Fortunately, patients with respiratory distress experiencing a medical emergency usually remain conscious and are able to assist the healthcare provider in making a definitive diagnosis for treatment.[10]

A. Airway obstruction. Can occur from objects being swallowed in the oral cavity or the tongue occluding the airway, *which is the most common cause of air obstruction,* when the patient becomes unconscious.

1. Mode of entrance of swallowed objects.
   a. Usually enters the gastrointestinal (GI) tract. Rare for the aspiration to occur into the trachea and lung.
   b. Esophagus. Most common site of obstruction in GI tract.
   c. Obstructed objects can cause infection, lung abscess, and pneumonia.

2. Acute airway obstruction. Can involve partial airway obstruction with good airflow, partial airway obstruction with poor airflow, or complete airway obstruction (**asphyxia**).
   a. Partial airway obstruction with good airflow.
      (1) Signs and symptoms. Patient remains alert and wheezes between coughs—has ability to breathe.

(2) Treatment. Remain with patient and encourage patient to cough to expel object.

b. Partial airway obstruction with poor airflow.

(1) Signs and symptoms include:

(a) "Crowing" sound during inspiration.

(b) Patient:

i. Experiences a weak, ineffective cough reflex.

ii. Cannot talk or makes altered voice sounds.

iii. Gives choking sign—grasping throat with hand.

iv. May become cyanotic and disoriented.

c. Complete airway obstruction.

(1) Initial phase.

(a) Patient is conscious, but struggling to breathe; gives choking sign.

(b) No air exchange occurs, and therefore no voice sounds are heard.

(c) Increase in B.P. and H.R. due to a decrease in air exchange.

(d) Patient becomes cyanotic.

(2) Second phase.

(a) Patient loses consciousness.

(b) Initially a decrease in B.P. and respiration and pulse rates can cease.

(3) Last phase. Dilated pupils and absent vital signs, which lead to full cardiac arrest.

3. Dental emergency management.

a. Ask patient, "Are you choking?"

b. Perform abdominal thrust (Heimlich maneuver), which elevates the diaphragm, forcing air from the lungs. Use chest thrusts in later stages of pregnancy or for obese patients.

c. If an object enters oropharynx during dental treatment, place patient in a supine position.

d. Instruct patient to turn to left side and lean with head down and upper body over side of chair to try to dislodge the item and keep airway open. Check for respiratory sounds.

e. If patient swallows the object, a radiograph needs to be taken at the hospital to determine its location.

f. If patient loses consciousness, activate EMS and assess ABCDs.

4. Prevention. Measures can be taken in the dental office to prevent objects from dropping into the upper airway; these include using:

a. High-volume evacuation (HVE) and saliva ejector.

b. Rubber dam.

c. Ligature on rubber dam clamp (Figure 14–2).

B. **Hyperventilation.** Involves increase in frequency and/or depth of respirations (rapid breathing rate/panting) in excess of metabolic needs, producing respiratory alkalosis—excess exhalation of carbon dioxide (CO_2); *one of the most common emergencies dealt with in dentistry,* patient almost always remains conscious throughout episode. Usually a response to stress.

1. Precipitating factors include:

a. Almost always occurs in 15- to 40-year-olds because of extreme anxiety. Patients try to hide fears;[6] uncommon in those who admit to their fears, such as children. Rarely occurs in adults over 40 years of age.

Figure 14–2   Applying a ligature on a rubber dam clamp to prevent swallowing.

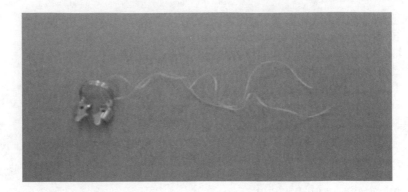

b. Head injury, severe bleeding, and hyperglycemia associated with diabetes.

2. Pathophysiology.
   a. Change in respirations due to an increased exchange of oxygen and carbon dioxide by the lungs.
   b. "Blowing off" of carbon dioxide results in a decrease below the norm—**hypocapnia.**
   c. As a result, blood pH rises, causing respiratory alkalosis. Alkalosis changes body chemistry, increasing the anxiety level even more, which triggers erratic behavior.

3. Signs and symptoms may last for any period of time and include:
   a. Feeling of chest tightness and/or suffocation.
   b. Lightheadedness or giddiness.
   c. Epigastric discomfort, palpitations of the heart, and lump in throat.
   d. Increase in R.R.

4. Dental emergency management.
   a. Terminate procedure and remove syringe or any other item that may cause anxiety from patient's view. Remove any materials from patient's mouth.
   b. Position patient upright.
   c. Use stress-reduction protocol and calm patient.
   d. Instruct patient to breathe slowly.
   e. Correct respiratory alkalosis. Use a small paper bag (over nose and mouth) or a clear resuscitation face mask and have patient breathe 6 to 10 breaths per minute (bpm) to enrich CO_2. If neither is available, have patient cup hands over nose and mouth.
   f. Subsequent dental treatment. Continue if patient and healthcare provider feel comfortable.

C. Asthma. Chronic lung condition characterized by shortness of breath due to bronchoconstriction and **bronchospasm** of the bronchi.
   1. Prevalence. Has increased in the past two decades.[11,12]
      a. Majority develop symptoms before the age of 5.
      b. Those at highest risk include:
         (1) Children: Twice as many boys as girls.
         (2) Young adults.
         (3) Racial and ethnic minorities living in urban areas.
   2. Precipitating factors (**allergens** or triggers) include:
      a. High emotional state, such as anxiety, stress, and nervousness.

CLINICAL TIP:

Protecting Your Knowledge: Basic life support (BLS) is rarely needed when treating a patient who is hyperventilating.

CLINICAL TIP:

Protecting Your Knowledge: Chronic obstructive pulmonary disease and asthma affect 25,000,000 Americans.[13]

  b. Tobacco smoke.

  c. Dust mites.

  d. Pollens.

  e. Mold.

  f. Animal fur.

  g. Other, such as viral respiratory infection, small birth size, and diet.

3. Pathophysiology.[12,14]

  a. Bronchoconstriction occurs when muscles of air passages squeeze and become narrow as a result of allergens (triggers).

  b. Bronchospasm is related to bronchiole inflammation caused when air passages produce extra mucus, making it harder to breathe by clogging the tubes; results in **tachypnea.**

4. Signs and symptoms include:

  a. Wheezing, often identified as hoarse.

  b. Shortness of breath.

  c. Coughing—sometimes this may be the only symptom.

  d. Production of sputum.

  e. Tachycardia.

5. Types of asthma.[12,14]

  a. Extrinsic (allergic or **atopic** asthma), history of an allergen.

   (1) Most common asthma of children.

   (2) Accounts for approximately 35 percent of all adult cases.

   (3) Triggered by certain allergens, such as:

    (a) Airborne: Includes house dust, feathers, and dander.

    (b) Food: Includes cow's milk, eggs, and fish.

    (c) Drugs: Includes aspirin, penicillin, nonsteroidal anti-inflammatory agents, cholinergics, and beta-adrenergic blocking drugs.

  b. Intrinsic asthma (nonallergic or nonatopic), no history of allergen.

   (1) Considered idiopathic or infective asthma.

   (2) Develops in adults after age 35 and attacks are more severe.

   (3) Can be precipitated by nonallergic factors such as:

    (a) Respiratory infection.

    (b) Physical exertion.

    (c) Environmental, such air pollution.

  c. Status asthmaticus: Persistent exacerbation of asthma.[6]

   (1) Life-threatening condition that does not respond to therapy; often drug-induced.

   (2) Patient experiences same symptoms as acute asthma, but manifestations may continue for a prolonged period; patient experiences:

    (a) Extreme fatigue.

    (b) Dehydration.

    (c) Severe **hypoxia** (oxygen deprivation).

6. Prevention.

  a. Determine factors that may trigger asthma episodes; remove patient from local irritants.

  b. Use stress-reduction protocol. Administer nitrous oxide for patient who has mild-to-moderate asthma. Nitrous is contraindicated if patient has severe asthma because of potential airway obstruction or is claustrophobic.

7. Pharmacotherapy.[12,14]
   a. Bronchodilators (β-adrenergic aerosolized). Relax smooth muscle lining of the bronchioles; inhalers: Albuterol (e.g., Ventolin, Proventil)—patient takes two to three puffs every 4 to 6 hours.
   b. Anticholinergics (e.g., Ipratropium). Inhibit contraction of bronchial muscle and reduce the production and secretion of mucus.
   c. Inhaled corticosteroids. Added when a patient needs to use an inhaled beta agonist more than three times per week.
8. Dental management.[12,14]
   a. Place patient's inhaler in an accessible area; sometimes patient may need to take several puffs of the inhaler immediately prior to treatment.
   b. Appoint the patient in the morning and schedule shorter appointments, if possible.
   c. Use stress-reduction protocol to minimize anxiety-induced asthma attacks.
   d. Do NOT use barbituates and narcotics during dental procedure—may increase risk of bronchospasm.
   e. Use **anxiolytic** agents when the patient is anxious and nitrous oxide is contraindicated.
9. Dental emergency management of an acute asthmatic attack.
   a. Terminate dental procedure and remove any materials from the mouth.
   b. Position patient sitting with arms thrown forward to increase comfort of the patient.
   c. Calm patient.
   d. Prepare for basic life support: B.P. and H.R. will be increased.
   e. Administer bronchodilator.
   f. Discontinue treatment and reschedule patient.
10. Dental emergency management of an acute, severe asthmatic attack.
    a. Follow steps as a. through e. above.
    b. Administer oxygen, if patient shows any sign of hypoxia.
    c. Activate EMS, if bronchodilator fails.

D. Panic attack.
   1. Precipitating factor includes acute anxiety.
   2. Signs and symptoms include chest pain, hyperventilation, anxiety, nausea, and parasthesia.
   3. Dental emergency management.
      a. Position patient comfortably.
      b. Explain procedure(s) to be performed for the patient.
      c. Give frequent breaks.
      d. Avoid administering oxygen if hyperventilation is part of attack.

E. Heart failure. Condition by which abnormal cardiac function does not allow the heart to pump the amount of blood needed to meet the requirements of tissue metabolism.
   1. Precipitating factors include:
      a. Pulmonary circulation: Left ventricular heart failure.
      b. Systemic circulation: Right ventricular heart failure, which is caused by left heart failure.
      c. Congestive heart failure: Involves the combination of right and left ventricles.
   2. Pathophysiology. When a condition, such as high B.P. or stenosis, demands an increase in cardiac workload changes in the heart muscle occurs causing muscular weakness.

3. Signs and symptoms include:
   a. Left ventricular heart failure.
      (1) Weakness and undue fatigue.
      (2) **Dypsnea** and tachypnea.
      (3) Cough with expectoration.
      (4) **Orthopnea,** where the patient can only breathe in an upright or seated position.
   b. Right ventricular heart failure. Develops after left ventricular heart failure. Signs and symptoms include those mentioned with left ventricular heart failure plus:
      (1) **Cyanosis** and cold skin in extremities due to decreased blood flow.
      (2) Peripheral edema: Swelling of feet and/or ankles.
      (3) Clinical signs of nausea, vomiting, and anorexia.
      (4) Headaches and irritability.
      (5) Engorged jugular veins in neck, due to blood not being able to be delivered to the heart.
   c. Congestive heart failure. In severe cases, signs and symptoms may include an ashen-gray or grayish-blue coloration of the skin, prominent vein distention, and ankle edema.
4. Dental emergency management of heart failure: Patients cannot tolerate treatment in a reclined position.
   a. Terminate dental procedure and remove all dental materials from mouth.
   b. Position patient most comfortably: Usually in an upright position to alleviate breathing difficulties.
   c. Activate EMS.
   d. Calm patient. This is especially important, because increased apprehension leads to increased cardiac and respiratory workload.
   e. Assess ABCDs.
   f. Administer oxygen.
   g. Monitor vital signs.
F. Acute pulmonary edema. Excess of serous fluid found in the alveolar spaces or interstitial tissues of the lungs.
   1. Precipitating factors include:
      a. Stressful situations, either physical or psychological.
      b. Salty meal.
      c. Noncompliance with medication.
      d. Infection.
   2. Pathophysiology. When heart is unable to provide the body with the oxygen it needs, shortness of breath and fatigue result.
   3. Signs and symptoms include:
      a. All signs of heart failure previously listed.
      b. Tachypnea.
      c. Dyspnea.
      d. In severe cases, cyanosis and frothy pink sputum.
   4. Dental emergency management. Same as listed under heart failure.
G. Chronic Obstructive Pulmonary Disease (COPD). Example includes emphysema (means "air in tissue"); a chronic, irreversible, degenerative disease of the lungs; fourth leading cause of death in the United States.[11]
   1. Precipitating factors include heavy tobacco smoking and air pollution.

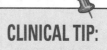

CLINICAL TIP:

Protecting Your Knowledge: Typically, the emphysematous patient is a 50- to 70-year-old male.

2. Pathophysiology.
   a. Alveoli (air sacs) in the lungs, where oxygen from air is exchanged for carbon dioxide in the blood, are destroyed.
   b. Walls of the air sacs become thin and fragile, creating permanent "holes" in the tissues of the lower lungs.
   c. As a result, the lungs transfer less oxygen to the bloodstream and the patient has difficulty exhaling.
   d. Since the patient inhales less oxygen, there is an increase in the level of carbon dioxide.
3. Signs and symptoms include:
   a. Dyspnea.
   b. Decrease in oxygen and increase in CO_2 levels, which results in:
      (1) Skin appearing pallor with gray hue and thick, like leather.
      (2) Facial expression appearing fatigued.
4. Dental treatment and emergency management.
   a. Reduce length of appointment with several rest periods because patient has difficulty tolerating long procedures.
   b. Patient position. May need to be in a modified or full upright position.
   c. If patient is having breathing problems and is coughing, then:
      (1) Stop treatment.
      (2) Administer oxygen at a low rate (2 to 3 liters), if needed, and *never* at 100 percent because patient could go into respiratory arrest.
      (3) If patient stops breathing, call EMS and prepare for ABCDs.

IV. Altered Consciousness

A. Diabetes Mellitus (DM). A metabolic disease of the endocrine system characterized by hyperglycemia, resulting from defects in insulin secretion, insulin sensitivity, or both. It is associated with several systemic complications, such as cardiovascular disease, stroke, kidney disease, blindness, and nervous system damage.
   1. Prevalence. An estimated 17 million people (6 percent of the population) have diabetes; 6 million cases are undiagnosed.[15]
   2. Normal glucose levels = 60 to 110 milligrams per deciliter (mg/dL).[15]
   3. Predisposing factors.
      a. Genetics.
      b. Destruction of the islets of Langerhans in the pancreas, which produce the insulin.
      c. Endocrine disorders, such as hyperthyroidism and hyperpituitarism.
      d. Long-term use of steroids.
   4. Classifications.
      a. Type 1 (Insulin-Dependent Diabetes Mellitus [IDDM]). Autoimmune disorder caused by the destruction of the insulin-producing β cells of the pancreas.[15,16]
         (1) Pathophysiology.[15]
            (a) Pancreas produces little or no insulin, therefore requiring exogenous insulin—injections on a daily basis to control blood glucose levels and to prevent **ketoacidosis.**
            (b) Since there is no or minimal insulin produced, there is a decreased entry of blood glucose into the cells, via receptors, creating an increase in blood glucose levels.

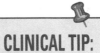

CLINICAL TIP:

Protecting Your Knowledge: Patients with type 1 DM are more prone to other autoimmune disorders, such as Graves' and Addison's disease.[15]

CLINICAL TIP:

Protecting Your Knowledge: Gestational diabetes mellitus (GDM) can occur during pregnancy. Most commonly, glucose levels return to normal after delivery. However, women who experience GDM are at increased risk in developing type 2 DM later in life.[16]

(c) As a result, the kidneys are not able to absorb the excess glucose, and the glucose spills over into the urine (glycosuria), causing a loss of energy.

(d) Because there is excess fluid accumulation in the plasma, there is a frequent need to urinate.

(e) Excess urination (**polyuria**) causes an increase in thirst (**polydipsia**)—essentially the body is dehydrating.

(f) Since glucose provides energy to the body, and there is a decrease in glucose, the body breaks down fats and/or protein for energy.
   i. Fats leave a waste product called **ketones.**
   ii. Ketones build up, causing ketoacidosis.

(2) Signs and symptoms include:[15,16,17]

(a) Hyperglycemia. High level of glucose—126–130 mg glucose/dL, results from eating too much, taking too little insulin, exercising too little, or if the patient is ill or under stress. Can lead to ketoacidosis.

(b) Polydipsia, polyuria, and **polyphagia.** Increased thirst, urination, and eating respectively.

(c) Weight loss and weakness (general fatigue) due to continual urinary loss of calories and inadequate cellular uptake of glucose.

(d) Increased irritability.

(e) Acetone breath (fruity, sweet smell on breath) due to ketoacidosis from abnormal and fast metabolism of fats and amino acids (proteins), which results in production of ketone bodies.

(f) Skin appears flushed and dry (NO sweating).

(g) Decrease in blood pressure.

(3) Oral manifestations include:[15]

(a) Xerostomia, which causes an increase in caries rate.

(b) Gingival hyperplasia.

(c) Burning mouth or tongue.

(d) Periodontitis.

(e) Opportunistic infections, such as candidiasis.

(4) Dental management considerations.[16]

(a) Medical history. Inquire from patient regarding:
   i. Recent blood glucose levels.
   ii. Frequency of hypoglycemic episodes—most common emergency experienced by a diabetic.
   iii. Medications, dosages, and times of administration.
   iv. When last meal was eaten.

(b) Scheduling appointments.
   i. Use stress-reduction protocol, because stress increases insulin needs.
   ii. Schedule morning appointments because endogenous cortisol levels are higher in the morning—cortisol increases blood sugar levels. Avoid scheduling appointments to coincide with peaks of insulin activity, which is the period of maximal risk of developing hypoglycemia.

> **CLINICAL TIP:**
>
> **Protecting Your Knowledge:** A diabetic can start hyperventilating when the blood level of ketoacids rise, and the blood pH drops. In a severe state it is called **Kussmaul's respirations,** which describes deep respirations.

CLINICAL TIP:

Protective Your Knowledge: Type 2 DM is more prevalent among African American, Hispanic, and Native American populations.[15]

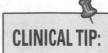

CLINICAL TIP:

Protecting Your Knowledge: Ketoacidosis is uncommon with type 2 DM.[15]

     (c) Diet. Confirm that patient has not only taken medications as usual, but also eaten normally; this decreases the risk of hypoglycemic episodes.

  b. Type 2 (Noninsulin-dependent diabetes mellitus [NIDDM]). Most common form of diabetes—approximately 90 to 95 percent of DM cases caused by impaired insulin function, due to a defect in the insulin molecule or from altered receptors for insulin.[15,16]

    (1) Signs and symptoms include:[15]

      (a) Increased appetite.

      (b) Polydipsia.

      (c) Xerostomia.

    (2) Pathophysiology. The pancreas may not produce enough insulin, the insulin produced may not be able to open the cells (receptors) for the glucose, or there are too few receptors available for the glucose to get through, thus creating hyperglycemia—high blood glucose.

    (3) Treatment. May require insulin injections or oral administered medications, but sometimes can be controlled by making the following recommendations, which will reduce the blood glucose level:

      (a) Weight reduction.

      (b) Mild or moderate exercise.

      (c) Caloric restriction.

    (4) Dental management. Most type 2 diabetics can be seen in the dental office without alteration in treatment.

B. Hypoglycemia. Low blood sugar or insulin shock; most acute complication in the office, which can result in a loss of consciousness and be life threatening.[16,17]

  1. Precipitating factors include:

    a. Omission or delay of foods.

    b. Excess exercise before meals.

    c. Overdose of insulin.

  2. Pathophysiology. Diminished cerebral function due to a lack of nutrition to the brain cells.

  3. Signs and symptoms include:

    a. Inability to perform simple tasks.

    b. Cold, wet (clammy) appearance.

    c. Increase in blood pressure.

    d. Mood change and mental confusion.

    e. Blood glucose levels below 60 mg/100 dL.

  4. Dental emergency management.[16]

    a. Terminate procedure.

    b. Sit patient comfortably, usually upright.

    c. Administer oral carbohydrate, such as canned frosting or tube frosting gel in the oral vestibule, juice, candy bar, or glucose tablets.

    d. Assess ABCDs.

  5. Permit patient to recover for at least one hour. Depending on how the patient feels, dismiss the patient or have an escort take the patient home.

C. Cerebrovascular accident (CVA) = stroke. Neurological disorder that results from interference of blood supply to a part of the brain, which causes destruction of brain tissue. Signs and symptoms include unilateral weakness and numbness, or paralysis of face, arm, or leg; also difficulty in speech and breathing.

1. Prevalence.
   a. Most common in males 60 to 69 years of age, except embolism, which commonly occurs from 20 to 70 years of age.[6]
   b. Intracranial hemorrhage accounts for approximately ten percent of all CVAs, but has the highest mortality.[6]
2. Precipitating factors include:
   a. **Thrombosis** (clot).
      (1) Most prevalent form of CVA.
      (2) Results from atherosclerosis—coronary artery disease (CAD).
      (3) Signs and symptoms vary depending on the area of the brain involved and may include:
         (a) Headache, dizziness, and vertigo.
         (b) Sweating and chills.
         (c) Nausea and vomiting.
         (d) Weakness or paralysis in extremities.
      (4) Usually preceded by transient ischemic attacks (TIA) = temporary or mini stroke.
         (a) Brief interruptions of blood supply to the brain.
         (b) Signs and symptoms. Same as with stroke, except they only last a short time (few minutes to less than 24 hours); can have transient numbness or weakness of extremities.
         (c) Attacks. May occur several times a day or less frequently.
         (d) Indicate presence of CVA.
         (e) Patient remains conscious during TIA, but experiences confusion.
   b. Embolic infarction. Plug or clot obstructing blood flow in a small blood vessel; onset is abrupt.
   c. Hemorrhagic. Ruptured cerebral blood vessel.
      (1) Source of bleeding is usually from arteries, due to:
         (a) Walls of artery rupturing because of a sudden increase in B.P.
         (b) Head trauma.
      (2) Signs and symptoms include:
         (a) Violent headache.
         (b) Nausea and vomiting.
         (c) Possible seizure.
3. Risk factors include:
   a. Hypertension. Individuals with a B.P. higher than 160/95 mm Hg are six times more likely to develop a stroke than those with a B.P. lower than 140/90 mm Hg.
   b. Diabetes and myocardial disease. Increase cardiovascular activity.
4. Treatment. Use:
   a. Anticoagulant therapy, such as heparin, for treatment of embolic stroke.
   b. Antiplatelet therapy, such as aspirin,[18] for treatment of recurrent TIAs.
5. Dental treatment considerations.
   a. Avoid dental treatment if CVA attack was within one month.
   b. Use stress-reduction protocol.
   c. Use nitrous oxide-oxygen conscious sedation.
   d. Contact physician if patient is on antiplatelet or anticoagulant therapy when dental treatment will produce bleeding.

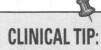

CLINICAL TIP:

Protecting Your Knowledge: CVA is most common in males, age 60 to 69 years.[6]

6. Dental emergency management.
   a. TIA.
      (1) Terminate procedure.
      (2) Place patient in upright or semi-upright position.
      (3) Assess ABCDs.
      (4) Monitor vital signs.
      (5) Activate EMS.
      (6) Administer oxygen.
      (7) Refer patient for medical evaluation.
   b. CVA (Conscious patient). Follow procedures 1 through 6 above. If symptoms persist, hospitalize patient.
   c. CVA (Unconscious patient).
      (1) Place patient in supine position; if B.P. is elevated, slightly elevate head and chest.
      (2) Activate EMS.
      (3) Assess ABCDs; prepare for BLS.

D. Thyroid gland dysfunction. Thyroid gland is located in the anterior portion of the neck below the thyroid cartilage.
   1. Function of thyroid. Produces and secretes three hormones important to the function of the body's tissues:
      a. Thyroxine (T_4).
      b. Triiodothyronine (T_3).
      c. Calcintonin.
   2. Types of thyroid dysfunction.[19]
      a. Hyperthyroidism (i.e., Graves' disease, thyrotoxicosis). Caused by excessive production of T_3 and T_4.
         (1) Pathophysiology. Result of excessive production of thyroid hormone by the thyroid gland or excessive administration of exogenous thyroid hormone.
         (2) Signs and symptoms include:
            (a) Increased metabolism rate, body temperature, heart rate, blood pressure, and weight loss.
            (b) Goiter. Enlarged thyroid due to pituitary releasing thyroid-stimulating hormone (TSH).
            (c) Nervousness, increased irritability, and insomnia.
            (d) Intolerance to heat and sweating.
            (e) Exophthalamus. Abnormal protrusion of the eyes.
         (3) Untreated hyperthyroidism may result in thyroid storm; rare occurrence yet can be life-threatening.
         (4) Dental emergency treatment and management of an unconscious patient with hyperthyroid disease.
            (a) Terminate procedure.
            (b) Place patient in supine position.
            (c) Activate EMS.
            (d) Assess ABCDs.
            (e) Administer oxygen.
      b. Hypothyroidism (i.e., myxedema).[19] Caused by a lack of thyroid hormones, which slow down body functions.
         (1) Precipitating factors include:
            (a) Advancing age.
            (b) Female.
            (c) Caucasians or Asians.

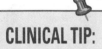

CLINICAL TIP:

Protecting Your Knowledge:
About 13 million people in the United States have thyroid disorders, but more than half remain undiagnosed.[19]

(d) Hashimoto's thyroiditis (autoimmune thyroiditis). Caused from the destruction of the thyroid gland by circulating antithyroid antibodies.

(2) Pathophysiology. Insufficient levels of circulating thyroid hormones.

(3) Signs and symptoms include:

    (a) Cretinism. Deficiency in thyroid hormones experienced during childhood; affects growth and development.

    (b) Increased weakness and fatigue.

    (c) Weight gain.

    (d) Puffy face and eyelids.

    (e) Cold intolerance.

    (f) Thick tongue.

(4) Severe case. Involves myxedema coma, which is rare, but is characterized by hypothermia, bradycardia, hypotension, and loss of consciousness.

(5) Dental emergency treatment and management of an unconscious patient with hypothyroid disease.

    (a) Terminate procedure.

    (b) Place patient in supine position.

    (c) Activate EMS.

    (d) Assess ABCDs.

    (e) Administer oxygen.

V. Seizure Disorder

Epilepsy. Common symptom of the underlying neurological disorder; can take a variety of forms.[20,21]

A. Partial seizures (focal seizures).

    1. Involve specific region of the brain and generally do *not* involve loss of consciousness.

    2. Involve psychomotor seizure, jacksonian epilepsy (a localized form of epilepsy with spasms confined to one part or one group of muscles), and self-induced seizure.

B. Generalized seizures. Originate from both brain hemispheres and cause loss of consciousness.

    1. Grand mal seizures (generalized **tonic-clonic seizure**). Most common form of seizure disorder.

        a. Precipitating factors include **idiopathic,** drug withdrawal, menstruation, fatigue, alcohol, and falling asleep or awakening.

        b. Phases.

            (1) Prodromal phase.

                (a) Occurs before seizure.

                (b) Increase in anxiety or depression.

                (c) Patient may also experience an aura (a visual, auditory, gustatory, or olfactory sensation immediately preceding the loss of consciousness), which is an actual part of the seizure and precedes the seizure.

                (d) May last a few seconds or several hours.

            (2) Preictal phase. Patient becomes rigid and pale, pupils dilate, and patient loses consciousness.

                (a) Flexion occurs: Myoclonic jerks.

                (b) Patient releases an epileptic cry: Sound produced when air is expelled through a partially closed glottis.

               (c) Changes in autonomic system occur: Increase in B.P. and heart rate due to the changes experienced by the body.

          (3) Ictal phase.

               (a) Tonic component involves muscles of respiration; therefore dyspnea and cyanosis may be evident. Lasts approximately 10 to 20 seconds and includes:

                   i. Tension or contraction of extremities.

                   ii. Dilated eyes.

                   iii. Distorted face.

               (b) Clonic component (convulsions). Involves alternating contraction and relaxation of muscles; lasts approximately 2 to 5 minutes and includes:

                   i. Frothing at the mouth.

                   ii. Appearance of blood due to patient biting the lateral borders of the tongue.

          (4) Postictal phase. Tonic-clonic movements cease.

               (a) Incontinence may occur.

               (b) Consciousness returns; patient is disoriented and confused.

               (c) Patient relaxes and sleeps deeply.

               (d) Patient fully recovers in approximately 2 hours.

     c. Onset is rapid from the initial symptom.

     d. Dental emergency management.

          (1) Preictal (prodromal) phase. Terminate procedure if an aura is evident; remove any dental appliances.

          (2) Ictal phase (seizure stage).

               (a) If not seated, place patient on floor in supine position with a padded item under head, if possible, and clear area surrounding patient. If patient is seated in dental chair, place in a supine position.

               (b) Activate EMS.

               (c) Assess ABCDs.

               (d) Try to gently restrain patient's extremities; DO NOT hold patient in a fixed position.

               (e) If possible, place a towel in patient's mouth to prevent biting lateral borders of tongue.

          (3) Postictal phase. Seizure has stopped, but be prepared in case another seizure occurs.

  2. Petit mal epilepsy. Absence of seizure.

     a. Signs and symptoms include:

          (1) Blank stare.

          (2) Transient loss of consciousness.

          (3) Does not include an aura or convulsions.

     b. Characteristics (can occur frequently).

          (1) Usually occurs between the ages of 3 and 15.

          (2) Most outgrow by adulthood.

     c. Dental emergency management.

          (1) Terminate procedure.

          (2) Reassure patient and determine level of alertness.

          (3) Consult physician.

          (4) Have an escort take patient home.

3. Status epilepticus. Same symptoms are present during convulsive stage of a grand mal seizure; however, it lasts longer with no recovery between episodes; major cause of death related directly to seizures.

VI. Chest Pain

A. **Angina pectoris** (ischemic heart disease [IHD]). Insufficient blood supply to the heart muscle, which may be precipitated by stress, anxiety, exercise, emotion, or heavy meal.[22] Sign of coronary artery disease (CAD).

1. Pathophysiology. Temporary inability of the coronary arteries to provide adequate oxygenated blood to the myocardium, resulting in ischemia.[22]

2. Types.
   a. Stable angina = chronic, classic, exertional angina.
      (1) Caused by CAD.
      (2) Triggered by strenuous activity.
      (3) Lasts between 1 and 15 minutes.
      (4) Relieved by nitroglycerin (sublingual tablets or translingual spray) and rest.
   b. Variant angina = Prinzmetal's, atypical angina.
      (1) Occurs while patient is at rest at any time, day or night.
      (2) Associated with dysrhythmias.
      (3) Relieved by nitroglycerin.
   c. Unstable angina = acute coronary insufficiency.
      (1) Syndrome between stable angina and myocardial infarction (MI).
      (2) Results from the progression of atherosclerosis.
      (3) Precipitating factors include any mentioned before or none.
      (4) Duration is up to 30 minutes with pain located substernally across both sides of chest and may include the neck and jaw.
      (5) Response to nitroglycerin is questionable.

3. Signs and symptoms.
   a. Early symptoms are often mistaken for indigestion or heart attack.
   b. As attack worsens, the primary clinical manifestation is chest pain, which usually originates substernally (thoracic pain) and patient may give **Levine sign**—clutching fist to chest. Patient may experience discomfort such as:
      (1) Squeezing and suffocating feeling.
      (2) Burning sensation.
      (3) Choking.
      (4) Dull ache.
      (5) Shortness of breath.
      (6) Nausea.
      (7) Diaphoresis.
   c. Pain. Resembles a heart attack, except there is a rapid response to rest, oxygen, and nitroglycerin.
      (1) Normally spreads across both sides of chest, but can also radiate to neck, mandible, stomach, and between shoulder blades.
      (2) Usually lasts throughout attack.

4. Dental emergency management.[22]
   a. Place patient's nitroglycerin in an accessible area.
   b. Terminate dental procedure.
   c. Position patient comfortably, usually upright or semi-upright.
   d. Administer oxygen.
   e. Assess ABCDs, if necessary.

CLINICAL TIP:

Protecting Your Knowledge:
After recovery of angina, dental care may be continued if both patient and dentist agree.[22]

    f. Determine diagnosis.

       (1) If patient acknowledges having angina on medical history, administer nitroglycerin—may repeat 3 times every 5 minutes, up to 15 minutes. Patient should feel better in 2 to 3 minutes. If no response to nitroglycerin, activate EMS immediately—*ALWAYS* have patient's nitroglycerin available within reach.

       (2) If patient has a history of angina, but attack does not feel like a typical attack, treat patient for myocardial infarction (MI) and activate EMS immediately.

       (3) If there is no cardiac history, activate EMS immediately.
           IF IN DOUBT OF ANGINA OR MI, ACTIVATE EMS AND TREAT FOR MI.

B. Myocardial infarction (MI) = heart attack. Results from a deficient coronary blood supply to the myocardium that results in cellular death and necrosis = myocardial ischemia. High incidence of mortality with death occurring within two hours of onset of signs and symptoms.

    1. Pathophysiology. Sudden occlusion of a major coronary vessel.

    2. Predisposing factors.

       a. Primary cause is atherosclerosis (CAD); most common site of thrombosis (blood clot) is left coronary artery.[22]

       b. Obesity.

       c. Males with a type A personality traits between the ages of 50 and 70.

       d. Undue stress.

    3. Modifiable risk factors. Some risk factors for MI are modifiable and include the following:

       a. Smoking.

       b. Blood lipids, especially low-density lipoproteins (LDLs).

       c. Blood pressure.

    4. Unmodifiable risk factors. Other risk factors for MI, which cannot be changed, include the following:

       a. Heredity.

       b. Male gender.

       c. Race: Nonwhite men and women.

       d. Age: By 55 to 64 years of age, 40 percent of deaths in males occur from CAD.

    5. Signs and symptoms.

       a. Pain: Experienced in 80 percent of MIs and lasts 30 minutes to several hours.[22]

        (1) Severe and described as pressing or crushing.

        (2) Located in the middle to upper one-third of sternum.

        (3) Rest or nitroglycerin do NOT reduce pain; morphine is usually needed.

        (4) Patient becomes restless and often uses Levine sign.

        (5) Nausea and vomiting may occur due to intense pain.

       b. Cold sweat.

       c. Patient is apprehensive, weak, and lightheaded.

       d. Dyspnea: Pain prevents normal breathing.

       e. Coughing and wheezing.

       f. Abdominal bloating.

       g. Skin: Ashen gray color, pale, cool, and moist.

       h. Nailbeds: Cyanotic, demonstrating difficulty with circulation.

CLINICAL TIP:

Protecting Your Knowledge:
Most MI deaths occur within the first two hours of coronary artery obstruction.[22]

i. Vital signs.
(1) B.P. may be normal, but usually low.
(2) Respirations: Rapid, yet shallow.
(3) Heart rate: Weak, thready, and rapid.
6. Medications. Patients will usually be on anticoagulant and antiplatelet (aspirin) therapy. If treatment involves risk of hemorrhage, contact physician first.
7. Dental treatment considerations.
a. Schedule short appointments.
b. Use supplemental oxygen to reduce the risk of hypoxia and myocardial ischemia.
c. Use nitrous oxide sedation to manage MI.
d. Avoid use of vasoconstrictors for any ASA IV cardiovascular-risk patient.
e. Avoid scheduling patient for at least one (1) month following heart attack, because there is an increased risk of reinfarction.
f. Contact patient's physician if in doubt of treatment or in case of needed emergency treatment.
8. Dental emergency management.
a. Terminate procedure.
b. Position patient comfortably.
c. Activate EMS.
d. Administer nitroglycerin.
e. Administer oxygen.
f. Monitor vital signs.

VII. Drug-Related Emergencies

A. Allergies. Involve a hypersensitive state acquired through exposure to a particular allergen, such as a food, drug, or other substance.
1. Types of allergies.
a. Type I (immediate hypersensitivity). Principle **antibody** = IgE, when a drug **antigen** binds to IgE antibody, the response yields edema and inflammation. Bronchioles are attacked, causing **anaphylactic shock.**
(1) Generalized. Results in an immediate response; most life-threatening and dramatic allergic reaction.
(2) Localized.
(3) **Urticaria** (skin).
(4) Bronchospasm (respiratory tract).
(5) Food allergy (GI tract).
b. Type II. Cytotoxic. Certain drug reactions.
c. Type III. Immune complex. Acute viral hepatitis.
d. Type IV. Delayed reaction (hours to days), such as contact dermatitis associated with latex gloves.
2. Common allergies experienced in dentistry.
a. Antibiotics, e.g., penicillin, tetracyclines, and sulfonamides.
b. Local anesthetics. Allergy is rare;[23] reactions can be a result to the drug itself; adverse reactions are highly correlated to medical status of patient.[24]
c. Latex. Classified under a Type IV allergic reaction—contact urticaria; principle areas affected are circumoral and facial skin and upper lip.[25]

3. Pathophysiology. Results from an antigen-antibody reaction, a reaction to the body's defense mechanism.
   a. Histiocytes (mast cells) may develop IgE receptor sites for the foreign antigen.
   b. When antigen is reintroduced to a sensitive individual, histamine, heparin, and other vasoactive amines are released as a result of the antigen-antibody reaction.
   c. Capillary bodies open throughout body, increasing intravascular space.
   d. If blood volume remains unchanged, there is insufficient blood to fill intravascular space.
   e. Blood pressure drops.
4. Reactions.
   a. Mild reaction includes urticaria, erythema, and itching.
   b. Severe reactions include **angioedema** and respiratory distress from swollen air passages.
   c. Life-threatening anaphylactic reactions—rare, but possible; include dyspnea, hypotension, and loss of consciousness.
5. Signs and symptoms.
   a. Skin reactions include warmth, tingling, urticaria, and **pruritus** to eyes and nose.
   b. Respiratory distress includes bronchospasms, cough, dyspnea, and throat tightness—angioedema.
   c. Cardiovascular collapse. Hypotension and loss of consciousness; anaphylactic shock—term used when there is a loss of consciousness due to hypotension from an anaphylactic reaction. Dental emergency management includes:
      (1) If patient is conscious, place in upright position; if patient is experiencing hypotension, place in supine position.
      (2) Assess ABCDs.
      (3) Activate EMS.
      (4) Administer oxygen.
      (5) Monitor vital signs.
      (6) Administer epinephrine (Epipen).[26] *Most important drug in treatment of allergy;* has vasoconstricting and bronchodilating properties.[22]
         (a) Counteracts the effects of histamine.
         (b) Reacts rapidly, but is also short acting.
         (c) Contraindicated in elderly and those with high B.P. and CAD.
         (d) Administer subcutaneously in side of thigh if reaction is mild; administer intravenously with more life-threatening allergic reaction.
6. Dental emergency management.
   a. If there is evidence of urticaria, pruritus, or wheezing, terminate procedure.
   b. Place patient in supine position.
   c. Assess ABCDs.
   d. Activate EMS.
   e. Administer epinephrine.
   f. Administer oxygen.
   g. Monitor vital signs every 5 minutes.

   h. May need to administer additional drugs, such as antihistamines and corticosteroids.
B. Drug-overdose reactions. Result from overly high blood levels of a drug (see Vasoconstrictor toxicity section in Chapter 1).
   1. In dentistry, there are four commonly used categories of drugs with significant overdose potential:
      a. Local anesthetics.
      b. Vasoconstrictors that narrow blood vessels.
      c. Sedatives, such as hypnotics.
      d. Narcotic analgesics.
   2. Pathophysiology. Results from high levels of a drug in various organs and tissues; entry into blood exceeds removal rate.
   3. Signs.
      a. Low-to-moderate overdose levels.
         (1) Confused and apprehensive.
         (2) Talkative.
         (3) Increased B.P., H.R., and R.R.
         (4) Nystagmus: Rapid, involuntary movement of eyeballs.
      b. Moderate-to-high levels.
         (1) Tonic-clonic seizures.
         (2) Depressed central nervous system (CNS).
         (3) Increased B.P., H.R., and R.R.
   4. Symptoms.
      a. Headache, dizziness, and lightheadedness.
      b. Ringing in ears.
      c. Numb tongue.
      d. Drowsiness.
   5. Dental emergency treatment.
      a. Mild reaction.
         (1) Administer oxygen.
         (2) Monitor vital signs.
      b. Severe reaction such as narcotic overdose. Treat with Naloxone, universal narcotic antagonist to reverse life-threatening respiratory distress.
         (1) Place patient in supine position.
         (2) Activate EMS.
         (3) Assess ABCDs.
         (4) Monitor vital signs.
         (5) Prepare to manage a seizure.

The healthcare provider must always be prepared to manage a medical emergency in an office setting. To help prevent medical emergencies from occurring, always obtain a thorough medical history, followed with complete dialogue. In addition, all vital signs should be taken to establish baseline readings. This provides the healthcare provider with "normal" readings, so abnormal readings can be recognized in an emergency situation. Also note any medications reviewed for possible dental/medical considerations (see Table 14–3).

Table 14-3   Treatment Review of Conditions During Episode

	Syncope	Orthostatic Hypotension	Angina	Acute M.I.	Acute Pulmonary Edema	CVA	Epilepsy	Hyperventilation	Asthma
Age	Young adults—male	↑ with ↑ age	40 + men	Elderly	Elderly	Over 40	<40	15–40 male	Under 10
Onset	Stress-related	Nonstress-related	Exertion Acute stress 3–5 min.	Stress 30 min. +	Acute stress Heart failure	Stress	Stress Aura	Stress	Stress
Signs & symptoms	Clammy, moist skin Pallor Sweating	Sitting up too fast Pregnancy Exhaustion Varicose veins	Levine sign Squeezing Cold sweat Nausea Radiating pain	Levine sign Radiating pain Not relieved by nitro	Pink frothy sputum Suffocating Panic Cyanosis Dyspnea Cough	Headache Nausea Vomiting Numbness Sweating Chills	*Petit* Blank stare (5–30 secs) *Grand* Tonic-clonic	Tingling and numbness of fingers/toes Chest pain Lightheaded Heart palpitations	Wheezing ↑ anxiety Sweating Coughing Dypsnea Bronchospasms
Vital signs	*Pre* ↓ B.P., ↑ H.R. Then H.R. ↓	↓ B.P. ↑ H.R.	↑ B.P. ↑ H.R.	↓ B.P. ↑ H.R. ↑ R.R.	↑ B.P. ↑ H.R. ↑ R.R.	↑ B.P. ↓ R.R. H.R. variable	↑ B.P. ↑ H.R. ↓ R.R.	↑ B.P. ↑ H.R. ↑ R.R.	↑ B.P. ↑ H.R. ↑ R.R.
State of consciousness	Should return to consciousness when in supine position	Should remain conscious	Remains conscious	Can become unconscious	No	Possibly with hemorrhage, but not usually	Yes	Should not occur	No
Tx Recommended	Supine A-B-C O$_2$ Ammonia	Same as syncope	Nitro Vasodilator O$_2$ Rest Relieved in 25 minutes	Nitro will NOT relieve	Upright High flow O$_2$ EMS	Ask if patient has had TIA (warning to not treat) Conscious—upright Unconscious—supine w/ elevated head	Dilantin Phenobarbital Supine—conscious Protect from injury Unconscious—flat	Upright Cup hands Breathe in paper bag 7% CO$_2$ + 93% O$_2$	Upright Bronchodilator
RDH Responsibilities	↓ stress O$_2$	Prevention—check medical history	↓ stress	↓ stress Nitro + O$_2$	↓ stress, ↓ panic, ↓ work load on heart			↓ stress DO NOT need O$_2$	Watch for S & S of side effects of inhaler

	Heart Failure	Emphysema	Hyper-thyroidism	Hypothyroidism	Acute Allergic	Hyperglycemia	IDDM	NIDDM	Hypoglycemia (Insulin shock)
Age	Elderly		20–40		Any		Adolescence	Over 40	
Onset	Slow	Smoker Environment	Slow Acute Anxiety	Slow Acute anxiety	Nonstress-related	Slow	Rapid	Slow	Rapid
Signs & symptoms	Jugular vein distension Dypsnea Orthopnea Fatigue	O₂ tolerant Dypsnea Gray hue Fatigue	Exophthalmus Nervous Sweating Hot and wet Rapid speech	Fatigue Cold intolerance Weak skeletal muscles	Skin Respiratory Anaphylaxis	Hot and dry Acetone breath Nausea ↑ thirst ↑ urine	Same as hyperglycemia	Same as hyperglycemia	Drunkeness like appearance ↑ anxiety ↓ weight
Vital signs	↑ B.P. ↑ H.R. ↑ R.R.	↑ R.R. Can stop breathing	↑ B.P. ↑ H.R. ↑ R.R.	↓ B.P. ↓ H.R. ↓ R.R.	↑ B.P. ↑ H.R.	↘ B.P. ↑ H.R. ↑ R.R.	↓ B.P.		↑ B.P. ↑ H.R. ↓ R.R.
State of consciousness		Possibly—NO 100% O₂	Yes, if uncontrolled	Yes, if uncontrolled		Should NOT happen			Yes
Tx Recommended	Meds.—diuretic Digoxin Antihypertensives Upright, EMS	Upright position	No epinephrine Antithyroid drugs Radiation	No CNS depressants No sedatives No narcotic analgesics Synthetic hormone	Epinephrine	Conscious—consult Unconscious—supine A-B-C-Ds EMS Glucose			Oral carbs EMS
RDH Responsibilities	↓ stress O₂—3–5L Upright	A-B-C-Ds EMS Short appts. Rest periods Modify position	A-B-C-Ds	A-B-C-Ds	A-B-C-Ds	Supine A-B-C-Ds EMS Insulin			

QUESTIONS

1. The MOST important measure for dental office personnel to take to prevent a medical emergency from occurring is to
   a. have the patient eat prior to appointment.
   b. have the patient schedule an early appointment.
   c. know the amount of medications(s) the patient is taking.
   d. take a thorough medical history.

2. The first step in CPR is to
   a. establish unresponsiveness.
   b. open airway.
   c. check breathing.
   d. give two slow breaths.

3. The emergency drug kit in a dental office should contain current medications likely to be used in an emergency. All members of the dental team should know what to do in case of a medical emergency.
   a. Both statements are TRUE.
   b. Both statements are FALSE.
   c. The first statement is TRUE. The second statement is FALSE.
   d. The first statement is FALSE. The second statement is TRUE.

4. Syncope refers to a(n)
   a. cardiac condition.
   b. allergic reaction.
   c. weight loss.
   d. lack of oxygen to the brain.

5. Which of the following signs and symptoms is NOT a sign of presyncope?
   a. Diaphoresis
   b. Dry skin
   c. Lightheadedness
   d. Warm feeling in the neck and face

6. The patient aspirates a crown into the oropharyngeal area. The first step the dental hygienist should make is to
   a. lower the back of the chair to assist the patient's effort to dislodge the object.
   b. try to remove the object.
   c. immediately administer four back blows.
   d. seat the patient upright.

7. Which one of the following patients is NOT predisposed to hyperventilation?
   a. The patient who hides his or her anxiety.
   b. A 5-year-old.
   c. One with high anxiety levels.
   d. A 25-year-old.

8. Which of the following is the MOST effective treatment for an asthmatic attack?
   a. Administer 100 percent oxygen.
   b. Place patient in a semi-supine position.
   c. Allow patient to use his or her inhaler.
   d. Sedate the patient.

9. The greatest risk factor in the development of all forms of CVAs is
   a. age.
   b. cancer.
   c. family history.
   d. hypertension.

10. A seizure can be caused by all of the following EXCEPT one. Which one is the EXCEPTION?
    a. Myocardial infarction
    b. Drug withdrawal
    c. Fatigue
    d. Alcohol

11. A patient suddenly complains of dyspnea, a suffocating feeling, a racing heartbeat, and is coughing up pink frothy sputum. Which condition is MOST likely to be present?
    a. Asthma
    b. Acute pulmonary edema
    c. Hyperventilation
    d. Partial airway obstruction

12. If during an emergency situation, a patient with emphysema is administered oxygen, the dental hygienist should observe for
    a. an increase in respiratory rate.
    b. decrease of dyspnea.
    c. respiratory arrest.
    d. return of pinkish color to the skin.

13. All of the following are classic signs and/or symptoms of hyperglycemia, as observed in the type 1 diabetic, EXCEPT one. Which one is the EXCEPTION?
    a. Polydipsia
    b. Cold and wet skin
    c. Polyuria
    d. Red face with dry skin

14. Exophthalamus, nervousness, tachycardia, heat intolerance, and hypertension are suggestive of which of the following conditions?
    a. Hypertension
    b. Hyperthyroidism
    c. Hyperparathyroidism
    d. Hypothyroidism

15. The MOST commonly encountered acute complication of diabetes in the dental office is
    a. hyperglycemia.
    b. hypoglycemia.
    c. Kussmaul's respirations.
    d. hypoparathyroidism.

16. The MOST important step in treating an anaphylactic reaction consists of administering
    a. oxygen.
    b. corticosteroids.
    c. antihistamines.
    d. epinephrine.

17. Angina pectoris pain is due to
    a. myocardial infarction.
    b. ischemia of the myocardium.
    c. failure of the left ventricle to pump blood sufficiently.
    d. spasm of the right ventricle.

REFERENCES

1. Morrison AD, Goodday, RHB. Preparing for medical emergencies in the dental office. *Journal of the Canadian Dental Association,* Vol. 65, 1999, 284–86.

2. ADA Council on Scientific Affairs. Office emergencies and emergency kits. *Journal of the American Dental Association,* Vol. 133, Number 3, 2002, 364–65.

3. Cooper, MD, Wiechmann L. In: *Essentials of Dental Hygiene: Preclinical Skills.* Upper Saddle River, NJ: Prentice Hall, 2005.

4. Spolarich AE. Drugs used to manage medical emergencies. *Access,* Vol. 14, Number 9, 2000, 42–43.

5. Haas DA. Emergency drugs. *Dental Clinics of North America,* Vol. 46, Number 4, 2002, 815–30.

6. Nunn P. Medical emergencies: The oral health care settings. *The Journal of Dental Hygiene,* Vol. 74, Number 2, 2000, 136–51.

7. Grimes, EB. The syncopal patient in the dental office. *The Journal of Practical Hygiene,* Vol. 10, Number 6, 2001, 39–42.

8. Findler M, Elad S, Garfunkel A, Zusman SP, Malamed SF, Galili D, Kaufman E. Syncope in the dental environment. *Refuat Hapeh Vehashinayim,* Vol. 19, Number 1, 2000, 27–33, 99.

9. Schafer DM. Respiratory emergencies in the dental office. *Dental Clinics of North America,* Vol. 39, Number 3, 1995, 541–54.

10. Galili D, Garfunkel A, Elad S, Zusman SP, Malamed SF, Findler M, Kaufman E. Respiratory distress. *Refuat Hapeh Vehashinayim,* Vol. 19, Number 1, 2002, 34–46, 100.

11. Day MD. Managing the patient with the severe respiratory problem. *Journal of the California Dental Association,* Vol. 28, Number 8, 2000, 585–89, 591–93, 595–98.

12. Spolarich AE. Drugs used to manage asthma. *Access,* Vol. 10, Number 15, 2001, 38–41.

13. McIvor A, Chapman KR. Diagnosis of chronic obstructive pulmonary disease and differentiation from asthma. *Current Opinion of Pulmonary Medicine,* Vol. 2, Number 2, 1996, 148–54.

14. Steinbacher DM Glick M. The patient with asthma: An update and oral health considerations. *The Journal of the American Dental Association,* Vol. 132, 2001, 1229–39.

15. Lalla RV, D'Ambrosio JA. Dental management considerations for the patient with diabetes mellitus. *Journal of the American Dental Association,* Vol. 132, 2001, 1425–31.

16. Silverstein LH, Brown AD. Diabetic dental patients: Management of medical emergencies. *Journal of Practical Hygiene,* Vol. 7, Number 5, 1998, 11–14.

17. Ring T. Diabetes. An epidemic on the rise. *Access,* Vol. 6, Number 15, 2001, 25–31.

18. Arnold M. Stroke as an emergency. *Schweiz Rundsch Med Prax,* Vol. 91, Number 36, 2002, 1421–27.

19. Goldsmith C. Hypothyroidism: Often overlooked, easy to treat. *Access,* Vol. 5, Number 17, 2003, 30–37.

20. Kennedy BT, Haller JS. Treatment of the epileptic patient in the dental office. *Journal of the New York State Dental Association,* Vol. 64, Number 2, 1998, 26–31.

21. Fiske J, Boyle C. Epilepsy and oral care. *Dental Update,* Vol. 29, Number 4, 2002, 180–87.

22. Malamed SF. Emergency medicine: Beyond the basics. *The Journal of the American Dental Association,* Vol. 128, 1997, 843–54.

23. Findler RL, Moore PA. Adverse drug reactions to local anesthesia. *Dental Clinics of North America,* Vol. 46, Number 4, 2002, 747–57.

24. Kaufman E, Garfunkel A, Findler M, Elad S, Zusman SP, Malamed SF, Galili D. Emergencies evolving from local anesthesia. *Rufuat Hapek Vehashinayim,* Vol. 19, Number 11, 2002, 13–18, 98.

25. Burke FJ, Wilson MA, McCord JF. Allergy to latex gloves in clinical practice: Case reports. *Quintessence International,* Vol. 26, Number 12, 1995, 859–63.

26. Becker DE. Management of immediate allergic reactions. *Dental Clinics of North America,* Vol. 39, Number 3, 1995, 577–86.

Chapter 15

Dental Implants

Sheri Granier Sison, RDH, BS

MediaLink

A companion CD-ROM, included free with each new copy of this book, supplements the procedures presented in each chapter. Insert the CD-ROM to watch video clips and view a large collection of color images that is also included. This multimedia library is designed to help you add a new dimension to your learning.

KEY TERMS

edema	masticatory efficiency	subperiosteal implant
edentulous	osseointegration	surgical guide
embrasure	periimplant	tin oxide
endosteal implant	prosthodontics	transosteal implant
exudate	provisional restoration	

LEARNING OBJECTIVES

After reading this chapter, the student will be able to:

- discuss the benefits of dental implants;
- identify the different types of dental implants;
- assess patient suitability for dental implants;
- state the importance of plaque control in the implant patient;
- explain the rationale of using a surgical guide;
- list the provisions for home care in the initial placement of the implant;
- list the provisions for home care following exposure of the implant;
- contrast the plaque control devices available for the implant;
- discuss the selection of plaque control devices;
- discuss the use of chemotherapeutic agents with dental implants;

- describe osseointegration;
- contrast the periimplant environment with the natural tooth;
- identify the indications for radiographs in patients with implants;
- assess the frequency of recall visits for patients with implants;
- describe an adequate implant prosthesis;
- evaluate the health of the periimplant tissue;
- discuss the types of instruments that can be safely used on the implant;
- identify the stages of disease in the periimplant environment;
- contrast the ailing, failing, and failed implant.

I. Introduction

Missing teeth can impact a patient's self-esteem and social interaction.[1] **Masticatory efficiency** can also diminish and compromise nutritional status, placing patients at risk for chronic illnesses such as diabetes, hypertension, and heart disease.[2] Dental implants have been successfully used as replacements for natural teeth.[3] They are used to replace teeth in a variety of situations, including single tooth replacement, partially **edentulous** cases, or in the patient who is completely edentulous. The **osseointegration** of the implant provides support for function of the dental prosthetic. Years of research indicate that dental implants are a superior method of tooth replacement in patient satisfaction, comfort, stability, and ability to chew.

Implant therapy involves complex treatment planning and dynamic plaque control. The dental hygienist can function as a principal member of the dental implant team and perform an essential service for the patient who requires **prosthodontic** treatment.

II. Types of Implants
A. **Transosteal** or transmandibular **implant** (TMI).
  1. Placement: Placed through the mandibular bone.
  2. Indications: Only in the severely resorbed mandible.
B. **Subperiosteal implant** (Figure 15–1)
  1. Placement: Placed against the bone, under the periosteum.
  2. Indications: Only for severely resorbed edentulous areas.
      a. Historically, this implant has been removed due to complications related to changes in the edentulous jaw, causing implant mobility, decreased stability, and infection that causes damage to the alveolus.
      b. Patients must be closely monitored and the implant removed upon infection.
  3. Requires two surgeries.
      a. First surgery: Allows for fabrication of the implant.
      b. Second surgery: Involves delivery of the implant.
C. **Endosteal implant** (Figure 15–2).
  1. Placement: Placed within the bone. A blade or plate-form implant can be placed in the mandible or maxilla, in a variety of bone widths and heights (Figure 15–3).
  2. Indications: For the patient with inadequate bone for a root-form implant.

III. Patient Assessment
Prior to determining the placement of implants, the patient's physical health, dental history, and psychological status should be evaluated.
A. Physical health. The patient must be in good physical health and should be able to tolerate necessary surgical procedures with good healing potential.[4] Determine patient's health by thoroughly evaluating medical history.

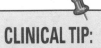

CLINICAL TIP:

Stabilizing Your Knowledge: A root-form implant is similar to the shape of a natural tooth; it can be placed in the mandible or maxillae with adequate bone. The root-form implant has been studied more than any other implant form and has proven to be a safe and effective means of replacing missing teeth.[3]

Figure 15–1   Subperiosteal implant.

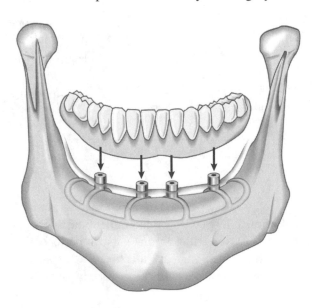

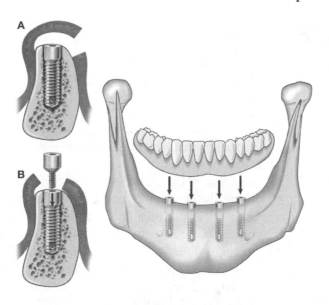

Figure 15–2   Endosseous implant.

1. Vital signs. Evaluate blood pressure along with pulse and respiration rates prior to treatment to determine baseline readings.
2. Complete basic lab work to rule out any systemic complications; these include:
   a. Complete blood count (CBC).
   b. Urinalysis.
   c. Sequential multiple analyzer of blood chemistry (SMAC).
3. Classify any existing presurgical risks using the American Society of Anesthesiology Classification (ASA).
   a. ASA I indicates no systemic illness and a normal lifestyle; therefore, a good candidate for dental implants.
   b. ASA II indicates well-controlled systemic illness and the ability to engage in normal daily activity, qualifying candidates for dental implants.
   c. ASA III indicates an impaired activity because of a chronic condition or multiple medical problems; systemic problems must be stabilized to be a candidate for dental implants; e.g., hypertension, type 1 and 2 diabetes mellitus, and epilepsy.
   d. ASA IV and V indicate serious medical complications and are therefore not appropriate implant candidates.[5]
4. Determine if patient has compromised healing from:
   a. Bleeding disorders, such as coagulation disorders, chronic leukemia, and thrombocytopenia.

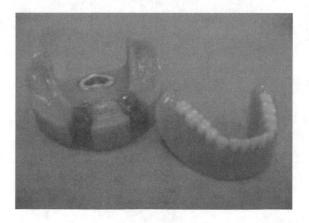

Figure 15–3   Endosseous implant.

CLINICAL TIP:

Stabilizing Your Knowledge: Uncontrolled plasma glucose levels can have an adverse effect on the healing potential of the implant and is a contraindication for treatment. The well-controlled diabetic, however, has no higher incidence in implant failure than a non-diabetic.[6,7]

CLINICAL TIP:

Stabilizing Your Knowledge: Tobacco use has been statistically associated with implant failure. The patient should be aware of the negative impact smoking has on the implant environment. The operator may opt not to place implants for patients who smoke.[8]

b. Connective tissue disorders, such as scleroderma, osteogenesis imperfecta, and fibromyalgia.
c. Chronic steroid therapy.
d. Immunosuppression therapy.
e. Uncontrolled diabetes.
f. Tobacco use.

B. Psychological evaluation. The implant candidate must be able to participate in necessary maintenance, which assists with the success of the implant. The patient should:
1. Understand the usefulness of the restoration and aesthetic value.
2. Know the procedures, transitional restorations, and time-frame involved.
3. Appreciate the financial commitments in implant placement, ancillary procedures, restorative fees, and ongoing maintenance.
4. Recognize the importance of good oral health and plaque control.

C. Dental history. The implant candidate must be etiology-controlled and free of dental disease.[9] In addition, there must be adequate alveolar bone for placement of the implant.
1. Identify tooth loss. The patient who has lost teeth due to disease or neglect may not be as compliant in home care as the patient who has lost teeth due to trauma.[10]
2. Evaluate:
a. Gingival tissues. Periodontally involved teeth in the partially edentulous patient can act as a reservoir for periodontal pathogens.[11] Implants require adequate and healthy gingival tissues.
b. Bone width and height. Examine adequacy of the alveolar bone with radiographs, such as the panoramic and the computer axial tomograph (CT) scan.[12] Implants require adequate bone width and height.
c. Position of anatomical landmarks. Anatomical landmarks, including the floor of the nose, maxillary sinus, mandibular canal, or submandibular fossa, must be considered in determining implant placement.
d. Position of teeth. The natural dentition must be considered in the evaluation of implant sites, including adequacy of space, root proximity, and the relationship of opposing dentition.

IV. Collaborative Treatment Planning

A. Good oral health and plaque control. Success of the implant is dependent on the health of the environment; a patient who cannot demonstrate adequate home care should be presented with alternative treatment options.

B. Complete preliminary treatment such as periodontics, orthodontics, and restorations.

C. Develop **surgical guide.** Working with the oral surgeon, the restoring dentist should fabricate a surgical guide to facilitate proper alignment and placement of the implant.
1. Device is typically made of clear acrylic resin and is positioned over the teeth or edentulous ridge.
2. Holes or slots in the guide are used to position the surgical drill in implant placement.

V. Surgical Placement, Restoration, and Home Care

A. Implant placement can be achieved by two different loading modalities.
1. Immediate functional loading. A functional prosthesis is connected to the implant immediately after placement.

2. Delayed loading. Implant is submerged under the gingiva and is left without function; implant is exposed after a healing period of approximately three months for the maxilla and six months for the mandible.

B. Initial placement. Following surgical preparation, the general steps in implant placement are as follows:

1. An incision is made and a full thickness flap is reflected; bony ridge is evaluated and augmented, if needed.
2. By using a surgical guide to indicate the implant site, the cortical bone is penetrated by a series of round burs, and the opening is enlarged by a predrill; depth of the implant site is prepared by a trephine.
3. After the site is prepared, the implant is tapped or screwed into position.
    a. If loading of the implant is delayed, the tissue is sutured to cover the area.
    b. If it is to be immediately loaded, an abutment cylinder is placed on the implant to expose it for restoration.

C. Home care following initial placement (24 hours after surgery). Advise the patient of the need for gentle and thorough homecare. Retention of plaque at the implant site has been linked to vertical crestal bone defects.[9]

1. Gently debride surgical site.
2. Instruct the patient in effective home care around the **provisional restoration** by using one or more of the following auxiliary aids:
    a. Interdental brush.
    b. End-tuft brush.
    c. Interproximal oral health aid.
    d. Superfloss or floss threader.
3. Apply chlorhexidine gluconate to the site with swab or brush twice a day.

D. Exposure of the implant. An implant that has been submerged will be exposed after a healing period of approximately three months in the maxilla and six months in the mandible before beginning the restoration. Following surgical preparation, the general steps in implant exposure are as follows:

1. An incision is made and the implant is exposed.
2. A healing cuff, which is exposed to the oral cavity, is placed.

E. Home care following implant exposure.

1. Mechanically debride the implant by using the auxiliary aids previously mentioned.
2. Apply chlorhexidine gluconate directly to the implant with auxiliary aid.
3. In the two weeks following implant exposure, rinse with chlorhexidine gluconate twice daily.

F. Restoration of the implant. Regardless of the type of restoration, the same general steps are used to fabricate a prosthesis.

1. Remove the healing cuff.
2. Place an impression coping on the implant.
3. Take impressions.
4. Fabricate the crown or prosthesis.
5. Deliver the prosthesis.

G. Home care of the final restoration.

1. Reinforce importance of home care and tailor instruction to the patient's needs based on:
    a. Access to the implant.
    b. Dexterity of patient.
    c. Design of the restoration.

CLINICAL TIP:

Stabilizing Your Knowledge:
To prevent scratching the implant surface, interproximal brushes must be "implant-safe." The core of the brush should be made with plastic or nylon-coated wire.

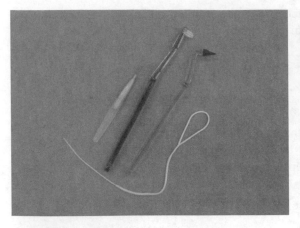

Figure 15–4   Auxiliary aids for implants. Interdental brush, end-tuft brush, interdental tip stimulator, and Proxi-floss.

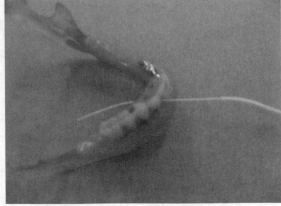

Figure 15–5   Using Superfloss to clean implant.

2. Perform primary plaque-control by using one of the following toothbrushes: Soft manual, power-assisted, and/or sonic.
3. Auxiliary aids. Use one of the following aids for cleaning around implants; use of interdental aids should be determined from the size and shape of **embrasure** space (Figure 15–4).
   a. Superfloss (Figure 15–5).
   b. Floss threader with floss.
   c. Gauze strips.
   d. Yarn.
   e. Proxi-floss (Figure 15–6).
   f. Dental tape.
   g. Interproximal brush with plastic or nylon-coated wire center (Figure 15–7).
   h. End-tuft brush.
   i. Foam tips.
   j. Disposable wooden picks.
   k. Rubber tip stimulator (Figure 15–8).

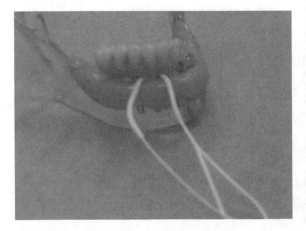

Figure 15–6   Using Proxi-floss to clean implant.

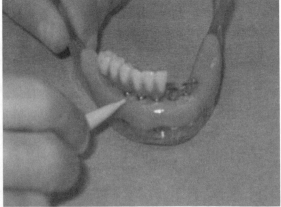

Figure 15–7   Using interdental brush to clean implant.

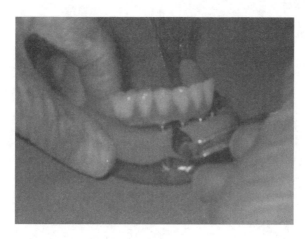

Figure 15–8   Using a rubber tip stimulator to clean implant.

4. Chemotherapeutics can be utilized as well. The following are recommended:
   a. Chlorhexidine gluconate: Delivered locally by floss or interdental aid.
   b. Rinse with four-essential oil mouth rinse, such as Listerine®, twice a day.[13]

VI. Implant Environment

The clinical appearance of the tissues surrounding natural teeth and dental implants are similar, but there are distinct differences in the organization and type of connective tissues.

A. Following implant placement. The healing process begins with the formation of a blood clot.
   1. Many complex histological events occur that result in bone formation and regeneration, and ultimately osseointegration.
   2. Osseointegration is the structural and functional connection between living bone and the dental implant—this bond lends stability to the implant and allows it to function as a natural tooth.
B. Perimucosal seal. A delicate barrier formed by the connective tissues. Compared to the periodontium around the tooth, it is a less effective barrier to bacteria than the attachment of a natural tooth.
C. Connective tissues.
   1. **Periimplant** tissue lacks a periodontal ligament, is less vascular, and has fewer fibroblasts than a natural tooth.[14]
   2. Collagen fibers run parallel to the implant surface without true attachment rather than inserting into the cementum of the tooth.
D. Bacteria. The same anaerobic, Gram-negative pathogens around natural teeth in the form of plaque are present in the implant sulcus and can affect the health of the tissues.[15]

VII. Maintenance of the Implant

A. Recare appointments. In the first year following restoration of the implant, three-month recare appointments are needed. Individual patient needs should dictate recare appointments thereafter.[14]
B. Radiographs. Take every three months in the initial year following restoration of the implant. Thereafter, take annual radiographs and compare to baseline radiographs.[14,16]
C. Examination of prosthesis and attachments.
   1. Prosthesis should provide adequate function.
   2. There should be no excessive occlusal stress that can contribute to peri-implant bone loss.

CLINICAL TIP:

Stabilizing Your Knowledge: A natural tooth has a periodontal ligament and is vascular. The connective tissue in the implant lacks a true attachment and has fewer blood vessels than the tooth. The result is the implant has less resistance to bacteria and the early inflammatory response is limited.

Figure 15–9   Plastic instruments.

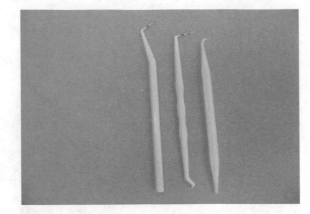

3. Surface of the prosthesis should be smooth to prevent the harboring of bacterial plaque.[16]

D. Evaluation of the health of the periimplant tissue.
   1. Clinically inspect tissue for signs of inflammation. Evaluate the tissue for the following:
      a. Color.
         (1) Healthy: Pale pink/coral pink.
         (2) Diseased: Acute, bright red.
         (3) Chronic: Bluish pink/bluish red.
      b. Consistency.
         (1) Healthy: Firm.
         (2) Diseased: Soft, spongy, smooth, shiny surface, and loss of stippling.
      c. **Edema:** Presence or absence.
      d. Bleeding, **exudate,** or tenderness.
   2. Note and quantify the presence, or absence, of debris, plaque, supra- and subgingival calculus as light, moderate, or heavy.
   3. Probing depth: Ideal pocket depths are less than 4 millimeters, with no bleeding.
      a. Use a plastic probe.
      b. Use a delicate probing technique, to avoid compromising the delicate barrier of the implant sulcus.
   4. Mobility. Indicates failure to achieve osseointegration.[14]

E. Deposit removal.
   1. Use implant-safe curettes and/or scalers that are:
      a. Plastic (Figures 15–9 and 15–10).
      b. Nylon.

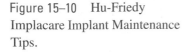

CLINICAL TIP:

Stabilizing Your Knowledge: Depending on the investigator, probing the implant sulcus is a debatable issue. The operator should use the best judgment when probing apparently healthy tissue. If the tissue appears inflamed, the operator should probe the implant sulcus.[14,15]

Figure 15–10   Hu-Friedy Implacare Implant Maintenance Tips.

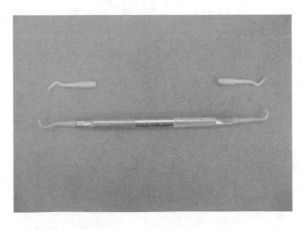

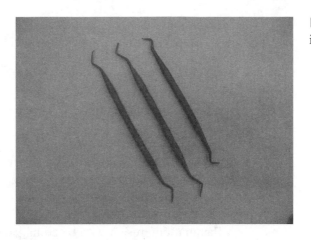

Figure 15–11 Graphite instruments.

  c. Graphite (Figure 15–11).
  d. Gold-tipped.
 2. Hand Instrumentation.
  a. Use a short working stroke with light pressure.
  b. Insert the instrument and close the blade against the abutment.
  c. Open the instrument past the deposit and engage it apically with the stroke extending coronally.
  d. Depending on the location of the deposit, use a horizontal, vertical, or oblique stroke.
 3. Ultrasonic and sonic scalers must be covered with plastic tip.
 4. Air polishing units are contraindicated, according to some investigators, but several studies demonstrate the safety and efficacy of air polishing units in deposit removal for the dental implant.[17–20]
 5. Polishing should be performed to remove plaque from the implant using a rubber cup with:
  a. **Tin oxide.**
  b. Flour of pumice.[9,14,21]
  c. Nonabrasive toothpaste.
 F. Modification or reinforcement of home care.
 1. May be indicated if patient's plaque control is ineffective.
 2. Resolve any of the patient's issues regarding implant care, such as negligence or lack of comprehension.
 3. Change auxiliary aid and modify technique patient is using, if necessary.
 G. Examine and remove deposits on natural teeth in the partially edentulous patient.
 H. Notify dentist of any changes in implant health or developing problems.

VIII. Periimplant Problems
Causes of periimplant problems are multifactoral; bacterial infection and biomechanical overload are predominate factors.[22]
 A. Periimplant mucositis.
 1. Similar to gingivitis around a natural tooth.
 2. Reversible bacterial infection with observable inflammatory changes.
 3. If allowed to progress, it causes periimplantitis, which affects surrounding bone. Evaluate for the following signs:
  a. Bleeding on probing.
  b. Edema.
  c. Tenderness.

> 📌
> **CLINICAL TIP:**
>
> **Stabilizing Your Knowledge:** Gold-tipped instruments should be examined for exposure of the underlying metal surface. NEVER sharpen gold instruments.[14]

> **CLINICAL TIP:**
>
> **Stabilizing Your Knowledge:** The "ailing" implant could be caused by bone loss from trauma or an arrested inflammatory process.

B. Periimplantitis. Affects the bone surrounding the implant; symptoms include those of periimplant mucositis, such as:
1. Increased pocket depth.
2. Presence of exudate.
3. Bone loss.[9,14,23]

C. Ailing implant. Must be closely monitored at maintenance appointments; determine if there is:
1. Bone loss without inflammation.
2. Advanced pocket depth with the absence of bleeding.[15]

D. Failing implant. Demonstrates persistent deterioration. Successful intervention, such as detoxification of implant surface or surgical treatment, are possible. Determine if there is:
1. Inflammation present with bleeding, edema, and exudate.
2. Bone loss, but with no mobility.[15]

E. Failed implant. There is no treatment for the failed implant and it must be removed. Determine if there is:
1. Inflammation present with bleeding, edema, and exudate.
2. Bone loss, with mobility.[15]

The dental implant can be a predictable replacement for natural teeth and superior to removable prosthetics. Because of the nature of the periimplant tissues, implants require intensive monitoring and maintenance. The dental hygienist is a constant in a dynamic process that begins with educating potential implant candidates. Disruption of biofilm through scaling and calculus removal, evaluation and assessment of tissue health, and patient home care instruction and motivation are all elements of implant care that allow the dental hygienist to function as a key player on the implant team. Ultimately, the dental hygienist has the capacity to perform a great service for the patient requiring prosthodontic treatment.

QUESTIONS

1. The indication for the transosteal or transmandibular dental implant is for
   a. severely resorbed mandible.
   b. severely resorbed maxilla.
   c. mandible or maxilla with adequate bone.

2. According to the American Society of Anesthesiology (ASA) Classification for presurgical risk, which of the following ASA patients is NOT an appropriate candidate for dental implants?
   a. I
   b. II
   c. III
   d. IV

3. Considering the health history, which of the following conditions would make a patient an acceptable candidate for an implant?
   a. Steroid therapy.
   b. Bleeding disorder.
   c. Diabetes mellitus.
   d. Immunosuppressive therapy.

4. Immediately following surgical placement of an implant, the chemotherapeutic agent of choice is
   a. warm saltwater.
   b. hydrogen peroxide.
   c. chlorhexidine gluconate.
   d. four essential oil mouthrinses.

5. Ossointegration is
   a. collagen fibers attached perpendicular to the implant surface.
   b. the formation of a perimucosal seal.
   c. the structural connection between alveolar bone and the implant.
   d. connective tissue fibers attached to the implant surface in a multidirectional pattern.

6. In the implant environment, plaque and calculus
   a. have a different composition than on teeth.
   b. accumulate similarly to teeth.
   c. cannot attach to the implant surface.
   d. attach loosely to the implant surface.

7. Periimplantitis is
   a. marked by bone loss.
   b. a reversible bacterial infection.
   c. similar to gingivitis.
   d. diagnosed by bleeding on probing, edema, and tenderness.

8. Which of the following combinations of radiographs BEST indicates adequacy of alveolar bone?
   a. Periapical and occlusal.
   b. Panorex and computer axial tomograph (CT) scan.
   c. Occlusal and panorex.
   d. Periapical and panorex.

9. In dental hygiene care of the implant, scaling is
   a. identical to instrumentation of natural teeth.
   b. accomplished with light pressure and a short working stroke.
   c. accomplished with firm pressure and a long working stroke.
   d. only performed coronal to the gingival margin.

10. Which of the following home care aids should be recommended for implant patients?
    a. Chlorhexidine rinse only.
    b. Implant toothbrushes.
    c. Any interproximal brush.
    d. End-tuft toothbrushes.

11. Periimplant problems may be caused by all of the following EXCEPT one. Which one is the EXCEPTION?
    a. Bacterial infection
    b. Biomechanical overload
    c. Trauma
    d. Chlorhexidine gluconate

REFERENCES

1. Slade G, Spencer AJ. Social impact of oral conditions among older adults. *Australian Dental Journal,* Vol. 39, Number 6, 1994, 358–64.

2. Hutton B, Feine J, Morais J. Is there an association between edentulism and nutritional status? *Journal of the Canadian Dental Association,* Vol. 68, Number 3, 2002, 182–87.

3. Weiss CM, Weiss A. *Principles and Practice of Implant Dentistry.* St. Louis, MO: C. V. Mosby, 2001.

4. Chitwood W. Implant candidates: Who qualifies? *Journal of Oral Implantology,* Vol. 22, Number 1, 1996, 56–58.

5. Traber KB. Preoperative evaluation. In: Dripps RD, Echenhoff JE, Vandam LD (eds.), *Introduction to Anesthesia* (9th ed.). Philadelphia: WB Saunders, 1997, pp. 11–19.

6. Farzad P, Andersson L, Nyberg J. Dental implant treatment in diabetic patients. *Implant Dentistry,* Vol. 11, Number 3, 2002, 262–65.

7. Abdulwassie H, Dhanranjai PJ. Diabetes mellitus and dental implants: A clinical study. *Implant Dentistry,* Vol. 28, Number 2, 2002, 74–81.

8. VehementeV, Chuang S, Daher S, et al. Risk factors affecting dental implant survival. *Journal of Oral Implantology,* Vol. 28, Number 2, 2002, 74–81.

9. Eskow RN, Sternberg Smith V. Preventive periimplant protocol. *Compendium of Continuing Education in Dentistry,* Vol. 20, Number 2, 1999, 137–54.

10. Meffert R. Implantology and the dental hygienists' role. *Journal of Practical Hygiene,* Vol. 4, Number 5, 1995, 12.

11. Quirynen M, De Soete M, van Steenberghe D. Infectious risks for oral implants: A review of the literature. *Clinical Oral Implants Research,* Vol. 13, Number 1, 2002, 1–19.

12. Reddy MS, Wang IC. Radiographic determinants of implant performance. *Advances in Dental Research,* Vol. 13, Number 6, 1999, 136–45.

13. Ciancio SG, Lauricello F, Shibley O, et al. The effect of antiseptic mouthrinse on implant maintenance: Plaque and the peri-implant gingival tissues. *Journal of Periodontology,* Vol. 66, Number 11, 1995, 962–65.

14. Silverstein L, Garg A, Callan D, Shatz P. The key to success: Maintaining the long-term health of implants. *Dentistry Today,* Vol. 17, Number 2, 1998, 104–111.

15. Meffert R. Maintenance and treatment of the ailing and failing implants. *Journal of the Indiana Dental Association,* Vol. 73, Number 3, 1994, 22–24.

16. Huband ML. Problems associated with implant maintenance. *Virginia Dental Journal,* Vol. 73, Number 2, 1996, 8–11.

17. Augthun M, Tinschert J, Huber A. In vitro studies on the effect of cleaning methods on different implant surfaces. *Journal of Periodontology,* Vol. 67, Number 3, 1996, 229–35.

18. Mengel R, Buns CE, Mengel C, Flores-de-Jacoby L. An in vitro study of the treatment of implant surfaces with different instruments. *International Journal of Oral and Maxillofacial Implants,* Vol. 13, Number 1, 1998, 91–96.

19. Meschenmoser A, d'Hoedt B, Meyle J, et al. Effects of various hygiene procedures on the surface characteristics of titanium abutments. *Journal of Periodontology,* Vol. 67, Number 3, 1996, 229–35.

20. Homiak AW, Cook PA, DeBoer J. Effects of hygiene instrumentation on titanium abutments: A scanning electron microscopy study. *Journal of Prosthetic Dentistry,* Vol. 67, Number 3, 1992, 364–9.

21. Koutsonikos A, Federico J, Yukna R. Implant maintenance. *Journal of Practical Hygiene,* 1996, 11–15.

22. Jovanovic SA. Peri-implant tissue response to pathological insults. *Advances in Dental Research,* Vol. 13, 1999, 82–86.

23. Bader H. Implant maintenance: A chairside test for real-time monitoring. *Dental Economics,* Vol. 85, Number 6, 1995, 66–67.

Chapter 16

Perioral Piercings

Betsy Reynolds, RDH, MS and Shirley Gutkowski, RDH, BSDH

 MediaLink

A companion CD-ROM, included free with each new copy of this book, supplements the procedures presented in each chapter. Insert the CD-ROM to watch video clips and view a large collection of color images that is also included. This multimedia library is designed to help you add a new dimension to your learning.

KEY TERMS

Association of Professional Piercers (APP)	median groove	piercee
bail	perioral piercing	piercer
labret		

LEARNING OBJECTIVES

After reading this chapter, the student will be able to:

- understand the clinical implications of head and neck piercings;
- recognize the importance of proper jewelry selection;
- formulate an aftercare plan for the care and maintenance of intra- and extraoral piercings involving the head and neck area;
- appreciate the significance of membership in the Association of Professional Piercers;
- recognize the importance of downsizing jewelry involving intraoral structures;
- understand why the use of a piercing gun is never appropriate.

I. Introduction

Over the past several years, piercings involving perioral areas have become a popular trend. Men and women of all ages and economic status find piercing ornamentation of the head and neck acceptable today. Even dental care providers can be seen sporting epidermal embellishments due, in part, to societal acceptance, personal preference, new piercing techniques, and new jewelry designs. Because piercings involving the intra- and extraoral structures may impact dental therapy, oral care providers must understand the health implications of these procedures.

II. History of Oral Piercing

A. Piercing has been practiced throughout the world for thousands of years.
1. Artifacts of the Ice Age show evidence of piercing.
2. Mummified remains of Egyptians demonstrate piercings.
3. African, Mesoamerican, and South American cultures continue to practice tongue and other oral piercings in ritual form (Figure 16–1).
4. Mayans built temples devoted to ritual piercing ceremonies.

Figure 16–1 Examples of tribal jewelry.

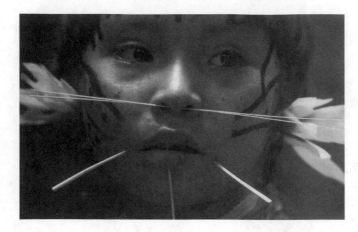

5. Wearing of labrets was widely practiced by the Eskimos and Aleutians of Alaska in prehistoric and early post-contact eras.

B. Tribal cultures around the world have made similar choices in piercing placements. This continuity in placement choices is not a result of lack of creativity but rather on the superior suitability of certain anatomy (such as the earlobe).

III. Present-day Demographics of Piercees

A. Any age or gender.

B. Persons exhibiting high or low self-esteem.

C. While some researchers suggest a link between body piercings in adolescents and increased risk-taking behaviors of these adolescents in the areas of gateway drug use, hard drug use, sexual activity, suicide and disordered eating behaviors, additional investigation is warranted.[1]

IV. Reasons for Piercing

A. Personal style statement.

B. Rite of passage.

1. Various cultures throughout the ages have used, and continue to employ, body modification procedures such as piercing to mark people who have achieved a certain age or level of bravery.

2. Piercing may also be used as part of an initiation rite into a club or gang.

C. Sense of community.

1. To some, piercing may help individuals fit in with peers who are also pierced.

2. To others, piercing may represent a way to stand out in a crowd.

D. Sexual enhancement.

E. An attempt to create one's own rituals and symbols of meaning. Efforts to revive ancient rituals that were shed long ago allow individuals to reconnect with the sacred.

V. Common Locations of Perioral Piercings

As piercing has resurfaced in the global community, new information on anatomy, jewelry, and asepsis has increased possible piercing placement locations;[3,4,5,6] all piercing placements should be decided by anatomical suitability and overall safety; piercing should be done by a professional trained in understanding anatomical impact on piercing sites.

A. Tongue—most common **perioral piercing;** placements include:

1. Dorsoventral—piercing is from the dorsum of the tongue through to the ventral surface; traditionally placed in the median groove of the tongue anterior to the lingual frenum (Figure 16–2).

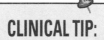

CLINICAL TIP:

Piercing Your Knowledge: When rendering health care, the "why" behind the piercing is of little significance. By questioning a dental patient's personal choice in matters such as piercing, trust between a patient and health care provider is often compromised. Do not ask about anything that does not have a bearing on how treatment will be rendered in the dental setting.

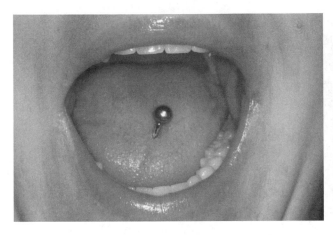

Figure 16–2   Dorsoventral median tongue piercing.

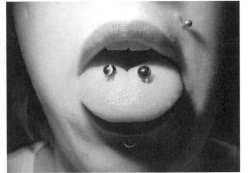

Figure 16–3   Dorsolateral lingual tongue piercing.

2. Dorsolateral lingual surface—piercing is from the dorsum of the tongue through to the ventral surface of the tongue lateral to the **median groove** (Figure 16–3).

B. Lip.
1. Second most popular form of intraoral piercing.[2]
2. Locations include both upper and lower lips (Figure 16–4).
3. Rings may be placed over either lip.

C. Midline **labret.** Piercing is centered at the midline above the upper lip in the philtrum or centered under the lower lip (Figure 16–5).

D. Cheek. May be performed to simulate a dimple or beauty mark—known as "Marilyn" or "Chrome Crawford" (Figure 16–6).

E. Frenum. Locations include:
1. Maxillary anterior frenum (Figure 16–7).
2. Mandibular lingual frenum. May be referred to as a "web piercing," especially if there is more than one frenal piercing.

F. Ear (Figure 16–8). Locations include:
1. Earlobe.
2. Ear cartilage, including tragus, anti-tragus, daith, conch, forward helix, anti-helix (snug), helix, and rook.
3. Industrial piercing: Binding two or more ear-piercing sites with a single piece of jewelry.

G. Eyebrow (Figure 16–9).

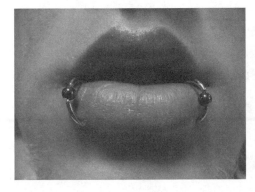

Figure 16–4   Lip piercings.

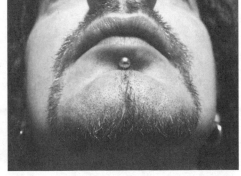

Figure 16–5   Labret piercing (chin).

Figure 16–6   Dimple piercing.

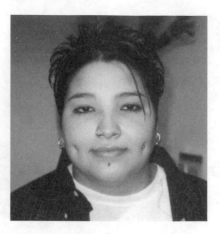

Figure 16–7   Maxillary frenal piercing.

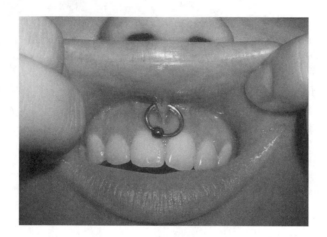

Figure 16–8   Examples of ear cartilage piercings.

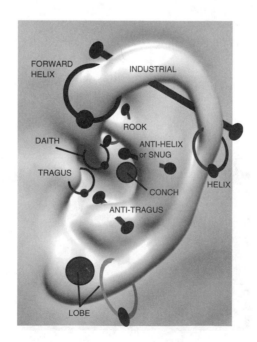

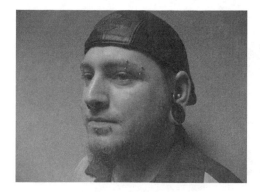

Figure 16–9   Eyebrow piercing.

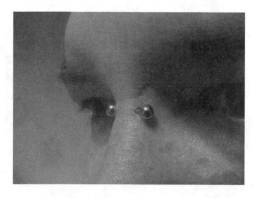

Figure 16–10   Nasion piercing. (Notice scarring superior to current placement. Scarring resulted from infection in previous piercing site.)

H. Bridge of nose ("Nasion") (Figure 16–10).

VI. Types of Piercing Jewelry

A. Barbell (Figure 16–11).
  1. A post or "bar" with a ball or **bail** on each end of a post; post is either internally or externally threaded to accommodate the bail.
  2. Remove both bails to allow for cleansing.

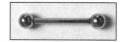

Figure 16–11   Barbell jewelry.

B. Ring.
  1. Not commonly used in tongue piercings.
  2. Most commonly worn in lip, nasal septum, supraorbital ridge, ear, and frenal piercings.
  3. Allows for better cleansing of a piercing when compared to a post and back piece of jewelry.
    a. Design of back locking mechanism of a post and back piece of jewelry traps bacteria and cellular debris in the area of the piercing making thorough cleaning difficult.
    b. For cleaning purposes, rings may be rotated through the piercing canal allowing the piercee access to the entire piece of jewelry; especially helpful when the jewelry should not be removed during initial healing of the piercing.

VII. Other Body Modification Procedures

A. Scarification: Cutting the skin to create an ornamental scar utilizing a medical grade scalpel.
B. Branding: Application of heated metal (either through cautery or strike metal) to skin to create visible designs.
C. Stapling: Although not common, epidermal staples may impact dental treatment if placed in an area that interferes with instrument placement.
D. Implanted jewelry: Spherical beads, jeweled casings, barbells or other types of jewelry placed subcutaneously.
E. Uvula piercing is dangerous piercing due to high risk of jewelry aspiration and gagging.
F. Side-to-side tongue piercing.
  1. Piercing that continues from one lateral border of the tongue to the other.
  2. Considered a dangerous piercing due to the risk of neural, vascular, and muscular damage.

Figure 16–12   Split tongue (notice both sides move independently).

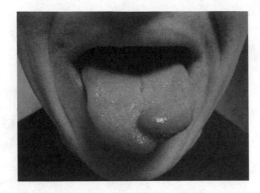

CLINICAL TIP:

Piercing Your Knowledge: The practices described in the section "Other Body Modification Procedures" represent a more extreme approach to body adornment. While members of the Association of Professional Piercers may practice body art forms (such as those described above) in areas where they are allowed by law, the APP does not address body modification procedures that do not involve piercing. Neither does the organization endorse unsafe, extreme piercing practices that may cause harm to the health and well-being of the **piercee.**

G. Tongue splitting (Figure 16–12).
1. Separates the tongue into right and left halves along the median groove.
2. Procedure may involve surgical cutting along the median groove or utilization of a laser or cautery unit.
3. Some states and several branches of the armed services prohibit the practice of tongue splitting.[7] Logging onto state websites allows interested individuals to keep abreast of legislation involving tongue splitting.

VIII. Jewelry Considerations

A. **Association of Professional Piercers (APP)** adopted broad minimum standards for jewelry to be placed into new piercings.
1. Due to biocompatibility, jewelry placed in new piercings must be made of one of the following metals:
   a. Surgical implant grade stainless steel (ASTM 316L [or LVM] F-138).
   b. Surgical implant titanium (ASTM Ti6A4VF-136).
   c. Niobium.
   d. Platinum.
   e. 14-karat or higher solid white or yellow gold.
   f. High-density, low-porosity non-toxic plastics.
      (1) Includes Tygon™ tubing and polytetrafluoroethylene (PTFE).
      (2) Both materials are autoclavable and come in a variety of sizes very close to the gauges worn in body piercing.
      (3) Can be useful in dental and medical situations where no metal jewelry can be worn.
2. Other criteria for jewelry. Must:
   a. Be free of nicks, scratches, burs, and polishing compounds.
   b. Be internally threaded (no threads on posts) for 16 gauge and thicker.
   c. Have rounded ends on rings.
   d. Have threads of 1.2 mm for 14- and 12-gauge and 0.08 mm for 10-gauge threaded stem ends.
3. Jewelry to avoid.
   a. Gold-filled, gold-rolled, or gold-plated.
      (1) Only a very thin layer or very small percentage of gold is used in these products.
      (2) Underneath the gold is either an inferior metal (i.e., nickel or aluminum) or an underplating of nickel or copper.
      (3) These materials are completely unacceptable for wear in body piercings due to their nonbiocompatible nature and ability to induce allergic reactions.
   b. Silver.
      (1) Reacts with the sulfur in the body to break down and tarnish.

CLINICAL TIP:

Piercing Your Knowledge: With the burgeoning popularity of piercing, many manufacturers have poured into the piercing jewelry market, knowing little or nothing about piercing and the most basic requirements for safety and quality. At this point in time, there is a tremendous quantity of jewelry on the market that an ethical, knowledgeable **piercer** would find completely unusable.

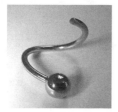

Figure 16–13   Bead ring jewelry in open position.

Figure 16–14   Captive bead ring jewelry.

Figure 16–15   Curved barbell jewelry.

(2) Many piercees find that even if they can wear silver comfortably in earlobe piercings, other areas of the body cause faster oxidation of the silver leading to more irritation of the piercing site.

  c. Other grades of stainless steel.

    (1) Include the 400 series, 302, 306, and high-carbon steel.

    (2) Many of these grades break down or corrode when in contact with saline (a main component of the human body and a common piercing aftercare solution).

    (3) Jewelry manufacturers are required by law to provide Mill Certificates to authenticate and confirm the composition of the stainless steel metal used in their products.

  d. Aluminum. Not suitably inert or biocompatible for use in the body.

  e. Organic materials. It is generally not appropriate to insert wood, bone, horn, leather, or other organic materials in a new piercing.

B. Jewelry styles.

  1. Bead ring (Figure 16–13).

    a. Has a bead fixed at one end of the ring.

    b. Opened and closed by bending.

    c. Suitable for piercings in which the jewelry will basically be left in place and not changed frequently.

    d. Sizes 12-gauge or thicker can require padded or brass-jaw pliers to bend for insertion and removal if the diameter is small.

  2. Captive bead ring (Figure 16–14).

    a. Most popular ring style in piercing jewelry.

    b. Held in place by spring pressure of the metal.

    c. Opened using either hand pressure on smaller gauges or using ring opening pliers for heavier rings.

  3. Barbell (Figure 16–15).

    a. Straight or curved piece of body jewelry with a ball or bead on each end.

    b. Most common location for a straight barbell is in the tongue; curved barbell is ideal for navels and other piercings that experience problems with friction.

    c. 14-gauge ⅝″ is the standard size for most tongue piercings.

      (1) Piercers generally use a 14-gauge ¾″ or ⅞″ barbell initially to allow for swelling.

      (2) Once tongue swelling has reduced, it is highly recommended to replace the longer barbell with a shorter one to minimize damage to oral tissues.

    d. It is recommended to remove both threaded bails for ease of cleaning and versatility.

CLINICAL TIP:

Piercing Your Knowledge: By various estimations, the number of allergic reactions to nickel, a metal often found in piercing jewelry, is increasing in this country. Although allergic reactions to metals are not a new phenomenon, many health care researchers are suggesting that there are more nickel allergies simply because more people are getting pierced and are using nickel-containing, nonbiocompatible jewelry.[8] Oral health care providers must be aware that the signs and symptoms of nickel allergy in a piercing site (redness, swelling, burning and itching) may often mimic those found in conjunction with a low-grade localized infection. If symptoms are present at more than one piercing site, it is more likely to be an allergy. Once a nickel allergy is diagnosed, it can be treated with topical creams and replacement of the offending nickel-containing jewelry with biocompatible jewelry. To avoid potential problems, experts agree that using only high grade, biocompatible products such as ASTM 316L (or LVM) F-138 stainless steel, surgical-implant jewelry is prudent. Although there is a small amount of nickel contained in implant grade stainless steel, the ionic bonds between the alloys contained in this stainless steel material prevent the nickel from interacting directly with the body.[1]

Figure 16–16   Labret flat back jewelry.

4. Labret (Figure 16–16). Available as a labret stud ("flatback") or a fish-tail labret.
   a. A labret stud ("flatback") is essentially a barbell with one of the bails replaced with a flat disc; designed for use for labret piercings but may also be appropriate for other piercings that can accept a barbell, such as tongue piercings.
   b. Unlike the disc back of a labret stud, the fishtail labret allows the jewelry to be custom bent to fit along the mucogingival margin; designed to minimize gingival recession.
5. Nostril jewelry.
   a. Nostril screw.
      (1) Design is based on ancient East Indian design.
      (2) Pre-bent end allows the stud to hug the inside of the nostril without injuring the septum or falling out easily.
      (3) Does not require a backing as does a regular stud earring.
      (4) Left- and right-bend designs are available, depending on whether the jewelry is to be worn in the right or left nostril.
   b. Nostril bone. Design is straight pin with a small rounded end to hold it in place once inserted into the nostril piercing.
   c. Nostril fishtail. Long straight jewelry which allows piercees to bend it to custom fit their piercing.
C. Jewelry removal. Can be difficult or impossible. Poor oral hygiene around intraoral piercings can lead to calculus deposit formation on the jewelry, making removal more difficult (Figure 16–17).
   1. Piercing needs to be fully healed before jewelry can be removed for any length of time.
      a. Prior to being fully healed, the piercing canal in areas such as the tongue may close in a matter of minutes.
      b. Should jewelry removal be necessary before the piercing has fully healed, the piercing canal must be kept open. This can be accomplished by threading sterile floss or sterile monofilament nylon into the piercing canal during procedures such as dental radiographs to keep the canal open and not distort the radiographic image.
   2. Jewelry threading. Jewelry can be either internally or externally threaded (Figure 16–18).
      a. Externally threaded jewelry has a threaded post which screws into the bail.
         (1) May cause trauma, especially in a newly pierced site, upon jewelry removal or insertion.
         (2) External threads may trap bacteria.

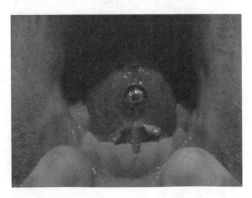

Figure 16–17   Calculus on barbell.

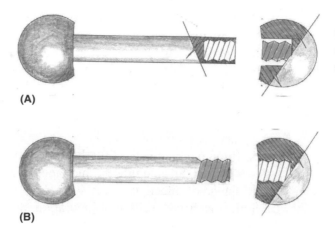

Figure 16–18   (A) Internally threaded jewelry. (B) Externally threaded jewelry (notice exposed threads).

b. Internally threaded jewelry has a threaded hole drilled into the shaft which is designed to receive the threaded post on the bail.
   (1) Because there are no exposed threads on the jewelry shaft insertion and removal is atraumatic and cleansing the jewelry is easier.
   (2) Generally superior in quality and finish and, therefore, more expensive to manufacture.
   (3) Highly recommended by professional piercers as being safer for piercings.
3. Jewelry removal instruments.
   a. Pliers.
      (1) Ring expanding or ring opening pliers are helpful for properly opening and installing captive bead rings.
      (2) Ring closing pliers are helpful in properly installing captive bead rings by tightening the gap of the captive ring to hold the bead in place.
   b. Hemostats.
      (1) Available in a variety of sizes and shapes.
      (2) Should be made of stainless steel to allow for repeated sterilization.
      (3) Assist in removing tightly attached bails from barbell jewelry.

IX. Complications of Perioral Piercings
A. Important health considerations.
1. Because piercing is an invasive procedure, any person requiring antibiotic premedication for invasive dental procedures will require antibiotic premedication prior to being pierced.
2. In certain situations, it is inappropriate to perform even the most standard piercing. Examples of when a physician consult may be warranted prior to receiving a piercing include:
   a. Positive history of heart valve disease, such as mitral valve prolapse.
   b. Positive history of heart murmur, diabetes, hemophilia, autoimmune disorders, or other medical conditions that may negatively influence the piercing procedure or the healing process.
   c. Signs of obvious skin or tissue abnormality that may include, but are not limited to, rashes, lumps, bumps, scars, lesions, nevi, macules, and/or abrasions.
   d. Potential piercee wishes to pierce irregular or surgically altered anatomy.

CLINICAL TIP:

Piercing Your Knowledge: Rarely is it necessary to remove jewelry for dental procedures. Unnecessary removal of jewelry in an inadequately or poorly healed piercing site can lead to cyst formation and possible infection in the area. Having the patient demonstrate how to remove his or her jewelry prior to beginning dental treatment is beneficial if the jewelry would interfere with CPR administration should a medical emergency occur. Be sure the piercee adequately washes his or her hands prior to touching the jewelry to minimize infection potential!

CLINICAL TIP:

Piercing Your Knowledge: Care, maintenance, and troubleshooting for body piercing is not yet a required course of study for most medical and dental professionals. Health care workers have tremendous knowledge and experience about issues relating to the human body. Relying on healing dynamic strategies in wound care treatment, the overall goal in health care delivery is to return the injured or diseased tissue to a state closely approximating the original structure and function. Wound closure is an integral component of this treatment strategy. Conversely, the creation of a piercing canal is dependent on establishing and maintaining a healthy opening within tissue structures. Therefore, when a medical or dental consultation is warranted for piercing concerns, it is recommended to seek advice from health care providers having specific knowledge, expertise, and experience in piercing dynamics.

e. Potential piercee is unsuited for the piercing due to occupational, recreational, or environmental factors.

3. It is advisable for a prospective piercee to refrain from piercing during pregnancy or if pregnancy is being planned for the near future.

4. Majority of troublesome piercings can be resolved without the piercing being lost or "abandoned."
   a. Advice to simply abandon the piercing is likely to be met with resistance from the piercee.
   b. If the piercing is not fully healed, or if there is localized infection in the area, abandoning the piercing may result in cystic formation or spread of infection.

5. Some localized swelling or induration, hardness, is not uncommon during healing of the piercing site (see Table 16–1).
   a. Not necessarily indicative of complications.
   b. Oral piercings, such as the tongue and lip, often swell significantly for three to five days following the piercing.
   c. Application of ice or use of an over-the-counter nonsteroidal antiinflammatory agent, according to package instructions, may help reduce swelling.

6. Healing piercings normally produce an exudate.
   a. Exudate contains various cellular components such as lysosomal enzymes, white blood cells (WBCs), blood plasma, and growth factors.
   b. Healing exudate is a clear, odorless, yellowish fluid that forms a crust on the jewelry at the openings of the piercing.
   c. Gently clean dried exudate from the piercing site daily to avoid irritation. Using warm water (distilled, if possible) and single-use paper products (instead of sponges or washcloths that may harbor bacteria) greatly decreases the risk of contaminating the piercing site.
   d. Differentiate healing exudate from purulent exudate.
      (1) Purulent exudate is an acute inflammatory exudate composed of dead and dying neutrophils and necrotic surrounding tissue; foul-smelling, milky, yellow-to-green in color.
      (2) Presence of purulent exudate indicates possibility of infection, never a sign of health; consultation with a physician is warranted, with possible antibiotic therapy.

7. Place piercings at a certain depth in order to be accepted and successfully healed by the body.
   a. Piercing(s) too deep or too shallow will likely be rejected by the body in much the same way the body rejects an unwanted splinter.
   b. If a piercing is shallow enough that the jewelry can easily be seen right through the tissue or if it encompasses less than ¼″ to 5/16″ of tissue, the jewelry will most likely need to be removed.[1]

Table 16–1   Average Healing Times for Various Head and Neck Piercings

Cheek	4–6 months or longer
Ear cartilage (all types)	2–3 months or longer
Earlobe	4–6 weeks or longer
Eyebrow	6–8 weeks or longer
Labret	6–8 weeks or longer
Lingual frenulum	6–8 weeks or longer
Tongue	4–6 weeks or longer

8. Importance of aftercare procedures.
   a. Wash hands thoroughly prior to contact with or near the area of a healing piercing.
   b. Educate the piercee about the importance of maintaining a clean environment in the piercing site and to provide information and instructions on the appropriate care for healing the piercing. A well-positioned piercing fitted with high-quality, biocompatible jewelry and performed under hygienic conditions can still go awry if proper after care procedures are not observed.
   c. Cleaning Protocol
      (1) Intraoral piercing care.
         (a) Rinse mouth four to five times daily with an alcohol-free antibacterial solution and/or a saline rinse; saline rinses should be either a sterile saline solution prepackaged with no additives or a noniodized sea salt mixture consisting of dissolution of 1/8 to 1/4 teaspoon of iodine-free sea salt into eight ounces of warm, distilled or bottled water.
         (b) Rinse mouth for thirty to sixty seconds after meals and before bedtime during the entire healing process.
      (2) Exterior of labret piercings.
         (a) Soak the piercing site in a saline solution and/or wash with a liquid antibacterial or germicidal soap; perform saline soaks two to three times daily utilizing fresh gauze or a cotton ball saturated with the saline solution.
         (b) Limit the use of soap on the exterior of the piercing to no more than once or twice daily; when antibacterial soap is used, it is recommended that the piercee lather a pearl-size drop of soap and apply the cleansing agent to the jewelry and the piercing site for no more than thirty seconds.
         (c) Rinse all traces of soap from the piercing site and jewelry to minimize tissue irritation.
         (d) Dry area thoroughly with a disposable product, such as gauze or tissue, following the cleaning procedure.
   d. In establishing appropriate aftercare protocol, dental health care providers can offer additional hints and tips to share with piercees healing intra- and extraoral piercings.
      (1) For labret or cheek piercings, care for both the inside of the mouth and facial surface areas.
      (2) For ear, ear cartilage, and facial piercings, shield piercing sites from hair spray, cosmetics, lotions, and other foreign substances to minimize the risk of infection or irritation. Disinfect telephone receivers and keep pillowcases clean and changed frequently to minimize the risk of developing infection in piercings involving exposed areas of the head and neck.
      (3) Avoid rotating jewelry while the piercing site is healing, except during cleansing.
         (a) Rotating jewelry during the healing stage risks tearing incompletely healed tissue and may lead to infection and possible cyst formation.
         (b) Because piercings heal from the outside in, a piercing site may appear healed on the surface, but the underlying tissue remains fragile.

CLINICAL TIP:

Piercing Your Knowledge: If infection is present in a pierced site, the jewelry should remain in place to allow for drainage of the purulent exudate. If the jewelry is removed when infection is present, the piercing canal may rapidly close leading to abscess formation and possible further spread of the infection. Use a new, disinfected, soft bristle toothbrush to gently debride the jewelry of foreign material while the infection is resolving. Especially in the case of an infected intraoral piercing, the piercee should employ oral home care strategies including use of a mild saline or alcohol-free commercial rinse, regular flossing, and thorough brushing to minimize further bacterial contamination in the infected area.

(4) In the case of threaded jewelry, such as barbells, check jewelry twice daily with clean hands to ensure the bails are screwed on tightly.
   (a) Like all threaded objects, bails tighten to the right and loosen to the left.
   (b) Tightening the bails on intraoral barbells will minimize the chance of accidental aspiration or swallowing of any portion of the jewelry.
(5) While a piercing is healing, avoid submerging the pierced area in water that could be contaminated, such as water found in hot tubs, lakes, swimming pools, or inadequately cleaned bathtubs.
   (a) During the healing process, showering is safer than taking a bath because bathtubs harbor a wide variety of microbes.
   (b) To bathe safely, thoroughly clean and rinse the bathtub with a bleach product prior to each bath; a running water rinse of the piercing site is recommended after bathing.
(6) Avoid over-cleaning the piercing because it can delay healing by creating tissue dryness and irritation.
(7) Once initial swelling of an intraoral piercing has subsided, generally after three to five days, it is important for the piercee to replace the original, longer post portion of barbell-style jewelry with a shorter post (Figure 16–19).
   (a) Shortening the barbell post is the best way to prevent damage to oral structures including bone, teeth, and gingival tissues.
   (b) Because this necessary jewelry change may occur during healing, it should be done by a qualified piercer in an aseptic environment.
(8) Avoid excessive play with oral jewelry because it can result in permanent damage to oral structures.
   (a) Undue trauma to the piercing site may result in the formation of scar tissue, piercing migration, and other complications.
   (b) If the piercing jewelry is intentionally placed against the teeth on a regular basis, the resulting pressure exerted against the underlying bone will lead to bony resorption and possible tooth loss.
   (c) If the barbell post is not downsized appropriately, the bail can rest between the mandibular and maxillary arches on the occlusal or incisal surfaces of opposing arches; if the piercee exerts biting pressure in this situation, chipping and fracture of the involved teeth can occur.
(9) Leave jewelry in the piercing canal at all times because healed piercings can shrink or close in minutes after having been in place for years.
(10) Avoid certain practices and products by the piercee during healing; the piercee should avoid the following:
   (a) Using any mouthwash containing alcohol to minimize irritation to the piercing site that may delay healing.
   (b) Using isopropyl alcohol, hydrogen peroxide, and iodine because they are overly drying and may cause irritation to the piercing site.
   (c) Applying antibiotic ointments to the piercing site because they prevent oxygen from reaching the wound and also form

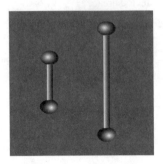

Figure 16–19 Comparison of longer healing barbell (right) and shorter post-healing barbell (left).

a sticky residue which can trap particulate matter, bacteria, and other debris which may irritate the area.

  (d) Chewing on foreign objects such as fingernails, gum, and pencils.
  (e) Sharing plates, cups, and eating utensils.
  (f) Consuming aspirin, alcohol, and excessive caffeine.
  (g) Practicing oral sexual contact, including wet kissing, during healing.
  (h) Causing undue trauma to the piercing site.
  (i) Touching the piercing site with unclean hands.
  e. Additional tips.
    (1) When eating
      (a) Eat slowly and place small bites of food directly onto the occlusal surfaces of the posterior teeth to avoid accidental cheek or tongue trauma.
      (b) Avoid spicy, salty, acidic, or hot temperature foods during the first few days post-piercing.
      (c) Eat or drink cold food or beverages to soothe and help reduce swelling.
      (d) For tongue piercings, keep the tongue level in the mouth while chewing and swallowing to avoid accidental trauma.
    (2) For cheek and lip piercings, use caution when opening the mouth wide because this can result in the jewelry backing catching on the teeth or gingival tissues.
    (3) Recommend piercee to carry a clean, spare bail should breakage or loss occur while the piercing is healing.
    (4) Contact a professional piercer if jewelry must be temporarily removed, such as for a medical procedure, during healing; the piercer will have suitable non-metal, sterilized material to place in the piercing canal.
    (5) If a piercee decides that he or she no longer wants the piercing, it is highly recommended to seek assistance with jewelry removal from a professional piercer if the piercing is not fully healed; also, the piercee must continue to clean the piercing site after jewelry removal until the piercing canal has completely closed.
9. Proper piercing protocol.
  a. According to the Association of Professional Piercers' "A Piercee's Bill of Rights," every person being pierced has the right to:
    (1) Be pierced in a scrupulously hygienic, open environment by a clean, conscientious piercer wearing a fresh pair of disposable gloves.
    (2) A sober, friendly, calm, and knowledgeable piercer who will guide the patient through the piercing experience with confidence and assurance.
    (3) Peace of mind, which comes from knowing that the piercer knows and practices the highest standards of sterilization and hygiene.
    (4) Be pierced with a brand new, completely sterilized needle, which is immediately disposed in a medical sharps container after single use on the piercee.
    (5) Be touched only with freshly sterilized, appropriate implements, properly used and disposed or resterilized in an autoclave prior to use on anyone else.

CLINICAL TIP:

Piercing Your Knowledge: Unfortunately, piercing guns are used by several piercing and retail establishments and are available for purchase by the general public. Because it is impossible to adequately sterilize a piercing gun between uses, it is unsafe to have any piercing procedure performed utilizing a piercing gun. Infections caused by the use of any unsterilized, contaminated equipment can result in permanent disfigurement. Further, the spring loaded mechanism of the piercing gun can result in tissue impingement in the piercing site, which delays or prevents proper healing, especially in areas of cartilaginous tissue.

(6) Be fitted only with jewelry which is appropriately sized, safe in material, design, and construction, and which best promotes healing; gold-plated, gold-filled *and* sterling silver jewelry is never appropriate for any new or unhealed piercing.

(7) Be fully informed about proper aftercare and to have continuing access to the piercer for consultation and assistance with all piercing-related questions.

(8) Know that piercing guns are never appropriate and often dangerous when used on anything, including earlobes.

b. Piercing should be done by a reputable professional piercer who is a member in good standing of the APP.

(1) APP membership is comprised of piercers and non-piercers who meet both personal and environmental criteria, companies who provide crucial goods and services to the piercing industry, and members of the health care community who support the efforts of the association.

(2) To be considered for membership in the APP, applicants must meet specific environmental and personal criteria. These include:

(a) Environmental criteria. The best standards of sanitation are observed in the piercing establishment—all surfaces in the piercing room must be cleanable, all equipment and products must be stored safely, and biohazard/sterile areas are well-managed.

  i. A level of safety and documentation within the applicant's studio must be demonstrated in addition to verification that every piercing client fills out a release form and is provided with both written and verbal aftercare instructions; the APP applicant must submit a walk-through 360 degree video of the entire facility including store front, foyer, piercing room(s), biohazard area, sterilization area, restroom, inside drawers, and closets.

  ii. A photograph of the autoclave with make, model, and serial number printed on the back of the photo; a copy of the two most recent spore test results for the applicant's autoclave from a biological monitoring service (the applicant will be required to submit monthly spore test documentation to maintain APP membership).

  iii. A business license, business card, and one or more samples of advertising the applicant has used.

(b) Personal criteria. As part of the APP application procedure, applicants must submit completed answers to a questionnaire provided by the Association of Professional Piercers (Figure 16–20).

  i. A copy of current CPR and First Aid certification: To maintain APP membership, these certifications must be kept current.

  ii. A copy of current Bloodborne Pathogens Training certificate, which must be renewed annually to maintain APP membership.

  iii. Proof of the length of time the piercer has been piercing professionally—a notarized statement, dated business

Questionnaire

The following questions are intended to determine your level of awareness of health and safety requirements for responsible piercing. Please type your responses.

1. Give a brief definition of the term "sterile".
2. Describe methods whereby objects in your studio could be made sterile.
3. What materials, equipment, or surfaces in your studio are sterile?
4. Give a brief definition of the term "disinfect".
5. Describe the methods and products used to disinfect objects or surfaces in your studio.
6. What materials, equipment, or surfaces in your studio are disinfected?
7. Give a brief definition of the term "contaminated".
8. Describe the concept of cross-contamination.
9. What kind of gloves do you wear?
10. Under what conditions is it necessary to change your gloves?
11. List three bloodborne pathogens:
12. In the context of piercing, what are the practical distinctions between Hepatitis and HIV?
13. How is new, unused jewelry cleaned in preparation for insertion in a fresh piercing?
14. How is previously worn jewelry cleaned in preparation for insertion in a fresh piercing?
15. How is the skin and other tissue to be pierced cleaned in preparation for a piercing?
16. How and with what are your piercing needles prepared for piercing, and how are they stored?
17. How many times are piercing needles used before being disposed?
18. How are piercing needles disposed?
19. What is the procedure in your studio for dealing with a needle stick?
20. What objects or areas in your studio are clearly marked with a biohazard sticker or sign?
21. Do you use a gun for any type of piercing? If so, please elaborate:
22. If you use a gun, how is it cleaned between uses?
23. Do you use any type of anesthetics? If so, please describe the method, product(s), and types of piercings involved:
24. What other services are offered in the room used to perform piercing? Please describe:
25. What are the specifications for the jewelry that you insert into new piercings? List all acceptable materials:
26. Where did you receive your training/apprenticeship/information? How long did you train?
27. Are you certified, licensed, or otherwise legally qualified or regulated by any source or authority? Please elaborate:
28. List any sources of continuing education directed towards improving your piercing knowledge and skills:
29. List the qualities that you feel are important in a piercer's bedside manner:
30. What is your policy on piercing persons under eighteen?
31. Under what circumstances related to yourself or to the customer would you refuse to perform a piercing?
32. We all make occasional mistakes. If a piercing does not come out as planned, how do you deal with this situation?

Figure 16–20   Questionnaire provided by the Association of Professional Piercers.

Health and Safety Agreement

The APP requires a signed agreement on record from each individual member. Violation of these basic, critical health and safety requirements is grounds for immediate revocation of membership. Please initial each numbered line as indicated to show that you have read and fully understand each point.

1. _____ I agree not to use ear-piercing guns in my studio due to the impossibility of properly sterilizing the equipment and the inappropriateness of ear piercing gun jewelry.

2. _____ I agree that all needles will be pre-sterilized, used on one person only in one sitting, and will be immediately disposed of in a medical sharps container.

3. _____ I agree that all forceps, tubes, etc. are to be pre-sterilized. If they are not used immediately, they will be stored in sterile bags and used on only one person in one sitting. After one such use, instruments will be appropriately decontaminated and then sterilized in an autoclave.

4. _____ I agree that all reusable, non-sterilized implements, such as calipers, will be nonporous and disinfected after each use with an FDA-approved commercial hard surface disinfectant.

5. _____ I agree that as many supplies as possible including corks, rubber bands, toothpicks etc., should be pre-sterilized in an autoclave, and if not used immediately, stored in a clean, closed container and disposed of immediately after a single use. In addition all skin prep products will be single use, and will be disposed of after one use.

6. _____ I agree that a new pair of medical-grade (sterile and/or non-sterile) gloves will be donned appropriately and worn for every procedure and that gloves will be changed frequently, and whenever there is the slightest chance for cross-contamination.

7. _____ I agree that the room used for piercings will be an enclosed room and used exclusively for piercing and jewelry insertion. This room must also be kept separate from the sterilization area. Piercing room, biohazard room, bathrooms and other common areas, will be kept scrupulously clean and shall be disinfected frequently. All surfaces shall be non-porous, allowing them to be cleaned with an FDA-approved disinfectant solution throughout the day and whenever cross-contamination might occur.

8. _____ I agree that all jewelry for initial piercings will be autoclaved prior to insertion.

9. _____ I will use only appropriate jewelry in initial piercings. Appropriate jewelry is made of Surgical Implant grade Stainless Steel 316L, 316L or LVM ASTM F-138, solid 14 karat or higher white or yellow gold, Niobium (Nb), Surgical Implant grade Titanium Ti6A4V ELI, ASTM F-136, solid platinum, or a dense low porosity plastic such as Tygon or PTFE. Threaded jewelry for initial piercings must have internal tapping (no threads on posts) starting from 16 gauge. Jewelry must be free of nicks, scratches, burrs, and polishing compounds. Ring ends should be rounded.

10. _____ I agree that it is important to be open, available and not under the influence of legal or illegal substances which might compromise my abilities. I agree to maintain my certification in First Aid/CPR, and Bloodborne Pathogen training. I agree to meet or exceed all health, safety and legal standards as required by my state and local authorities. I understand that it is important not to misrepresent myself, my abilities, or my standards in any way. I agree to consider all new health and safety suggestions, as they become known to me and to make appropriate changes in my technique as applicable. I agree that it is the moral, ethical, and professional responsibility of all piercers to continue to seek out, absorb and share health and safety information relevant to the craft throughout my career. I also agree to APP logo specifications and guidelines.

NAME (please print): _____ Studio name: _____

Address: _____

Business phone: _____ Fax:_____

Web: _____ Email: _____

Signature _____ Date _____

Witness _____ Date _____

Figure 16–21 The APP Health and Safety Agreement form.

document, or newspaper article are examples of acceptable proof.

(3) Types of APP membership.

   (a) Professional business member. This is a piercer who works full-time in a piercing studio and has more than one year of professional experience; must meet both personal and environmental criteria for membership.

   (b) Professional member at large. The applicant works full- or part-time at one or more studio locations and has more than three years professional experience; applicants must meet personal and environmental criteria, at all studio locations, for membership.

   (c) Associate member. This individual has less than one year of professional experience or is a non-piercing worker in a piercing establishment; if working as a piercer, the personal and environmental criteria must be met; if person is a non-piercing employee, the environmental criteria must be met.

   (d) Corporate associate member. This category applies to individuals who are associated with the body piercing industry; applicants are required to provide a letter describing in what way their services or products benefit the profession of body piercing; examples of corporate associate members include jewelry manufacturers, medical suppliers, insurers, and educators.

   (e) Patron member. Members of this category are not actively involved in the body piercing industry but support the APP and its goals; there are no requirements for membership other than to support the efforts of the APP.

(4) As part of the APP application process, the applicant must sign the Health and Safety Agreement form (Figure 16–21), agree to the basic tenets contained in the agreement and keep the document on record for every individual APP member; violation of these basic, critical health and safety requirements is grounds for immediate revocation of APP membership.

B. Prevention of piercing complications.

1. Piercing professional must use proper sterile, disposable equipment in a hygienic environment to prevent disease contamination during a piercing procedure.

2. Piercee must demonstrate strict adherence to proper aftercare protocol following the piercing procedure; without compliance, even the best piercing may become infected or irritated.

3. Use properly fitted and sized jewelry made of biocompatible materials to significantly decrease permanent damage to orofacial structures and minimize hypersensitivity reactions, such as allergic reactions to inferior grade metals.

CLINICAL TIP:

Piercing Your Knowledge: Occasionally, a non-APP studio and/or individual piercer falsely claims membership in the Association of Professional Piercers. In order to ensure that a piercer is indeed an APP member in good standing, potential piercees are urged to visit the Association of Professional Piercers' website at: www.safepiercing.org to verify the piercer's membership. Should a piercer be deceitfully claiming association with the APP or is using the APP name and/or logo (Figure 16–22) in advertising or otherwise, it is critical to report such transgressions directly to the Association of Professional Piercers in order to safeguard the reputation of the association's membership.

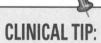

CLINICAL TIP:

Piercing Your Knowledge: Knowing the APP members in your locality will enable you to work closely with these professionals in dealing with your intra- and extraoral piercing concerns.

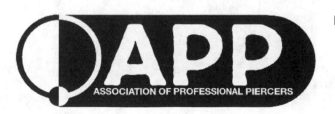

Figure 16–22   The APP logo.

4. Seek medical assistance for piercees demonstrating signs and symptoms of infection in a timely manner; antibiotic therapy may be warranted; remember that the jewelry must be kept in place if infection is suspected to avoid closure of the piercing canal, possible abscess formation, and further spread of infection.

5. Use of internally threaded jewelry is less likely to tear the fragile lining of a healing piercing canal; tearing of the canal lining may introduce epithelial cells into a connective tissue environment leading to cyst formation at or near the piercing site.

6. For intraoral piercings in which threaded barbells are used, the piercee is advised to check the tightness of the bails daily to minimize the chance of accidental aspiration or swallowing of the jewelry.

7. Avoid use of an abrasive paste (prophylaxis paste of all grits) or airpolisher for a piercee with head and neck piercings, including those involving the ears, until the piercee has completely healed.

   a. The aerosolized particulate material used in these procedures may cause irritation and infection in a newly pierced site.

   b. Utilize ultrasonic and hand instrumentation instead.

C. Clinical strategies for detecting intraoral damage from improper piercings.

   1. Routinely taken, on an annual basis, periapical radiographs in the mandibular and maxillary anterior regions when patients with tongue, lip, and frenal piercings present for dental hygiene care. Severe bone loss requiring bone grafting or extraction(s) can result if the jewelry has not been downsized; appropriate referral to a dental specialist may be warranted.

   2. Oral health care providers need to carefully check teeth for chips and fractures, especially the lingual surfaces (Figure 16–23).

   3. Evaluate the piercing site for signs of infection such as the presence of purulent exudate, irritation, or improper healing on a regular basis.

   4. Recession and abrasion are common results of improperly placed piercings involving the lips, frenums, tongue and cheek (Figure 16–24); similar damage may also result from using inappropriate jewelry in these areas; the dental hygienist needs to evaluate the cause of any gingival recession and/or tooth abrasion in the area of a piercing, make suggestions to prevent or minimize damage, and record significant findings in the piercee's record.

Figure 16–23   Chip due to improper barbell length.

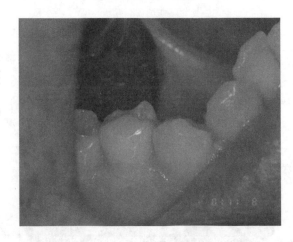

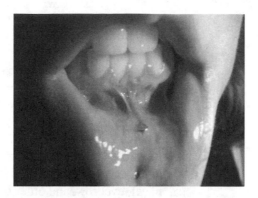

Figure 16–24   Recession due to improper labret placement.

X. Regulatory Control of Piercing Industry

A. The piercing industry as a whole is not a highly regulated, licensed profession.

1. State laws vary in regard to piercing regulations. To research the laws in each state, do an Internet search for the state's home page; once there, search for legislation using keywords such as "body piercing" or "body+piercing".

2. This method also works for county and city searches. If local areas and states both have regulations, the stricter ones will apply.

B. Occupational Safety and Health Administration (OSHA) compliance. As a federal agency, OSHA monitors and regulates worker safety for all businesses with one or more employees.

1. Whether piercing-specific legislation has passed in a given area, OSHA has explicit requirements that relate to piercing.

2. To comply with OSHA requirements, piercing establishments with one or more employees must meet the following standards:

   a. Observe Universal Precautions for Bloodborne Pathogens.

   b. List standard operating procedures detailing exposure control plan, exposure determination, engineering controls, work practices, housekeeping, personal protective work clothing and equipment, regulated biohazard waste disposal, communication of hazards to employees (both written and verbal), recordkeeping/documentation, appropriate information and training, adequate decontamination and disinfection, employer-provided Hepatitis B vaccine, and accurate reporting of all exposure incidents.

C. Piercing of minors.

1. Laws regarding the piercing of minors vary by location.

2. A minor's body is the legal responsibility of his or her parent or legal guardian.

   a. For any piercing of a minor, a parent or legal guardian must be present to sign a consent form.

   b. Proof-positive, state issued photo identification is required from the legal guardian as well as a bona fide form of identification from the minor wishing to be pierced.

   c. In the event the parent has a different last name and/or address from the child, documentation is needed to prove the relationship such as divorce papers and remarriage certificate.

3. A child who cannot comprehend the piercing procedure and consequences should not be pierced under any circumstances.

a. In infants, the body is still developing. An immature immune system may develop life-long allergic reactions to the materials found in the piercing jewelry, such as nickel.

b. A baby is obviously unable to care for a piercing.

c. Health care providers should provide parents with all pertinent information regarding the health and safety issues involved in piercing infants.

4. Minors age sixteen or over, with the consent and release of the parent or legal guardian, may be eligible (depending on circumstances, studio policy, and local/state laws) for piercings of the ear cartilage and lobes, nostril, navel, eyebrow, and other oral/facial areas. Other piercings are either potentially dangerous, unethical to perform, or problematic to heal.

5. Many studios simply refuse to pierce anyone under the age of eighteen.

XI. Resources

The Website of the Association of Professional Piercers (APP), www.safepiercing.org, contains valuable information for piercees and healthcare providers interested in keeping their pierced patients healthy. Oral piercing aftercare guideline brochures are available for order and may be distributed to pierced patients in the dental setting.

Piercing practices involving the head and neck area present unique challenges to the dental healthcare provider. Understanding the oral and systemic ramifications of these procedures will greatly aid the dental hygienist in developing and implementing treatment strategies designed to treat the pierced dental patient in a safe manner.

QUESTIONS

1. When is it appropriate to pierce with a piercing gun?
   a. When just the earlobe is to be pierced.
   b. Piercing guns may be used in any piercing procedure.
   c. When piercing infants.
   d. It is never safe to use a piercing gun.

2. Which of the following materials should *not* be used for piercing jewelry?
   a. Niobium
   b. Titanium
   c. Gold-filled metal
   d. Platinum

3. When can piercing jewelry be removed?
   a. Any time following the piercing procedure.
   b. Only after the piercing has fully healed.
   c. Daily during the first three months following the piercing.
   d. When there is evidence of infection.

4. Which grade of stainless steel should be used in piercings?
   a. ASTM 316L F-138
   b. PTFE
   c. ASTM Ti6A4VF-136
   d. Any surgical grade stainless steel may be used.

5. The average healing time for a tongue piercing is
   a. four to six days.
   b. four to six weeks.
   c. four to six months.
   d. four to six years.

6. One of the best ways to avoid intraoral trauma from a tongue piercing is to
   a. use only sterling silver jewelry.
   b. increase the barbell length.
   c. increase the gauge of the jewelry.
   d. downsize the jewelry once initial swelling has decreased.

7. Intraoral piercings are
   a. a new fad embraced by adolescents.
   b. an ancient form of body modification.
   c. a sign of deviant social behavior.
   d. best performed by utilizing a piercing gun.

8. The professional organization dedicated to the safety of the piercing profession is the
   a. Association of Professional Piercers (APP).
   b. Association of Piercing Gun Users (APGU).
   c. Society of Radical Body Modification (SRBM).
   d. American Association of Piercing Professionals (AAPP).

9. Which type of threading is recommended for piercing jewelry?
   a. Externally threaded.

b. Laterally threaded.
c. Internally threaded.
d. Bails should be fixed and not removeable.

10. When cleaning an intraoral piercing site
    a. an alcohol-based antimicrobial rinse should be used several times a day.
    b. an alcohol-free antibacterial solution and/or a saline rinse should be used four to five times daily.
    c. full strength hydrogen peroxide should be used to flush the piercing site followed by rinsing with a prescription antimicrobial agent at least eight times daily.
    d. toothpaste with a whitening agent may be used to clean the piercing site and the jewelry.

REFERENCES

1. The Association of Professional Piercers. *Procedure Manual* (U.S. Edition). Self published. 2002.
2. Mercury M. *Pagan Fleshworks: The Alchemy of Body Modification.* Park Street Press. Rochester, VT. 2000.
3. Miller J-C. *The Body Art Book: A Complete Illustrated Guide to Tattoos, Piercings, and Other Body Modifications.* The Berkley Publishing Group. New York, NY. 1997.
4. Vale V and Juno A. *Modern Primitives: An Investigation of Contemporary Adornment and Ritual.* V/Search Publications. San Francisco, CA. 1989.
5. Rubin A. *Marks of Civilization: Artistic Transformations of the Human Body.* Regents of the University of California. Los Angeles, CA. 1988.
6. Bish B. *Body Art Chic.* Trafalgar Square Publishing. North Pomfret, VT. 1999.
7. Baird C. Forked tongues. *The Cleveland Free Times* (www.freetimes.com). June 11, 2003.
8. Salvatore S. Piercing woes: Allergic reactions to jewelry a pointed problem. In [cnn.com/HEALTH/9812/04/body.piercing/] December 4, 1998.

Chapter 17

Dentin Hypersensitivity

Mary D. Cooper, RDH, MSEd

MediaLink

A companion CD-ROM, included free with each new copy of this book, supplements the procedures presented in each chapter. Insert the CD-ROM to watch video clips and view a large collection of color images that is also included. This multimedia library is designed to help you add a new dimension to your learning.

KEY TERMS

A-δ (A-delta) pulpal fiber

abfraction

obturate

odontoblasts

odontoblastic process

repolarization

smear layer

LEARNING OBJECTIVES

After reading this chapter, the student will be able to:

- define dentin hypersensitivity;
- discuss the prevalence of dentin hypersensitivity;
- discuss the causative stimuli for dentin hypersensitivity;

- explain how dentin hypersensitivity can be managed/treated;
- competently apply fluoride varnish to patients' teeth to treat hypersensitivity.

I. Introduction

Dentin hypersensitivity is a short, sharp pain arising from exposed dentin in response to stimuli typically thermal, evaporative, tactile, osmotic, or chemical that cannot be ascribed to any other form of dental defect or pathology.[1]

II. Prevalence

A. In the general population, prevalence ranges from 8 percent to 57 percent;[2] prevalence can be as high as 80 percent of patients in periodontal practices.[3]

B. Although sensitive teeth are more prevalent in older patients, hypersensitivity is experienced by a significant number of young adults.[4] People between 30 and 40 years of age experience and report dentin hypersensitivity most frequently.[3]

III. Causes

A. Gingival recession due to occlusal problems, overcontoured crown margins, excessive brushing, and erosion due to improper diet, to name a few. Susceptible tooth surfaces include:

1. Receded gingival tissues, exposing the cementum and dentin.
2. Lost enamel or apically migrated junctional epithelium.

CLINICAL TIP:

Stimulating Your Knowledge: Some patients who have used anti-tartar dentifrices complain of increased tooth/dentin sensitivity.

3. Facial surfaces of maxillary canines, first premolars, followed by incisors, second premolars, and then molars due to more vigorous toothbrushing on the facial gingival surface, although any tooth in the dentition may experience pain associated with dentin hypersensitivity.

B. Root surface morphology. Approximately 10 percent of teeth have an area of exposed dentin at the cementoenamel junction (CEJ).

1. Cementum is thin or nonexistent on the cervical root; consequently, when attachment fibers are lost, the hard tissue exposed to the oral environment is dentin.

2. For sensitivity to be felt, exposed dentin must have dentinal tubules that are open to the oral cavity and pulp.

3. Nonsensitive tooth. Exposed root surface does not react to a triggering stimulus, has fewer open dentinal tubules at exposed surfaces, and the diameters of the tubules are much narrower than those in teeth that do react to triggering stimuli and experience sensitivity.[5]

   a. Average diameter of tubules in sensitive teeth is two times wider than tubules in nonsensitive teeth.[5]

   b. Difference in the diameter of the dentinal tubules significantly increases the rate of fluid flow within the tubule, which most likely contributes to pain stimulation.

IV. Explanation of Pain Mechanism

Although not well understood, the most accepted mechanism of action is the Brännström's hydrodynamic theory, which is based on fluid dynamics.

A. Theory suggests that when a stimulus—chemical, thermal, or tactile—contacts an exposed surface of a dentinal tubule, it alters the movement of:

1. Fluid in the dentinal tubule.

2. **Odontoblastic process** within the dentinal tubule.

B. Alterations in fluid and odontoblastic process movements exert pressure on the nerve endings in the pre-dentin and pulp, causing the nerve endings to deform and act as receptors (Figure 17–1).

C. **A-δ pulpal fibers** surrounding the **odontoblasts** are stimulated and send an impulse to the brain creating a painful response.

CLINICAL TIP:

Stimulating Your Knowledge: When there are more dentinal tubules with larger diameters, there is increased fluid movement within the tubules. Increased fluid movement increases hypersensitivity.

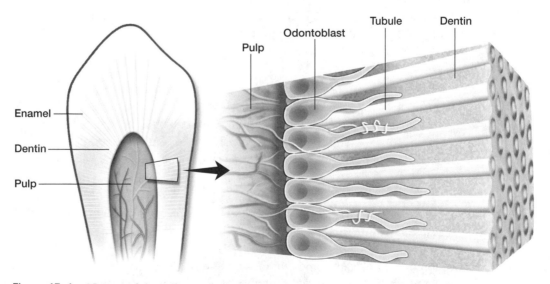

Figure 17–1   Nature of the pulp.

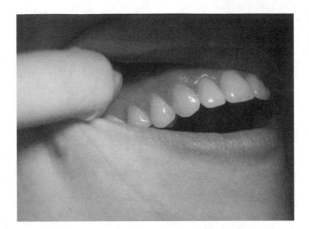

Figure 17–2   Exposed root surface due to recession.

V. Risk Factors Contributing to Hypersensitivity[3]

If an action or a clinical condition contributes to exposing and opening dentinal tubules, it is considered a predisposing factor for dentin hypersensitivity. Predisposing factors include:

A. Mechanical wear, such as:

1. Abrasion due to toothbrush, improper brushing, and/or abrasives in toothpastes.[3]
2. Attrition. Causes include:[3]
   a. Tooth-to-tooth wear.
   b. Bruxism initiated by occlusion or habit.
   c. Wear facets created by occlusal forces during chewing.

B. Abfraction.[3] Cervical stress-lesion as a result from eccentric forces; can create a wedge- or V-shape at the cementoenamel junction (CEJ).

C. Erosion. Loss of tooth structure caused by acids.

D. Gingival recession and periodontal therapy that results in gingival recession (Figure 17–2).

VI. Causative Stimuli

There are various stimuli that, when in contact with exposed and open dentinal surfaces, may elicit a painful sensation in a tooth.

A. Toothbrush abrasion and abrasive dentifrices. There is some controversy surrounding toothbrush abrasion or the use of "abrasive" dentifrices.

1. Aggressive scrub brushing and/or the use of abrasive pastes may erode cervical dentin, but this action produces a **smear layer**—protective surface layer—that may help to counteract sensitivity.[6]
2. If a dentifrice is too abrasive, if it is used too frequently, or if it is applied with too much force, the paste may remove the beneficial smear layer, resulting in open tubules and sensitivity.

B. Chemical erosion. Enamel and dentin are susceptible to chemical wear (erosion) from excessive acid attacks.[2] Sources of acids include:

1. Extrinsic (diet).
   a. Formed by plaque bacteria when dietary carbohydrates are ingested and digested.
   b. Naturally occurring in foods/beverages (i.e., citrus fruits, juices, ciders, carbonated drinks, and wines).
2. Intrinsic. Include gastric acids that are regurgitated into the oral cavity during excessive vomiting (i.e., bulimia, anorexia nervosa, antiretroviral

CLINICAL TIP:

Stimulating Your Knowledge: Predisposing factors for dentin hypersensitivity are not causative factors in pain production, but their role is one of increasing a tooth surface's susceptibility to stimuli.

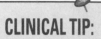

CLINICAL TIP:

Stimulating Your Knowledge: It is recommended that individuals with hypersensitive teeth be discouraged from bleaching. Over use of bleaching products increases the likelihood of sensitivity.[3]

CLINICAL TIP:

Stimulating Your Knowledge: If modifying the patient's self-care methods and/or diet does not relieve dentin hypersensitivity, desensitizing treatments should be recommended.

CLINICAL TIP:

Stimulating Your Knowledge: There are several desensitizing agents available. Only a few have been listed.

medications, and pregnancy) or from gastroesophageal acid reflux disease (GERD).

C. Thermal. Causes include:
  1. Hot and/or cold foods and beverages.
  2. Cold air on exposed dentinal surfaces; cold is the most common cause of hypersensitivity.[7]

D. Tactile. A foreign object touching an exposed dentinal surface may elicit sensitivity. Examples include toothbrush bristles, toothpicks, denture clasps, and dental instruments, such as explorers, periodontal probes, scalers, and curettes.

VII. Management of Dentin Hypersensitivity

A. Differential diagnosis needed to rule out other possible sources causing the pain, such as:
  1. Dental caries.
  2. Pulpitis.
  3. Tooth fractures.
  4. Fractured or leaking restorations.

B. Assess patient behavior. Educate patient to remove or modify risk factors.
  1. If applicable, limit dietary acids.
  2. Practice thorough plaque control; modify toothbrushing technique if existing technique uses too much pressure or if the direction of the strokes contribute to gingival recession.
  3. Recommend toothbrushing before eating meals because eating lowers the pH in the oral cavity—acid-exposed enamel is more susceptible to toothbrush abrasion than nonexposed enamel.[8]
  4. Evaluate periodontal condition.

C. Desensitizing Treatments.[3,9] Consist of either interrupting pulpal nerve activation **repolarization** and pain transmission or reducing the fluid flow within the dentinal tubules by creating a smear layer or by blocking (occluding) the tubule ends.
  1. Patient-applied treatments for home care include:
     a. Desensitizing dentifrices. Include active agents that have been accepted by the American Dental Association (ADA) Council on Dental Therapeutics as effective in relieving sensitivity.
        (1) Examples of active agents include:[3]
           (a) 0.24 percent sodium fluoride, i.e., Aquafresh Sensitive Teeth, Advance White for Sensitive Teeth, Crest Sensitivity Protection, Butler Sensitive, and Sensodyne Original Flavor.[3]
           (b) Potassium nitrate. Most widely available active agent in desensitizing dentifrices.
              i. 5 percent potassium nitrate, sodium monofluorophosphate, i.e., Orajel Sensitive Pain-Relieving toothpaste, Rembrandt Sensitive, and Sensodyne Extra Whitening).[3]
              ii. 5 percent potassium nitrate, 0.45 percent stannous fluoride, i.e., Colgate Sensitive Maximum Strength.[3]
           (c) Strontium chloride. Less commonly used agent. Mode of action—reduces sensitivity by occluding or sealing the open ends of the dentinal tubules.
        (2) Mode of action. Potassium nitrate depolarizes nerve fibers; fluoride forms precipitate within dentin tubules.

(3) Properties.
  (a) Easy availability; over-the-counter (OTC).
  (b) Typically requires two to four weeks use before patient notices a reduction in sensitivity.
(4) Application. For best results, brush twice daily brushing with a soft-bristled toothbrush; use proper toothbrushing techniques.

b. Self-applied fluoride rinses. Both stannous and sodium fluorides occlude dentinal tubules.
  (1) Examples include:[3]
    (a) 0.63 percent stannous fluoride (i.e., Gel-Kam Oral Care Rinse), daily prescription rinse.
    (b) 0.2 percent sodium fluoride (i.e., Fluorinse), weekly prescription rinse.
  (2) Mode of action. Fluoride forms precipitate within dentinal tubules.
  (3) Application. Follow manufacturer's directions.

c. Self-applied fluoride gels and pastes.
  (1) Examples include:[3]
    (a) 0.4 percent stannous fluoride (i.e., Gel-Kam Gel, Omni Gel, and Take Home Care); available OTC.
    (b) 1.1 percent sodium fluoride (i.e., Control Rx); available by prescription.
    (c) 0.2 percent neutral sodium fluoride (i.e., Prevident 5000 Plus); available by prescription.
  (2) Mode of action. Fluoride forms precipitate within dentin tubules.
  (3) Application. Follow manufacturer's directions.

2. Professionally applied treatments. Many agents and/or dental materials are available that can be topically applied to exposed dentinal surfaces to block (occlude/**obturate**) dentinal tubules. The most common include:

a. Fluorides.
  (1) Examples of active ingredients include:[3]
    (a) 0.4 percent stannous fluoride, 1.09 percent sodium fluoride, 0.14 percent hydrogen fluoride (i.e., Gel-Kam Dentin Bloc).
    (b) 0.63 percent stannous fluoride (i.e., PerioMed).
  (2) Mode of action. Fluoride forms precipitate within dentin tubules.
  (3) Properties. Useful chairside for before and after scaling procedures.
  (4) Application. Follow manufacturer's directions.

b. Varnish. 5 percent sodium fluoride (i.e., Duraphat®).[3]
  (1) Mode of action. Forms a protective layer (blocks) of calcium fluoride that prevents fluid flow in the tubules.
  (2) Properties.
    (a) Sets in the presence of moisture.
    (b) Provides immediate fluoride uptake.
    (c) Remains on teeth until brushed off.
    (d) Promotes remineralization during cariogenic challenges.
    (e) Because the sodium fluoride in the varnish may interact with other fluoride preparations, avoid applying a professionally applied topical fluoride gel treatment (i.e., tray or isolation) after fluoride varnish is applied.
    (f) If the patient is taking daily fluoride supplements, they should not be taken for several days after fluoride varnish application.

CLINICAL TIP:

Stimulating Your Knowledge: There is no evidence to support the effectiveness of "dabbing" the dentifrice directly on exposed dentinal surfaces as a topical ointment.

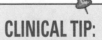

CLINICAL TIP:

Stimulating Your Knowledge: Tooth surface isolation is not required when using Duraphat® varnish. The varnish is moisture tolerant, adheres well to moist dentinal surfaces, and sets in the presence of saliva.

Figure 17–3 Professional application of fluoride varnish.

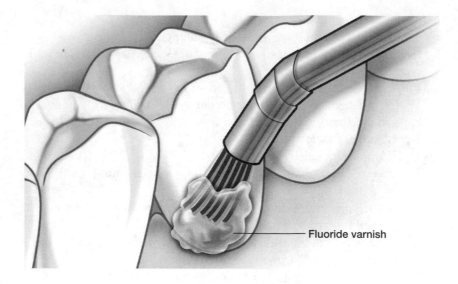

Fluoride varnish

(3) Application.
   (a) Use brush to apply varnish (Figure 17–3).
   (b) Instruct patient to rinse; varnish can be removed by brushing.
(4) Postapplication instructions. After varnish is applied, the patient should avoid eating hard foods and/or toothbrushing for at least two hours—this recommendation is necessary because any early mechanical cleansing/rubbing of the treated tooth surface can remove the varnish.
c. Chemical desensitizers.
   (1) Examples of active ingredients include:[3]
      (a) 36.1 percent HEMA, 5 percent gluteraldehyde (i.e., GLUMA).
      (b) 6.9 percent Copal resin, 0.145 percent strontium chloride (i.e., Zarasen Desensitizing).
      (c) Benzalkonium chloride, HEMA, 0.5 percent sodium fluoride (i.e., Hurriseal).
      (d) 35 percent HEMA, 5 percent gluteraldehyde (i.e., Hamaseal G Desensitizing Solution).
   (2) Mode of action. Penetrates tubules precipitating plasma proteins to seal them.
   (3) Properties.
      (a) Use caution with those containing gluteraldehyde, which is a soft tissue irritant; avoid tissue contact.
      (b) Use sparingly.
      (c) Some are available with no etch step.
   (4) Application. Use manufacturer's directions; may require multiple steps.
d. Dentin bonders.
   (1) Example of active ingredients includes methacrylate polymer and 2 percent chlorhexidine (i.e., All-Bond 2).[3]
   (2) Mode of action. Contain hydrophilic resin primers that penetrate and seal tubules.
   (3) Properties. Can be followed with composite restorations for significant cervical lesions; many products available.
   (4) Application. Requires light cure; follow manufacturer's directions.

e. Oxalates.
(1) Example of active ingredients includes:[3]
(a) 2.7 percent potassium mono-oxalate (i.e., Protect).
(b) 2.9 percent potassium oxalate (i.e., Sensiblock).
(c) Oxilic acid and copolymer with sulfonic group (Pain-Free Desensitizer).
(2) Mode of action. Potassium mono-oxalate forms precipitate within dentin tubule; low pH supports formation of calcium oxalate precipitate; potassium depolarizes nerve fibers.[3]
(3) Properties. Useful chairside for before and after scaling procedures.
(4) Application. Follow manufacturer's directions.
f. Surface sealers/self-etch primers.
(1) Examples of active ingredients include:[3]
(a) Urethane dimethacrylate, fume silica, Triclosan, aminofluoride (i.e., Seal and Protect).
(b) Acetone-ethonal primer, phosphate monomer (i.e., Clearfil SE Bond).
(2) Mode of action. Seals tubule lumen.
(3) Properties. Requires a light cure.
(4) Application. Follow manufacturer's directions.

A differential diagnosis should be made to eliminate causes of sensitivity such as caries and fractures. Once these causes are eliminated, treatment can be determined. Often treatment can be as simple as using a desensitizing dentifrice.

QUESTIONS

1. All of the following factors can contribute to causing gingival recession EXCEPT one. Which one is the EXCEPTION?
   a. Periodontal surgery.
   b. Erosion.
   c. Placing an occlusal restoration.
   d. Improper toothbrushing method.

2. Which of the following recommendations can be made to the patient to help alleviate the discomfort caused by root sensitivity?
   a. Use a sodium bicarbonate rinse.
   b. Rinse with a nonfluoridated mouth rinse.
   c. Brush with a dentifrice that contains potassium nitrate.
   d. Floss the area.

3. All of the following stimuli can elicit discomfort in a receded area EXCEPT one. Which one is the EXCEPTION?
   a. Toothbrushing.
   b. Eating sweets.
   c. Drinking an iced beverage.
   d. Applying a potassium nitrate dentifrice with a cotton tip applicator.

4. Before undergoing any treatment for hypersensitivity, the patient should have a differential diagnosis completed, because other conditions can cause similar types of discomfort associated with dentinal hypersensitivity.
   a. Both statement and reason are correct.
   b. Both statement and reason are incorrect.
   c. The statement is correct, but the reason is incorrect.
   d. The statement is incorrect, but the reason is correct.

5. All of the following are desensitizing agents EXCEPT one. Which one is the EXCEPTION?
   a. Tetracycline
   b. Potassium nitrate
   c. Fluoride
   d. Sodium citrate

6. The MOST common sites and teeth affected with dentin hypersensitivity are the
   a. lingual cervical surfaces of the molars.
   b. facial cervical surfaces of the canines and premolars.

c. lingual cervical surfaces of the anterior teeth.

d. facial cervical surfaces of the anterior teeth.

7. All of the following are in-office procedures used to treat dentin hypersensitivity EXCEPT one. Which one is the EXCEPTION?

a. Bonding agents

b. Glass ionomer

c. Potassium nitrate

d. Oxalate

REFERENCES

1. Holland, GR, Narhi, MN, Addy, M. Guidelines for the design and conduct of clinical trials on dentine hypersensitivity. *Journal of Clinical Periodontology,* Vol. 24, Number 11, 1997, 808–13.

2. Dababneh RH, Khouri AT, Addy M. Dentine hypersensitivity—an enigma? A review of terminology, epidemiology, mechanisms, aetiology and management. *British Dental Journal,* Vol. 187, Number 11, 1999, 606–11.

3. Tilliss T. Understanding dentin hypersensitivity. *Dimensions of Dental Hygiene,* 2003, 22–31.

4. Canadian Advisory Board on Dentin Hypersensitivity. Consensus-based recommendations for the diagnosis and management of dentin hypersensitivity. *Journal of the Canadian Dental Association,* Vol. 69, Number 4, 2003, 221–26.

5. Absi EG, Addy M, Adams D. Dentine hypersensitivity: A study of the potency of dentinal tubules in sensitive and non-sensitive cervical dentine. *Journal of Clinical Periodontology,* Vol. 14, Number 5, 1987, 280–84.

6. Adams D, Addy M, Absi EG. Abrasive and chemical effects of dentifrices. In: Embery G, Rolla G, eds., *Clinical and Biological Aspects of Dentifrices.* Oxford, UK: Oxford University Press, 1992, pp. 345–55.

7. Dowell P, Addy M. Dentine hypersensitivity—a review. Aetiology, symptoms and theories of pain production. *Journal of Clinical Periodontology,* Vol. 10, Number 4, 1983, 341–50.

8. McAndrew R, Kourkouta S. Effects of toothbrushing prior and/or subsequent to dietary acid application of smear layer formation and the potency of dentinal tubules: An SEM study. *Journal of Periodontology,* Vol. 66, Number 6, 1995, 433–48.

9. O'Neill-Smith K. Diagnosing and managing dentin hypersensitivity. *Contemporary Oral Hygiene.* Vol. 4, Number 6, 2004, 12–13.

DESENSITIZATION PERFORMANCE COMPETENCY

Student _____

Date _____

Instructor _____

Patient's Name _____

	S	U	Comments	Re-evaluation		
				Instr: _____		
				Date _____		
				S	U	Comments
1. Selects appropriate patient with exposed root surface sensitivity.						
2. Completes prophylaxis procedures prior to requesting competency.						
3. Prepares desensitizing solution and armamentarium for procedure.						
4. Isolates appropriate teeth using cotton rolls.						
5. Inserts saliva ejector to maintain a dry field.						
6. Applies desensitizing solution to tooth surface, yet stays away from soft tissues.						
7. Applies solution continuously for 30 seconds and lets it dry. Repeats process for a second time.						
8. Gives patient warm water for gentle rinsing.						

Courtesy of Indiana University Purdue University Fort Wayne Dental Hygiene Program.

Glossary

A-δ (A-delta) pulpal fiber   A myelinated, sensory nerve fiber located where the pulp and dentin meet. The fiber functions to sense pain, touch, and temperature when a relatively low sensory stimulus is applied to the tooth.

abfraction   A loss of enamel and dentin at the cervical area caused by traumatic lateral forces on a tooth.

abrasion   Wearing away of the surfaces of the teeth by friction. Excessive wear can be caused by the sand or grit present in spit tobacco.

absorbable suture   Suture material prepared from a substance that exhibits progressive loss of mass and/or volume through breakdown by tissue enzymes; results in loss of tensile strength within 60 days.

acoustics   Energy associated with sound waves.

active tip area   Frequency of the ultrasonic scaler determines the size of the active tip area. In the 25 to 30 kHz range, the active tip area is approximately 4.3 millimeters; in contrast, the active tip area in the 40 to 50 kHz range is generally less than 2.4 millimeters.

addiction   Compulsive use of a habit-forming drug or substance accompanied by increasing frequency and intensity to experience the desired effects.

administration   Means by which the drug or agent is introduced into the body.

air embolism   Abnormal presence of air in cardiovascular system causing an obstruction of blood flow through the vessels.

air polisher   A powered, powder-abrasive device.

alginate   A sea-kelp by-product supplied as a flour-like powder; used to obtain a negative reproduction of the teeth.

allergen   An antigen that can elicit an allergic response.

alternate fulcrum   Point of stabilization other than the incisal or occlusal tooth surface; used to enhance instrumentation. Examples include:

> **cross arch**   Fulcrum placed in the opposite quadrant of the same arch.
>
> **extraoral**   Fulcrum placed on a point outside of the mouth, such as the border of the mandible, cheek, or chin.
>
> **finger on finger**   Fulcrum placed on index finger of nondominant hand to increase access of deeper pockets or to provide an alternate fulcrum rest as in the case of missing teeth.
>
> **opposite arch**   Fulcrum placed on the arch opposite of the one being instrumented.

> **reinforced**   Supplemental fulcrum applied with index finger of nondominant hand to dominant hand to gain additional force in a stroke when needed.

amplitude   Distance the ultrasonic insert tip travels in one single vibration—also referred to as a tip displacement.

anaphylactic shock   Type of allergic reaction that affects the entire body; results from an antigen/antibody reaction.

anchor tooth   Usually the most posterior tooth that anchors the rubber dam clamp and the rubber dam material.

angina pectoris   A severe constricting pain in the chest, due to ischemia of the heart muscle.

angioedema   Noninflammatory, localized swelling involving skin, subcutaneous tissue, underlying muscle, and mucous membranes; related to allergy.

antibody   Substance found in the blood or tissues that respond to or react with an antigen.

antigen   Substance that causes formation of an antibody.

anxiolytic   Antianxiety agent.

apnea   Absence of breathing.

approximate   To bring together, as in the edges of a wound.

area-specific curette   Instrument designed to adapt to a specific tooth surface; has one useful cutting edge per working end, a rounded back and toe, forming a half-moon shape.

articulating paper   Thin paper strips coated with blue or red ink used to check and adjust occlusion.

asphyxia   Impaired exchange of oxygen and carbon dioxide; leads to hypercapnia, hypoxia, and loss of consciousness.

aspirate   Gentle retraction of the thumb ring after the needle has reached the deposition site; aids in preventing intravascular deposition of solution.

Association of Professional Piercers (APP)   An international nonprofit association dedicated to the dissemination of vital health and safety information related to body piercing to piercers, health care providers, and the general public.

atopic   Genetically determined state of hypersensitivity to environmental allergens.

Atraumatic Restorative Treatment (ART)   Developed in third-world countries to accommodate the need for restoring teeth in areas where no electricity was available. Specific tools are used to remove decay, and specific materials are used to restore the teeth and bonds to the tooth with minimal preparation.

automatically-tuned scaling unit   Ultrasonic scalers that are designed to automatically tune the frequency of each insert tip to correlate specifically with the selected amplitude.

bacterial wicking   Tracking of bacteria along the suture strands into the wound.

bail   Ball at the end of a barbell that may be fixed or removable.

bidi   (sometimes spelled *beedies* or *beadies*). Hand-rolled, often unfiltered cigarettes, filled with finely flaked tobacco bundled in a fuzzy leaf and bound tightly with a colored thread. Imported from India, the stubby sticks are about half the diameter of cigarettes, come in flavors, and have twice the nicotine.

biofilm   Complex community of living microorganisms found on inert and living things.

biotransformation   Process by which a drug is converted to a less active form.

bonding agent   Liquid placed onto the tooth after the etching stage to increase the bond strength between the sealant material and the tooth.

bradycardia   Decreased heart rate.

bronchospasm   Contraction of the smooth muscle in the walls of the bronchi and bronchioles; associated with asthma.

carbon monoxide (CO)   Colorless, odorless, highly poisonous gas found in tobacco smoke.

carcinogenic   Any cancer-causing agent.

carcinoma   Cancer that originates from epithelial cells.

caries risk   Determination of an individual's propensity for caries experience.

cast   A positive reproduction of the teeth and oral tissues made from gypsum products; used in fabricating dental appliances, i.e., dentures, mouthguards, and bleaching trays, or for diagnostic purposes.

cavitation   Describes the action of liquid when it comes in contact with the intensely vibrating oscillating tip of an ultrasonic insert. This spray, found at maximum vibrating points along the working end, consists of small air cavities, commonly called bubbles, which are rapidly formed and then implode.

cavosurface   Area where the walls of the cavity preparation meet the external surface of the tooth.

chemical cure dressing   A mode of self-cure or setting of a dressing in which the ingredients unite in a chemical process that starts as soon as the blending is complete. Setting time is influenced by warm temperature and the addition of an accelerator; in contrast with light-cured dressing.

chewing tobacco   Smokeless tobacco sold in pouches as loose-leaf, plugs, bricks, and twists. It is held in the mouth between the cheek and gingiva and is chewed or sucked to extract the nicotine.

chlorhexidine gluconate   Chemotherapeutic mouth rinse with broad antibacterial and antifungal action; supplied in the United States as a .12% mouth rinse.

chronic obstructive pulmonary disease (COPD)   Progressive disease process that most commonly results from smoking. COPD is characterized by difficulty in breathing, wheezing, and a chronic cough. It includes both chronic bronchitis and emphysema. Treatment includes use of bronchodilators and oxygen for those with advanced disease and absolute avoidance of smoking. Complications include bronchitis and pneumonia.

cleoid-discoid carver   A hand instrument used to carve anatomy into an amalgam restoration; can be used to remove excess set amalgam; cleoid end is teardrop shaped, discoid end is disk shaped.

contra angle handpiece   A slowspeed handpiece with the working end bent at an angle to improve access to tooth surfaces. Uses contra-angle finishing burs that are attached by way of a latch. Contra-angle attachments that fit slow speed handpiece may be latch-type or friction grip.

contralateral   Opposite side.

corrosion   The irreversible deterioration of a metal by a chemical or an electrochemical reaction resulting in a pitted, rough surface.

craving   Powerful, even uncontrollable, desire for a drug or other substance.

curing   The process of a dental material's changing state, usually a liquid to the final state—a solid.

cyanosis   Blue or gray coloring of skin and mucous membranes caused by insufficient oxygen.

cycle   One complete linear or elliptical stroke path of the ultrasonic insert.

dead space   Space left in the body as the result of a surgical procedure.

debridement   Use of hand or mechanical subgingival instrumentation to remove root surface irritants to promote healing; aimed to remove toxic substances without overinstrumentation or intentional removal of cementum; use with gentle, yet thorough, light, overlapping strokes.

dependence (physiological)   Condition in which the body relies upon a drug or substance; results in specific body cell alterations and in a state where continued use is necessary to maintain the body's state of normalcy and balance.

deplaquing   Removal of bacterial plaque and its toxins following the completion of supragingival and subgingival debridement; performed at reevaluation and maintenance appointments using curettes and/or ultrasonic instrumentation.

diaphoresis   Profuse sweating.

dipping   Act of placing moist snuff in the mouth.

disc   A thin, flat, circular piece of material that has abrasive particles impregnated to its surface. Used to smooth restorative surfaces; fastened to a slowspeed handpiece.

distribution   Transportation of a drug or agent to all parts of the body by the blood stream.

ditching   Abrading or notching the tooth structure adjacent to a restorative margin.

drug   A substance that can alter mood, perception, or consciousness.

dyspnea   Difficulty in breathing.

edema   Swelling from excessive fluid in cellular tissue beneath the mucous membrane.

edentulous   Without teeth.

elastic   A flexible material that can be stretched without permanent change in shape.

elasticity   Ability of suture material to regain its original length and form after stretching.

embrasure   V-shaped space between two teeth.

enameloplasty Surgical removal of tooth structure usually carried out by the dentist in preparation for a sealant placement.

endodontic therapy Procedures including pulp removal, cleansing and enlarging root canal, and obliteration of root canal(s) with a filling material.

endoscopy A computerized fiberoptic camera, resembling a periodontal probe, that uses magnification to visualize root surfaces; allows subgingival calculus to be located and removed.

endosteal implant Type of dental implant placed within the alveolar bone.

etchant Low pH substance placed on the tooth to prepare it to accept a sealant.

eugenol Analgesic organic liquid that is colorless or pale yellow, oily, with a pungent, spicy taste; it is the main component in clove oil.

excretion Removal of the drug and its breakdown products from the body.

extended terminal shank Additional 3 millimeters added to the shank of the instrument to enable access into deeper periodontal pockets, 5 millimeters and above.

exudate Fluid that is released from blood vessels, usually the result of an inflammatory process. Fluid may contain cells, proteins, and inflammatory components such as leukocytes, antibodies, and fibrin.

file A periodontal debridement instrument resembling a Naber's-style furcation probe with 360-degree diamond coating; allows for access in furcations, as well as deep narrow vertical pockets, and can be used with push-pull strokes.

finishing Process of producing the final shape and contour of a restoration.

finishing bur A small rotary abrasive instrument used in a handpiece to remove excess restorative material and/or to smooth the surface of the restoration; available in a variety of sizes and shapes, typically with twelve or more flutes.

flash A thin, overextension of the dental amalgam beyond the cavosurface margin onto the tooth surface.

frequency Number of cycles per second of the ultrasonic scaler insert; affects the speed of the moving tip.

fulcrum Point of stabilization used during instrumentation—usually the tip of the ring finger.

gel A semisolid material.

gelation The process of a sol setting to a gel.

gelation time Length of time that elapses from the beginning of mixing a solution until gel setting occurs.

glass ionomer Type of material, with the benefit of high fluoride release, used as a sealant in high caries risk individuals; used as a temporary filling material in the United States and for ART.

green stone An abrasive stone inserted into a slowspeed handpiece; used to recontour/reshape an amalgam.

gypsum Mined calcium sulfate that has been processed, i.e., stone and plaster.

halitosis Unpleasant breath.

hemostasis Stoppage or sluggishness of blood flow; to arrest bleeding; various mechanical, thermal and chemical methods are available to decrease flow of blood into wound site.

hookah Pipe with hose that filters and flavors tobacco by using a glass water chamber.

hydrocolloid A suspension of solid particles in water; water-based impression material.

hydrophilic Water loving.

hydrophilicity The ability to be water loving.

hydrophobic Water hating.

hyperemia Excess blood supply in a body tissue.

hyperventilation Increased ventilation exceeding metabolic needs.

hypocapnia Decrease level of carbon dioxide.

hypoxia Lacking oxygen in tissue.

idiopathic Cause is unknown.

imbibition A swelling of an impression material due to water absorption.

in phase Condition that creates a precise correlation between frequency and amplitude of the ultrasonic scaler tip.

inelastic Rigid, nonflexible.

inverting instrument Used to invert or tuck the edges of the rubber dam material around the teeth.

irreversible pulpitis An inflammatory response of the pulp—acute or chronic—resulting in pulpal death.

ischemic Deficiency of blood supply in a body tissue.

isolation Making teeth visible through the rubber dam material and separating them from oral fluids.

Jet Shield™ An aerosol-reduction device.

ketoacidosis Acidosis due to an excess amount of ketone bodies.

ketones Compounds produced during oxidation, or the breakdown, of fatty acids.

key punch hole Largest punch/hole made in the rubber dam material which is placed over the anchor tooth.

kretek Clove cigarettes made with 60% tobacco and 40% cloves.

Kussmaul's respirations Abnormally deep, rapid sighing respiration.

labret A piercing involving the lip or cheek.

leukopenia Decrease in the number of circulating leukocytes.

leukoplakia Formation of white, irregularly shaped, thickened patches in the oral cavity. Often found at the site of spit tobacco placement and may become squamous cell carcinoma (3 to 5% of cases).

Levine sign Patient places fist against the sternum when suffering from chest pain associated with angina.

ligate To tie; to unite firmly.

light-cured dressing A dressing that is chemically activated through blue-light energy from an external source, in contrast with self-cured dressing.

linen abrasive strip A long, thin strip of linen-like material with a fine abrasive glued onto it; pulled through interproximal areas to polish amalgam or composite resin.

local anesthesia Loss of sensation in a localized area of the body by an anesthetic agent caused by depression of excitation in nerve endings or an inhibition of the conduction process in peripheral nerves.

magnetostrictive ultrasonic scaler Method of creating mechanical movement using a low voltage signal. Handpiece contains wire coils that activate magnetic strips or rods, causing the scaler tips to vibrate.

mandrel A cylindrical, metal locking device that fits into a slowspeed handpiece; used to hold finishing and polishing discs.

manually-tuned scaling unit Allows the operator to adjust the frequency setting for each insert via a tuning or frequency control knob.

margination Process of using instruments and various abrasives on an overcontoured dental amalgam surface to produce a restorative surface that is flush with existing tooth surface.

masticatory efficiency Measure of how well a person chews to break down food particles.

mechanical retention Means by which the sealant material is held onto the tooth. After the tooth is prepared with an etchant, the microscopic enamel rods act as a mechanical retention for the resin material to adhere.

mechanical therapy Refers to debridement of the roots by meticulous use of hand- and/or power-driven scalers to remove plaque, endotoxin(s), calculus, and other plaque-retentive local factors; refers to both supra- and subgingival scaling as well as root planing.

median groove Centrally located on the dorsal surface of the tongue; groove extends from the tip to the base of the tongue and represents the site of fusion of the distal tongue buds during embryonic development.

memory Ability of the suture material to return to its original unknotted state; its tendency to not lie flat and to return to its shape set by packaging.

metabolism Continuously occurring chemical and physical processes in living organisms and cells by which a living substance is formed and maintained; releases energy for all vital processes.

mixing pad Small pad of coated paper glued on two or more sides; used as a disposable area for mixing components of dental materials.

modeling compound Used to secure the rubber dam clamp to the tooth.

necrosis Death of a tissue.

needle holder Metal instrument shaped similarly to a hemostat, with locking beaks that contain ratchets that hold the needle securely in place for suturing.

nicotine ($C_{10}H_{14}N_2$) An alkaloid derived from tobacco that acts as the addictive agent in both smoking and spit tobacco. It is a colorless, transparent, oily liquid, having an acrid odor and burning taste; it is intensely poisonous.

N-nitrosamines Cancer-causing chemicals found in cured tobacco products.

nonabsorbable suture Suture material that exhibits little loss of mass/and or volume and is relatively unaffected by tissue enzymes; results in retained tensile strength greater than 60 days.

nonsurgical periodontal therapy Involves plaque removal, plaque control, supra- and subgingival scaling, root planing, and the adjunctive use of chemical agents with the goal of returning the gingival tissue to a healthy, noninflammed state that can be maintained easily by the patient and the operator.

obturate Obstructs/blocks the passage through dentinal tubules.

odontoblast Cell responsible for forming dentinal tissue; located in the pulp next to the predentinal tissue in the pulp periphery.

odontoblastic process Cellular process of the odontoblast that extends and fills the dentinal tubule. Odontoblastic processes move outward when subjected to cold temperatures and inward when exposed to heat.

open margin A space between the dental amalgam margin and the cavity preparation generally caused by poor condensation, amalgam fracture, or erosion.

operating field Also known as the treatment area—clinical site where treatment is being rendered.

operculum Tag of tissue remaining over the occlusal surface of the tooth as it erupts.

oral cancer Cancer of the oral cavity, including lips, tongue, gingival tissue, hard and soft palate, floor and roof of the mouth, mucosal membrane, and oropharynx.

orthopnea Difficulty in breathing when lying down.

osseointegration Structural and functional connection between living bone and the dental implant.

out of phase Condition where the frequency of the ultrasonic scaler insert tip is offset with respect to the amplitude.

overhang An area of a restoration that does not meet the adjacent tooth surface smoothly. A dental amalgam restoration that has an area that extends beyond the cavosurface margin; usually occurs in the interproximal area due to improper placement of the matrix band or wooden wedge.

palm grasp Operator's palm is firmly placed on the handle of the rubber dam forceps so the thumb is placed on the posterior end of the handle while the fingers grip the arc.

periimplant Periodontal tissue surrounding the implant.

periodontal debridement An all-encompassing term used to denote removal of hard and soft deposits, by-products, and toxins from the coronal tooth surfaces, root surfaces, sulci or pockets, used to treat periodontal and gingival inflammation where tissue response measures treatment success.

periodontal dressing A protective material applied postoperatively to the necks of teeth and to the surface of a wound created by a periodontal surgical procedure.

periodontal surgery Surgical procedure used to modify the periodontium in an attempt to treat or prevent periodontal disease; often requires sutures.

perioral piercing A piercing involving the head and neck area.

piercee An individual who receives a piercing procedure.

piercer An individual who performs piercing procedures.

piezoelectric scaling tip The scaling tip that threads into a piezoelectric ultrasonic handpiece.

piezoelectric ultrasonic scaler Method of creating mechanical movement using a high voltage electric signal; handpiece contains nonremovable crystals or ceramic discs that create vibration in the scaler tip.

plaque Biofilm that is a complex arrangement of multiple species of bacteria cohabitating in an impenetrable muccopolysacharide substrate.

pliability Ease of handling suture material.

polishing Creating a lustrous, smooth, and shiny finish to a dental restoration.

polydipsia Increase in thirst.

polymerization Process of curing initiated by light energy.

polyphagia Increase in eating.

polyuria Increase in urination.

power Electrical energy in the ultrasonic scaler handpiece used to generate insert vibration.

Preterm Low Birth Weight (PLBW) Birth less than 37 weeks in utero with weight less than 2,500 grams (5 pounds, 8 ounces) with tobacco being one of the risk factors.

primary intention healing Rapid process of healing in a clean wound that has been closed promptly, usually after injury or operation, and where tissue damage is minimal (i.e. surgical incision); this type of healing is associated with minimal tissue loss.

prosthodontics Branch of dentistry that specializes in the restoration and replacement of teeth.

provisional restoration Stable temporary restoration that is used during the surgical healing period and completion of the final prosthesis.

pruritus Itching.

pumice A silica-like volcanic glass abrasive; used as a polishing agent for amalgam.

recement Process of cementing if the original cementation did not hold or if the cemented crown was removed.

repolarization Recovery of an excited cell.

resin Type of sealant material that is comprised of polymers; does not release any therapeutic agents.

retarder A product or agent (chemical agent) that slows the gelation time.

reversible pulpitis Transient inflammatory response in the pulp tissue.

root detoxification Removal of endotoxins, plaque, and stain from root surfaces.

root planing Definitive treatment designed to remove residual calculus, cementum, and other toxic material to smooth root surfaces, generally with hand instruments; an extension of scaling usually used to smooth the root surface(s).

rubber dam clamp Metal clamp used to anchor and stabilize the rubber dam material.

rubber dam forceps Metal instrument used to carry the rubber dam clamp to and from the tooth; aids in placement of the clamp around the tooth.

rubber dam frame/holder Plastic or metal frame that is used to stretch the rubber dam material away from the operating field.

rubber dam material Flexible sheet of latex or latex-free material used to isolate teeth, to protect the patient and operator and to improve visibility of the operating field.

rubber dam napkin An absorbable material used to separate the rubber dam material from the patient's skin.

rubber dam punch A metal instrument designed with a stylus and punch plate that allows for holes to be made in the rubber dam material.

rubber dam stamp or template Stamps or templates used to aid in the accurate punching of the rubber dam material.

scaling Mechanical removal of hard and soft deposits from the tooth.

sealant Mechanical or therapeutic barrier placed on teeth to block the toxic effects of biofilm formation.

secondhand smoke Breathing in smoke created by someone who is smoking.

self/auto-cured dressing A dressing that has a setting reaction through a chemical activation when two components are mixed, in contrast with light-cured dressing.

septa/septum Portion(s) of the rubber dam material located interproximally between the punched holes.

sharps container A puncture-resistant container used to store sharp objects such as needles after use, prior to their disposal minimizing accidental injury and/or infection.

shortened blade curette Instrument designed with half the blade length of a regular curette.

slurry A mixture of dry, powder particles and water.

smear layer Collagen and calcified tissue on exposed dentin that occludes dentinal tubule openings.

smokeless (spit) tobacco Tobacco that is not smoked.

snuff A dry, powdery tobacco product that is usually sniffed into the nose; if moist, finely cut and ground tobacco product sold in small tins and placed in the mouth between the teeth and gingiva or lip.

sol Agar particles suspended in water; dispersed phase is solid, and the continuous phase is liquid.

sonic scaler Scaling device that operates in the audible range; operates at 3 to 8 kHz (3,000 to 8,000 cycles per second). Sonic scaler tip vibration is created by the passage of compressed air over a series of metal plates housed in the handpiece.

spoon excavator A hand cutting instrument primarily used to remove carious material from a cavity preparation; can be used to remove small amalgam overhangs.

square knot Formed by weaving two strands of suture together with two tight throws in opposite directions (one throw in one direction and another throw in the opposite direction); easiest and most reliable method of surgical tying.

stroke Maximum distance the ultrasonic scaler tip moves during one cycle; controlled by either a power control knob on the ultrasonic scaling unit or through an adjustable footswitch.

study model A positive reproduction of the teeth and oral tissues for the purpose of studying and/or demonstrating dental symmetry and tooth relationships.

subperiosteal implant Type of dental implant with a framework that is placed over the mandibular bone, under the periosteum.

surgeon general Chief medical officer of the United States Army, Air Force, or Public Health Service.

surgeon's or friction knot   Formed in the same fashion as the square knot except there are two throws in one direction and another throw in the opposite direction.

surgical guide   Custom-fabricated acrylic sheet prepared by the restoring dentist to guide the surgeon in the preferred placement of the implant.

surgical knot tying   An interlacing of the suture material by fastening the material together in a series of loops or throws to prevent its spontaneous separation; two most common knots used are the square knot and the surgeon's knot.

suture (v)   To stitch with material to secure wound tissue in apposition until it has healed.

suture (n)   Strand of material used to ligate (tie) blood vessels and to approximate (sew) tissues together until healing has occurred; a sterilized medical device consisting of a surgical needle, strand, and package.

syneresis   Shrinkage of an impression material due to water loss by evaporation.

syringe   A device to which a needle is attached that allows an anesthetic solution to be injected into a desired area.

tachycardia   Rapid beating of the heart.

tachypnea   Rapid breathing.

tag   Finger-like depression created on the tooth surface by etching solution in preparation for sealant placement.

tarnish   A reversible discoloration on the surface of a metal.

temporary   Not permanent; has a short expectancy for efficacy; for this discussion a temporary restoration can last 8 to 52 weeks.

tensile strength   Measure of a material or tissue's ability to resist deformation and breakage; a measure of the strength of the material throughout the healing period.

thermoplastic   Ability of a material to change its physical characteristics when exposed to temperature changes, i.e., softens when heated, hardens when cooled.

thrombosis   Clot.

throws   Loops created with the suture strand around the beaks of the needle holder and then sliding the loops off the instrument while grasping the loose ends of the suture material.

tin oxide   Superfine polishing agent used on teeth and restorations.

tip   Portion of the ultrasonic insert that is adapted to the tooth surface.

tobacco   A plant widely cultivated for its leaves, which are used primarily for smoking. The tabacum species is the major source of tobacco products.

tolerance   The capacity to assimilate a drug, such as nicotine, continuously or in increasing larger doses to achieve a constant effect.

tonic-clonic seizure   Movement marked by alternating contractions and relaxation of muscles.

transducer   Converts electrical energy into mechanical energy, causing vibration of ultrasonic scaling tip working end. In magnetostrictive units, the transducer is an integral part of the ultrasonic insert; in contrast, the transducer in a piezoelectric scaler is housed in the scaler handpiece.

transient   Temporary.

transitional sealants   Used to seal a tooth temporarily; this term is usually used for glass ionomer sealants.

transosteal implant   Type of dental implant placed through the alveolar bone.

triturator   Machine used for mixing certain dental materials; also known as an amalgamator.

ultrasonic scaling insert   A device placed in the handpiece of a magnetostrictive ultrasonic scaler, which contains a transducer that converts electrical energy to mechanical energy, causing the working end of the insert tip to vibrate.

ultrasonic scaler   Range of acoustical vibrations that cannot be heard by the human ear; ultrasonic dental scalers are manufactured with frequencies ranging from approximately 20,000 to 50,000 vibrations per second (vps); these ultrasonic vibrations are a unit of frequency often referred to as cycles per second (cps) or hertz (Hz).

universal curette   Instrument designed to use in all areas of the mouth.

uptake   Absorption of the agent or drug through the tissue into which it was introduced in preparation for distribution to other parts of the body.

urticaria   Vascular skin rash; smooth, slightly elevated patch with severe itching.

utility wax   A soft, flexible, rope-like material used to improve impression tray fit.

vasodilation (vasodilatation)   A drug causing dilation of the blood vessel.

withdrawal syndrome   Intense physiological disturbances that occur when abruptly discontinuing the administration of a drug that, by its prolonged use, induced physical dependence. Signs and symptoms include nausea, irritability, insomnia, restlessness, and headaches.

wound   Injury to any tissue, usually by physical means, that disrupts its continuity.

Index